Keynotes in
Hysteroscopy

Learn Hysteroscopy
It is an amazing technology
With innovations in optics, instruments and energy
Became useful ornament in Gynecology
Incredible diagnostic modality
Giving 'See and Treat' Opportunity
Truthful Friend in Infertility
Rewarding results in Septoplasty
Bringing hope in Bad Obstetrics History
Dynamic in Submucous Myomectomy
Asherman and Polypectomy
And useful in many many
Emerged as a wonderful magic stick truthfully
For all ages 'Good Luck' surgery
But use it skillfully and Artistically
Handle with care and judiciously
The magic follows automatically
You will love it ultimately !

Dr Sushma Deshmukh

Keynotes in
Hysteroscopy

Editors

Sushma Deshmukh MD, DGO

Director, Central India Test Tube Baby Centre
Head, Department of Obstetrics and Gynecology
Get-Well Hospital and Research Institute
In-Charge, Deshmukh Hospital
Nagpur, Maharashtra, India

Rahul Manchanda MD, FICOG FICMCH, FICS

Director, Manchanda's Endoscopic Centre and
Head, Gynae Endoscopy Unit
PSRI Hospital
New Delhi, India

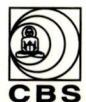

CBS

CBS Publishers & Distributors Pvt Ltd

New Delhi • Bengaluru • Chennai • Kochi • Kolkata • Mumbai

Bhopal • Bhubaneswar • Hyderabad • Jharkhand • Nagpur • Patna • Pune • Uttarakhand • Dhaka (Bangladesh)

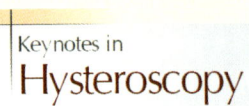

Keynotes in
Hysteroscopy

ISBN: 978-93-88527-71-2

Copyright © Editors and Publisher

First Edition: 2019

Published by Satish Kumar Jain and produced by Varun Jain for

CBS Publishers & Distributors Pvt Ltd
4819/XI Prahlad Street, 24 Ansari Road, Daryaganj, New Delhi 110 002, India.
Ph: 23289259, 23266861, 23266867   Fax: 011-23243014   Website: www.cbspd.com
e-mail: delhi@cbspd.com; cbspubs@airtelmail.in.
Corporate Office: 204 FIE, Industrial Area, Patparganj, Delhi 110 092
Ph: 4934 4934   Fax: 4934 4935   e-mail: publishing@cbspd.com; publicity@cbspd.com

Branches

- **Bengaluru:** Seema House 2975, 17th Cross, K.R. Road,
  Banasankari 2nd Stage, Bengaluru 560 070, Karnataka
  Ph: +91-80-26771678/79   Fax: +91-80-26771680   e-mail: bangalore@cbspd.com
- **Chennai:** 7, Subbaraya Street, Shenoy Nagar, Chennai 600 030, Tamil Nadu
  Ph: +91-44-26680620, 26681266   Fax: +91-44-42032115   e-mail: chennai@cbspd.com
- **Kochi:** 42/1325, 1326, Power House Road, Opposite KSEB Power House,
  Ernakulam 682 018, Kochi, Kerala
  Ph: +91-484-4059061-65   Fax: +91-484-4059065   e-mail: kochi@cbspd.com
- **Kolkata:** 6/B, Ground Floor, Rameswar Shaw Road, Kolkata-700 014, West Bengal
  Ph: +91-33-22891126, 22891127, 22891128   e-mail: kolkata@cbspd.com
- **Mumbai:** 83-C, Dr E Moses Road, Worli, Mumbai-400018, Maharashtra
  Ph: +91-22-24902340/41   Fax: +91-22-24902342   e-mail: mumbai@cbspd.com

Representatives

• **Bhopal**	0-8319310552	• **Bhubaneswar**	0-9911037372	• **Hyderabad**	0-9885175004	• **Jharkhand**	0-9811541605
• **Nagpur**	0-9021734563	• **Patna**	0-9334159340	• **Pune**	0-9623451994	• **Uttarakhand**	0-9716462459
• **Dhaka (Bangladesh)**	01912-003485						

Printed at HT Media Ltd., Greater Noida, UP, India

to

My Hystero-Friends
Dr Osama Shawki
Who is full of Hystero-energy
Who loves and lives with Hysteroscopy
With mission of spreading Gynoscopy
&
Dr Sergio Haimovich
Who is Academy, that is Hystero-rich
Wonderful friend always with solution
With angelic smile and affection!

Dr Sushma Deshmukh

to

---

my mother Dr Prabha Manchanda

Dr Rahul Manchanda

Foreword

Hysteroscopy, the unique way to look inside the uterine cavity, has revolutioned the gynecological daily practice, eliminating the incorrect diagnosis due to the use of "blind" techniques.

During the last twenty years of technical evolution, together with the relate upgrade of the original technique, has created a new approach to the uterine cavity, defined as "office hysteroscopy", a real "see and treat" procedure.

Today we are able to examine most of genital tract, from the vagina to the uterine cavity, and to treat benign pathologies without the need of the operative theatre.

The success of office hysteroscopy is a "team play" procedure where all the components influencing the result play a big role: Do not think that it is enough to use a latest-generation hysteroscope or to participate in a workshop to become an expert in office hysteroscopy! Training is the milestone but the knowledge about physics and physiology, as well as the use of all the possible methods to reduce patient's discomfort are fundamental to win the game. You miss one of them and the procedure will be unsuccesful!

And "last but not least", remember, we have to work in the interest of the patient, both from the point of view of the diagnosis and of the comfort.

This handbook will drive through all the different aspects of office hysteroscopy in a "practical" way, with a wide use of suggestion and "tips & tricks", necessary to better understand the different procedures.

Enjoy it!

Stefano Bettocchi
Head, "Minimal Invasive Gynecological Surgery Unit"
University of Bari, Italy

Foreword

It has been 150 years since Pantaleoni, widely considered the first hysteroscopists, introduced a surgical technique that has grown from being a diagnostic tool to one which offers a multitude of therapeutic uses.

While this publication was conceived as a way for thought leaders in the field to provide the readers with ways to improve their hysteroscopic practice, it really is much more. It is a collection of 150 years of experience that forms the basis of good gynecological care.

Today our patients can easily have intrauterine conditions not only diagnosed but also treated by hysteroscopy. It is the quintessential 'natural orifices surgery' which makes it readily adaptable to office care.

The location in the office brings benefits to all stakeholders—the patient, the gynecologist and the payors. These benefits are convenience, cost, and frequently the avoidance of a hysterectomy.

Abnormal uterine bleeding is a frequent problem encountered by gynecologists and is not adequately evaluated without direct visualization of the uterine cavity by hysteroscopy. Menorrhagia is a common indication for hysterectomies that can frequently be avoided by the removal of polyps or submucosal myomas or by endometrial ablation.

A command of hysteroscopy is mandatory to be a well-rounded gynecologist and this publication is resource for both the beginner and the expert.

Franklin D Loffer MD FACOG
AAGL Medical Director

Preface

As the name suggests, this book really contains *Keynotes in Hysteroscopy*. In today's world, operative video hysteroscopy is a concept that now seems almost prosaic in itself. The world is changing very fast with advanced technology, which has also blessed medical field. For hysteroscopy, it was like from rejuvenation to revolution in instruments, energy systems, optics and surgical techniques.

This handbook on hysteroscopy is designed in a simple way considering the expectations of reader. It will help the gynecologists in day-to-day surgeries of hysteroscopy.

There are different sections in book which provides systematic learning of the wonder technology of hysteroscopy. It is like an autolearning and upgradation.

One of the greatest transformations within the history of surgery has been the paradigmatic shift away from open surgery into the realm of operative video hysterolaparoscopy approach. This book will be beneficial for beginners as well as hysteroscopy.

Sushma Deshmukh

Dear friends, treat uterus
Solve mystery, though mysterious
Evaluate properly as it is precious
Understand various problems and focus
Apply TVS—2D, 3D, Doppler for diagnosis
Any abnormality
Try to look into uterus
Hysteroscopy—A Gold Standard Yes
So repair and save uterus, Be Generous!

Acknowledgements

Hysteroscopy is getting popularized day by day. Along with sonography, hysteroscopy is also taking amazing strides in obstetrics and gynecology to see, diagnose and treat the problems.

It was our wish to have handy book like *Keynotes in Hysteroscopy* for our Ob-Gy kingdom including us. Though it was difficult path with a lot of struggle, we have enjoyed this amazing experience. In this beautiful odyssey, my wonderful friend Dr Rahul Manchanda was always with me.

I must appreciate the support of CBS Publishers and their team especially Mr Prasun Bhattacharya, and Mr YN Arjuna Senior Vice-President—Publishing, Editorial and Publicity. Because of their persistent endeavor, this book has seen the light of today. All international and national faculties involved in this book also contributed their views and original research in a systematic way within the prescribed time limit. Thanks to all of them from the bottom of my heart.

My husband Dr Sudhir and sons Dr Sushant and Suyash (Final MBBS student) were always with me in this academic journey. In fact, my sons always solved the technical problems. My mother Dr Sarojini Deshmukh and my father Dr PR Deshmukh are the main energy sources for me.

I always thank to almighty God for making my world prosperous by adding beautiful people in my life!

Sushma Deshmukh

This book is a treatise on hysteroscopy and its practical aspects. It is being released to commemorate the First ever Regional Global Hysteroscopy Congress.

I would like to thank all the co-authors and my co-editor who have very kindly contributed to it.

This is the first book from our stables and is probably going to be the most important one.

I would like to dedicate this especially to my mother Dr Prabha Manchanda who at this time is fighting a battle with life. She had the foresight to put me on the path of hysteroscopy and has been in more ways than one, a lady before her times.

My family, my wife Bhavna and kids Anya and Anvi, who have stood by me in these most trying times and endured my many unsavoury moods. I thank them for being there.

I hope this book will help many people and ignite the same passion that I have for hysteroscopy in the young and the seasoned.

Rahul Manchanda

Contributors

Abhishek Chandavarkar DNB, DGO
Advanced Endoscopy Fellowship
(France and Mumbai)
Consultant Endoscopic Surgeon
Mumbai, India

Aditya Khurd DNB
Fellowship in Reproductive Medicine, IVF and ICSI
Fellowship in Minimal Access Surgery, Pune, India

Akila B MBBS, MS
Assistant Gynecologist
Paul's Hospital, Centre for Advanced
Endoscopy and Infertility
Kochi, Kerala, India
drakhila1987@gmail.com

Alka Kumar MBBS, MS
Director and Sr. Consultant Hysteroscopic
Surgeon
Women's Health Centre, Queen's Road, Jaipur

Alonso Luis MD
Centro Gutenberg. Malaga, Spain
Centro Gutenberg. Gynecology. Malaga, Spain

Amy L Garcia MD
Medical Director Center for Women's Surgery—
Garcia Sloan Centers, LLC
Minimally Invasive Gynecologic Surgery
Fellowship Trained in Minimally Invasive
Gynecologic Surgery
Assistant Clinical Professor
Department of Obstetrics and Gynecology
University of New Mexico
Albuquerque, New Mexico

Atul Kumar MS
Consultant Endoscopic Surgeon
Women's Health Centre, Jaipur, India

Carugno Jose MD, FACOG
Department of Obstetrics and Gynecology
Minimally Invasive Gynecology Unit
University of Miami. Miller School of Medicine
Miami, USA

Duan Hua
President of Gynecological Endoscopy Branch
of Beijing Medical Association
Vice-president of Chinese Society of
Gynecological Endoscopy (CSGE)
Professor of Capital Medical University
Director of Minimally Invasive Gynecology Center
Beijing Ob and Gyn Hospital, China

Esha Sharma MD
Gyne-endoscopic Consultant
Delhi

Geetha R MBBS, MS
Assistant Gynecologist
Paul's Hospital, Centre for
Advanced Endoscopy and Infertility
Kochi, Kerala, India
drgeethar03@gmail.com

George Paul MBBS, MS
Assistant Gynecologist
Paul's, Hospital, Centre for Advanced
Endoscopy and Infertility, Kochi, Kerala, India
drgeorge6@gmail.com

Giampietro Gubbini MD
Madre Fortunata Toniolo Hospital
Bologna, Italy

Hannah, Palin MD
Obstetrics and Gynecology Department.
Minimally Invasive Gynecology Unit. University
of Miami. Miller School of Medicine. Miami, USA

Haresh Vaghasia
MD, (Obgyn–Mumbai) DOH (Italy) DAE (Austria)
Registration Number–84381
Consultant Endoscopic Surgeon, Mumbai
Apollo Spectra Hospital, Mumbai and Bethany
Hospital, Thane

Ichnandy Arief Rachman
Course Director
Karmig Center
Indonesia

Jinyan Zhao
Department of Ob and Gyn
The Second Affiliated Hospital of Xi'an Jiao
Tong University
No 157, Xi Wu Road
Xi'an, 710004, China

José Jiménez
Clinica "Leopoldo Aguerrevere"
Caracas, Venezuela
Unidad de Fertilidad Unifertes
Caracas, Venezuela

José Metello
Hospital Garica de Orta, Almada, Portugal
Ginemed-Maloclinics, Lisbon, Portugal

Mamta Dighe
IVF Specialists
Pune, India

Manorhita Gaikwad MBBS, DGO
Director and Consulting Obstetrician and
Gynaecologist
Nirveda Nursing Home, Mahim and Mangal
Health Mediators, Charkop, Mumbai, India

Marie Hanna BSBA
University of Florida College of Medicine, USA

Mario Franchini MD
Regional Health Agency of Tuscany
Borgo Santa Croce 17, 50122
Florence, Italy

Maryam Iqbal
Consultant Gynecologist
Pakistan

Milind Telang MD, DGO, DNB OBGY, Dip in Endoscopy
(Germany, USA). Dip in Office Hysteroscopy (Naples, Bari)
Consultant Galaxy Care Laparoscopy Institute
Pune

Nagendra Sardeshpande
DNB, DCPS, DGO, DFP, MBBS
Consultant Gynecological Endoscopic Surgeon
Mumbai

Nash S Moawad MD, MS, FACOG
University of Florida College of Medicine
Gainesville, FL, USA

Neha Lalla MS, DGO, DPE
Consultant Gynec Endoscopic Surgeon
Apollo Spectra Hospital
Mumbai

Nidhi Chandil DGO, DNB
Fellow at Gynae Endoscopy Unit
Manchanda's Endoscopic Centre and PSRI
Hospital, New Delhi

Nitin Haresh Kumar Shah
MS, DNB (ObGy.), FCPS, DGO, DFP
Director Vardann Multispeciality Hospital
Hon. Scientific Secretary AFG
Executive Managing Council Member IAGE
Mumbai, India

Osama Shawki
Professor of Gynecologic Surgery
Department of Gynecology
Cairo University School of Medicine
Director of Ebtesama Centre for
Advanced Endoscopic Surgery
Cairo, Egypt

Pankaj Mate
Gynaec Endoscopic Surgeon
Ahmednagar, India

Paul PG
Paul's Hospital
Vattekkattu Road, Kaloor, Kochi 682017
Kerala, India

Péter Török MD, PhD
Assistant Professor in Ob/Gyn
University of Debrecen, Faculty of Medicine
Department of Obstetrics and Gynecology
92 Nagyerdei krt, H-4032 Debrecen, Hungary

PG Paul MBBS, DGO
Consultant Gynecologist and
Endoscopic Surgeon,
Paul's Hospital, Centre for Advanced
Endoscopy and Infertility
Kochi, Kerala, India
drpaulpg@gmail.com

Priyanka Pramod Sawadkar MBBS, DGO
Consultant–Vaishnavi Hospital and Endoscopy
Centre (PG Institute)
Latur, Maharashtra

Rahul Manchanda MD, FICOG FICMCH, FICS
Head of the Gynae Endoscopy Unit
Manchanda's Endoscopic Centre and PSRI
Hospital, Delhi, India

Rajesh V Darade
MBBS, DNB, FCPS, FICS (USA), FICOG, FICMCH, DGO, DFP,
MNAMS, New Delhi
Gynaec Endoscopic Surgeon
Infertility Specialist and Director
Vaishnavi Hospital and Endoscopy Centre
(Post Graduate Institute)
Latur, Maharashtra
IVF Specialist–New Hope Test Tube Baby Center
Latur, Maharashtra

Richa Sharma MS, MNAMS, FICOG, FICMCH
Fellow at Gynae Endoscopy Unit, Manchanda's
Endoscopic Centre, PSRI Hospital and Assistant
Professor at UCMS and GTB Hospital, Delhi, India

Riddhi Desai MS, OBGY, PGDMLS, Dip in Endoscopy
(Pune, USA). Dip in Office Hysteroscopy (Italy)
Consultant Advanced Multispecialty Hospital
Mumbai

Sadhana Khurd Dipl. In Vaginosonography (Germany)
and IVF–ICSI Certification (Singapore)
Pune, India

Sanjeev Khurd MD, FICOG, Dipl. in Laparoscopy Surgery
(Germany)
IVF Consultant, Pune, India

Sergio Haimovich MD, PhD
Director, Gynecology Ambulatory Surgery
Hillel Yaffe Medical Center. Technion–Israel
Technology Institute
Hadera, Israel
Head, Hysteroscopy Unit
Del Mar University Hospital
Barcelona, Spain

Sha Wang PhD
Beijing Obstetrics and Gynecology Hospital
Capital Medical University, Beijing, China

Shan Xu
Department of Obstetrics and Gynecology
The Second Affiliated Hospital of Xi'an Jiao
Tong University
No. 157, Xi Wu Road
Xi'an, 710004, China

Sumeetkaur Mehta MBBS, DNB, FRM
Assistant Gynecologist
Paul's Hospital, Centre for Advanced
Endoscopy and Infertility
Kochi, Kerala, India
drsumeetmehta@gmail.com

Sushma Deshmukh MD, DGO
Director, Central India Test Tube Baby Centre
Head, Department of the Obstetrics and
Gynecology
Get-Well Hospital and Research Institute
In-Charge of Deshmukh Hospital
Nagpur
Maharashtra, India

Vandana Khurd MS (Obst and Gyn) DNB
Khurd's Infertility, Endoscopic Surgery, ICSI and
Test–Tube Baby Centre
Pune, India

Vinati Kishor Maniar MBBS, DGO
Mumbai
Consultant, Vaishnavi Hospital and Endoscopy
Centre (PG Institute)
Latur, Maharsahtra

Xiang Xue
Department of Obstetrics and Gynecology
The Second Affiliated Hospital of Xi'an Jiao Tong
University
No. 157, Xi Wu Road
Xi'an, 710004, China

XiaoLi Ma PhD
Beijing Obstetrics and Gynecology Hospital
Capital Medical University
Beijing, China

Yehia Shawki
Hysteroscopic Surgeon
Egypt

Yousaf Latif Khan MD
Obs and Gynae
Senior Consultant Endoscopic Gynaecology
Hamid Latif Hospital
Lahore, Pakistan

Contents

Let's Begin with Hysteroscope and Hysteroscopy

Introduction to Hysteroscopy

Sushma Deshmukh

Every invention is a worldly creation,
it is like a newborn develops through its milestones,
with every up and down taken care by the concerned one,
blooms in a step-wise fashion, accepting critics and honors
resulting in an extraordinary outcome!

INTRODUCTION

Endoscopic viewing of uterine cavity, i.e. hysteroscopy is a wonderful technology with less invasive form of treatment. Step by step the operative hysteroscopic procedures have revolutionized the therapeutic aspect of gynecological surgeries.

In the present scenario, hysteroscopy ranks as one the top most modalities. This technique is minimally invasive, less morbid and maximally beneficial for the patient. In real sense, it is a rewarding day care procedure. All procedures related to it start with 'hystera', i.e. womb—a Latin word.

Knowing about Hysteroscopy

In today's modern medical practice, endoscopy has become the third eye of gynecologist. Hysteroscopy has achieved a prominent place in obstetrics and gynecology. The innovations in energy systems, optic, instruments and surgical techniques have given Midas touch to hysteroscopy.

A hysteroscope is an endoscope that carries optical and light channels or fibers. It is introduced in a sheath that provides an inflow and outflow channel for insufflations of the uterine cavity. In addition, an operative channel may be present to introduce scissors, graspers or biopsy instruments.

Along with visualization of uterine cavity, one can take the biopsy or treat the benign intra-uterine pathologies. It plays important role in unification of uterine cavity in case of septum.

Apart from its wonderful curative surgeries, the procedure is very friendly, cost-effective with minimal disturbance to the patient. Even one can do hysteroscopy without anesthesia. Hysteroscopy has become popular due to its philosophy, i.e. see and treat.

How to begin?

Train yourself and start with the basic set up. To begin with we have to consider two important aspects:
1. Office hysteroscopy procedures
2. Proper operation theatre with all facilities

In my opinion, we can have space for office hysteroscopy procedures but well-equipped back-up is always required.

Learn the required gadgets and one has to marry with the instruments to know every details. Also understand the other players of the orchestra like distention media, energy sources, recording system. To begin with, we can start diagnostic and small operative procedures like removal of small polyps. Then focus on the advanced surgeries of the hysteroscopy. It requires passion, dedication, thorough knowledge and skill.

Know your Instruments

In the last, few years, refinement in optical and fiberoptic instrumentation, along with operative accessories, has dramatically improved visual resolution and operative technique. Today, many hysteroscopic procedures have replaced older, more invasive techniques.

The hysteroscope consists of three parts: The eyepiece, the barrel, and the objective lens (Fig. 1.1). There also are different types of light sources. A xenon source with a liquid cable is considered the superior option (ACOG, 1994; Shapiro, 1988). Most hysteroscopes have the capacity to input media and drain media in order to control for volume and visibility in clearing bubbles from the view. The focal length of the instrument is important for visualization. The scopes also come in different styles—Rigid, contact, micro, and flexible.

The tip of the hysteroscope can have different angles, which allow for improved or specific visualization. The angle options are 0°, 12°, 15°, 25°, 30°, and 70°. Commonly used different viewing angles are 0°, 12°, and 30°. For diagnostic purpose, a 30° forward oblique telescope is ideal and a 12° telescope probably would be ideal for resectoscope which requires the loop electrode in the field of vision all the time. A 0° hysteroscope allows for a distant panoramic view, while an angled one might give a better view of the ostia in an abnormally shaped endometrium.

The hysteroscopes are available in various diameters 1.2 mm (flexible), 2 mm, 2.9 mm (Bettocchi), standard 4 mm. For all practical purposes, if you have a 2.9 mm (Bettocchi) and a 4 mm (standard and resectoscope) rigid telescope with 30° forward oblique angle, it would suffice for a complete hysteroscopic set-up. We can use 2.9 mm Bettocchi office hysteroscope for all diagnostic as well as many operative (like small polyps, thin septum, synechiae, tubal cannulation, etc.) procedures. In case of operative procedures like submucous myoma, the 4 mm scope needs to be combined with an operative sheath with a diameter of 7 to 8.5 mm. So you need to dilate cervix up to 9–10 mm.

Nowadays, small diameter size hysteroscopes from 1–2.9 mm are being used (without dilatation of cervix.) for office purpose.

Normal saline is commonly used for diagnostic as well as with bipolar energy in operative as a distension media but when we use monopolar energy then glycine is used.

For light source, one can start with halogen to LED, step by step, but xenon is the ideal with cable 4.5 mm diameter with 350 cm in length.

Cameras can be from single chip, 3 chip to high definition. Recording system should be perfect. Each and every video should be recorded.

Knowing Indications and Contraindications

Hysteroscopy is indicated for various reasons, viewing the uterus directly from inside confirms many conditions.

Patient can have variety of problems like structural, and pathological abnormalities with hormonal imbalance. This important

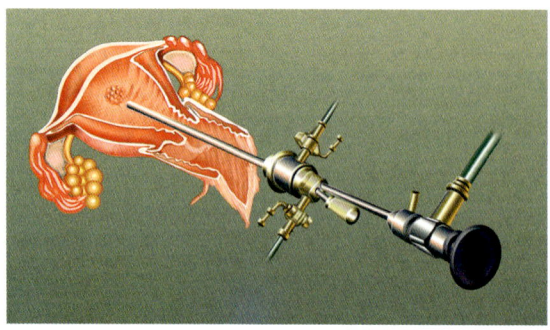

Fig. 1.1: Hysteroscope in the cavity

investigation can be used in all age group of patients.

1. *In Infertility*

- To treat polyps, myoma
- Cannulation for proximal tubal block
- To treat Mullerian anomalies
- To see endometrium before IVF
- Along with laparoscopy

2. *In Abnormal Uterine Bleeding*

- For treatment polyps and myoma
- Treatment of DUB
- Endometrial ablation

3. *In Asherman's Syndrome*

- To treat amenorrhea
- To create cavity by breaking adhesions

4. *In Recurrent Pregnancy Loss*

- To treat Mullerian anomalies, e.g. resection of uterine septum
- To break synechiae

5. *In Family Planning*

- For sterilization
- Misplaced intrauterine devices

6. *In Oncology*

- To diagnose endometrial carcinoma
- For targeted biopsy
- Any genital tract neoplasm

7. *Obstetrics*

- In isthmocele for diagnosis and treatment
- Cervical ectopic pregnancy
- Embryoscopy, and
- Nowadays, hysteroscopy is indicated in many obstetric and gynecological conditions.

Before starting the discussion, let us have revision about uterus.

ANATOMY

The mature, nongravid uterus is a thick-walled, muscular, hollow pear-shaped organ, tapering end being cervix which projects in upper vagina. It weighs 40–80 gm and about 8–9 cm in length, 4–5 cm in width and 2–3 cm in thickness. These measurements vary with age, phase of menstrual cycle and parity.

The uterus is made up of a body or corpus, isthmus and cervix (Fig. 1.2). The part of the body situated above the level of insertion of

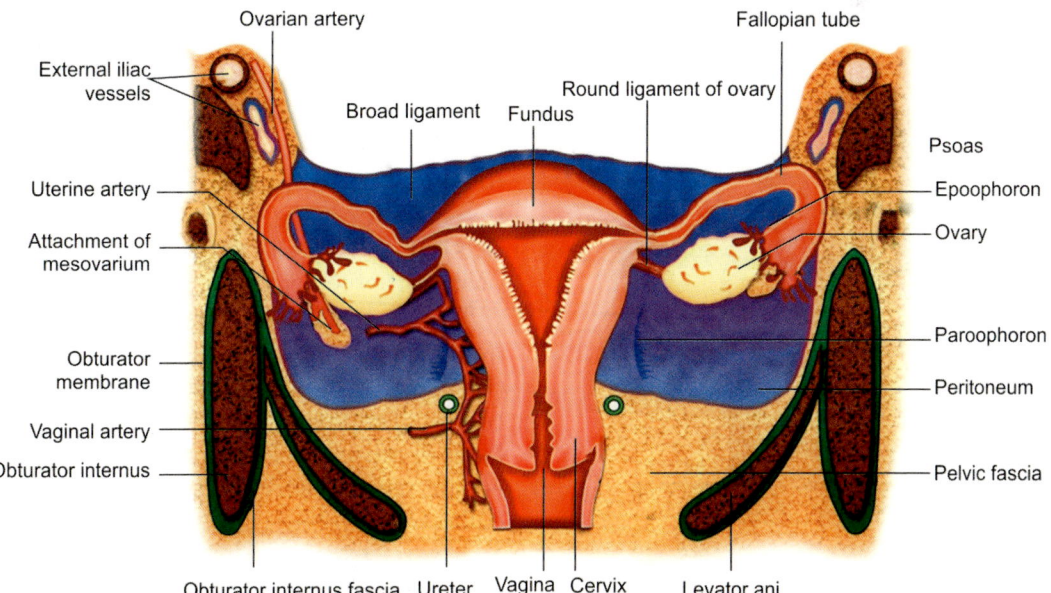

Fig. 1.2: Uterus—anatomical structure and coronal section of the pelvis

fallopian tubes is described separately as fundus. The area of insertion of each fallopian tube on fundus is termed the cornu (associated with the intramural portion of the fallopian tubes). The opening of the cervix into the vagina is the external os uteri.

The uterine cavity is triangular in shape, when seen from the front the length is approximately 4–5 cm and the lumen communicates with the lumina of the two fallopian tubes at the two cornua and with the vagina through endocervical canal at the internal os (Fig. 1.3). Uterine cavity is no more than a slit when seen from side.

Corpus (Including Fundus)

The corpus makes up two-thirds or three-quarters of the uterus of mature woman. The walls of the uterus (myometrium) are heavily muscled and measure about 2 cm thick. The myometrium consists of an outer longitudinal muscle layer, an inner circular submucosal muscle layer, and an interposed thick middle layer, richly populated by vessels. The myometrium is composed of smooth muscle cells. These are spindled, with blunt-ended

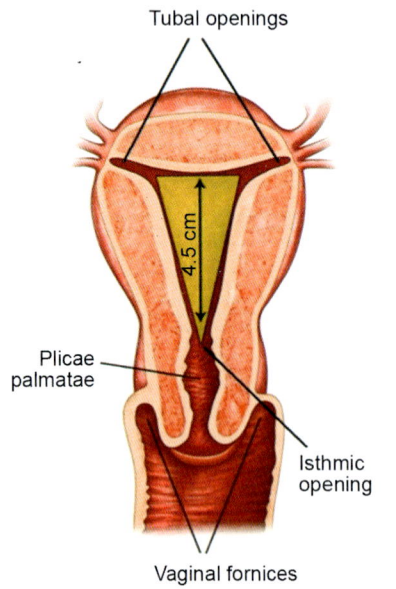

Tubal openings

4.5 cm

Plicae palmatae

Isthmic opening

Vaginal fornices

Fig. 1.3: Uterine cavity seen as inverted triangle

fusiform nuclei. The myometrium is lined by endometrium—a specialized form of mucous membranes. It varies in thickness, depending upon phase of the menstrual cycle and ranges between 1 and 8 mm, frequently is thickest in the fundus. It is covered by a single layer of cuboidal or low columnar epithelium. It is divided into a deep basal layer and superficial functional layer. The functional layer is composed of the superficial compact layer and deeper spongy layer. Basal layer constitutes the 'reserve cell layer' of the endometrium, lined by simple to pseudostratified epithelium in dark, compact stroma. The epithelium shows no evidence of secretory activity or mitotic activity in either glands or stroma.

Isthmus

The isthmus is an annular zone which lies between the cervix and body of uterus also called the lower uterine segment. It corresponds to the level of the internal os of the cervix. It is around 0.5–1 cm in length and very narrow in nulliparous woman. The mucosa is smooth compared to the highly folded endocervix.

Cervix

The cervix is cylindrical in shape measuring 2.5–3.5 cm in height and 2 cm in diameter. Half of the cervix projects into the vagina (portio vaginalis) while half is above vaginal attachment (supravaginal cervix). The terminus of the cervix is round and has a circular or transverse opening; the external os. There are two lips, the anterior shorter and thicker and posterior which is longer and thinner.

The upper part of the cervix is composed mainly of involuntary muscle, many of the fibers being continuous with those in the corpus. The lower half has a thin peripheral layer of muscle (the external cervical muscle) is otherwise entirely composed of fibrous and collagenous tissues.

The mucous membrane lining the canal (endocervix) is thrown into folds which consist of anterior and posterior columns from which radiate circumferential folds to give the appearance of tree trunk and branches, hence the name arbor vitae (Fig. 1.2). The irregularity of surface can make the passage of sound difficult in young nullipara. The endocervix is covered by a single layer of tall columnar epithelium. The mucosa is whitish pink and deeply clefted to form the plicae palmatae. Retention cysts are frequently visible within the canal. The vaginal part of cervix is covered with the squamous epithelium continuous with that of the vagina.

Blood Supply and Lymphatics

The uterine arteries, which arise from the internal iliac arteries, are the main blood supply to the uterus. The uterine veins ultimately open into the internal iliac veins. Uterine lymphatics drain from subserosal plexus into the pelvic and periaortic lymph nodes. A few lymphatics from the fundus along with round ligament drain into superficial inguinal nodes.

The myometrium has a rich autonomic innervations, and appears to be predominantly sympathetic.

Changes in Uterus with Age and Parity

In childhood, the cervix is longer than the corpus uteri, the proportion being 2:1. At one stage in intrauterine development, the proportions are 5:1 or 6:1. At and after puberty, the corpus grows faster than the cervix, and the later represents only one-third of the total length of the mature uterus, sometimes only one-quarter of the parous uterus. After climacteric, the uterus atrophies, its overall length is reduced and its walls become thinner, less muscular and more fibrous. The cervix shrinks so that the vaginal portion no longer projects and the external os becomes more or less flushed with the vaginal walls (Fig. 1.4).

Positions of the Uterus

When viewed from side, the adult uterus is seen to bend on itself (anteflexed/retroflexed) or at cervix (anteverted/retroverted). The normal position of the uterus is anteverted on the bladder (Fig. 1.5).

Characteristically, the uterus is anteverted over the urinary bladder. As a result of childbearing and stretching of main ligamentous supports, the uterus may be displaced backwards toward the sacrum (retroversion). Occasionally, uterus is flexed posteriorly on itself (retroflexion). At the time of examination of patient, it is important to know accurate anterior or posterior displacement of uterus as it helps in performing a successful hysteroscopic examination.

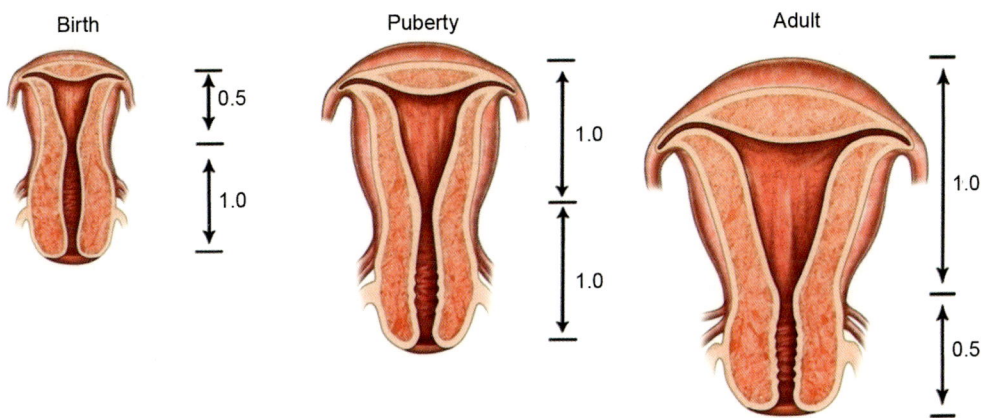

Fig. 1.4: Schematitc representation of the change in uterine length and cervix/corpus ratios at birth, puberty and adulthood

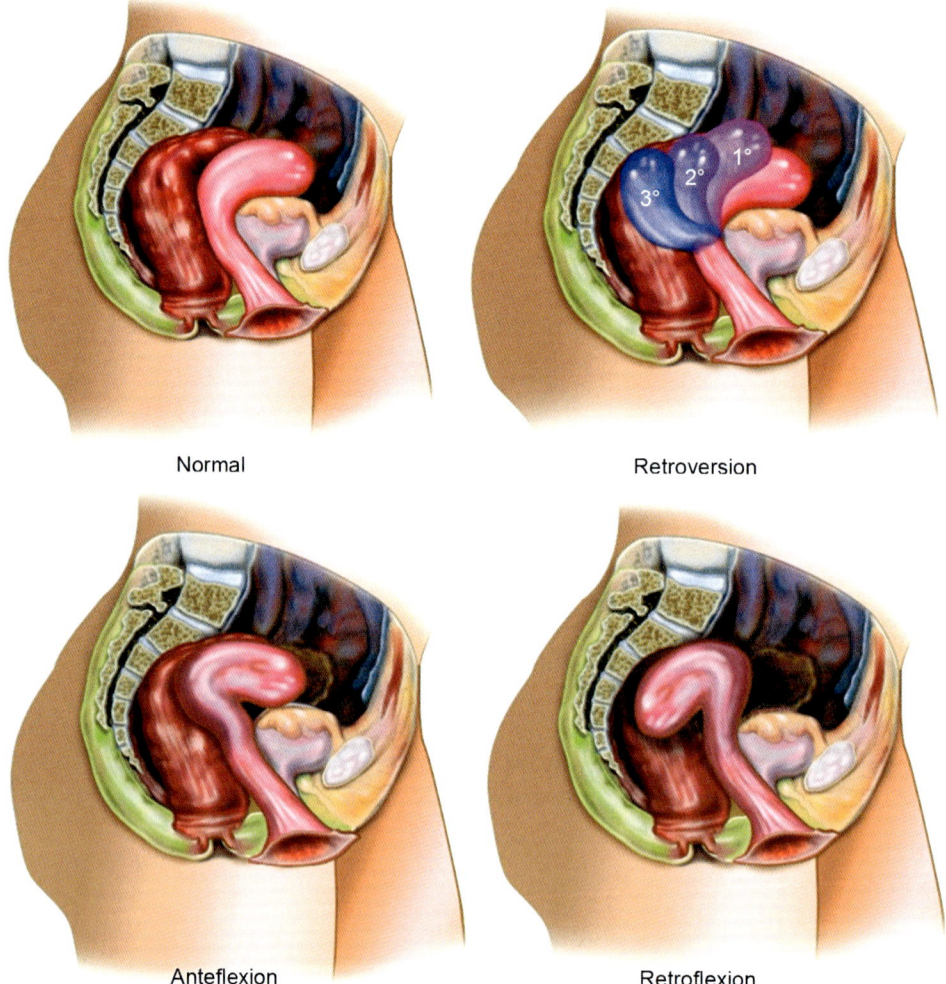

Normal   Retroversion

Anteflexion   Retroflexion

Fig. 1.5: Positions of uterus: Normal position of the uterus is anteverted on the bladder. Other variations are retroversion, anteflexion, retroflexion

Endometrium

It needs special attention. It is a composite tissue which gets viewed through hysteroscopy and we can assume a provisional diagnosis before the histopathology report. It is the endometrium which constantly changed according to the phases of menstrual cycle.

We study the endometrium in abnormal uterine bleeding and in infertile patients. Knowledge of the hysteroscopic appearance of the lesions is necessary. So we can take exact biopsy of that lesion.

Phase of the Menstrual Cycle and Appearance of Endometrium

Normal endometrium exhibits hues ranging from tan to pink.

a. *In proliferative phase*: It appears rather flattened. On contact hysteroscopy, it appears almost translucent with fine vessels (Fig. 1.6).

b. *In secretory phase*: The endometrium becomes velvety and magenta in color. Under contact hysteroscopy, it shows irregular polypoid patterns (Figs 1.7 and 1.8).

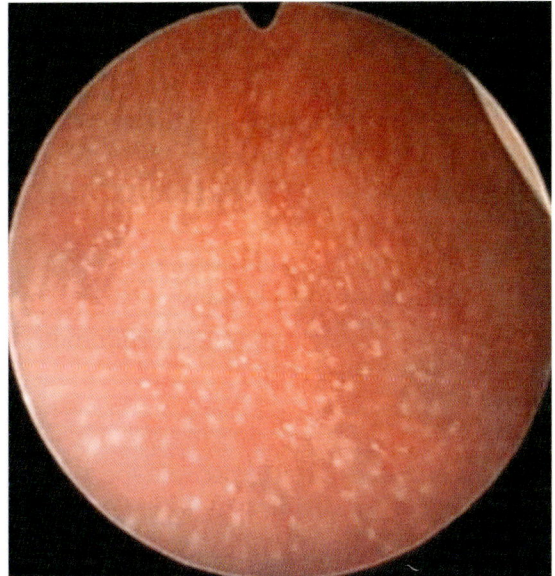

Fig. 1.6: Hysteroscopic view in proliferative phase (*Courtesy*: Dr Luis Alonso Pacheco)

Also one should appreciate the typical post-menopausal endometrium (Figs 1.9 and 1.10).

Dysfunctional or Abnormal Endometrium

1. Due to dysfunction of the hypothalamo-pituitary-ovarian axis.
   a. Hypogonadotropic hypogonadism: Seen in infertile patients, athletes, individuals with significant weight loss and anorexias.

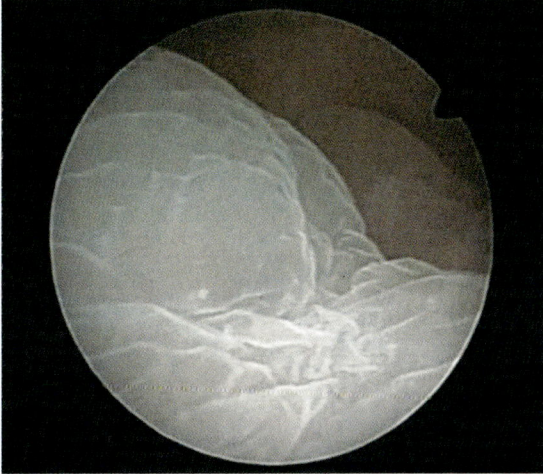

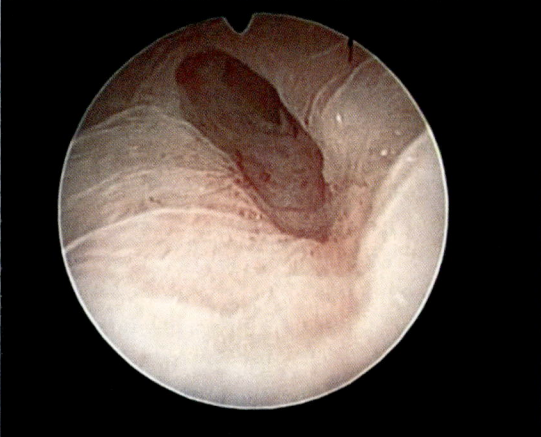

Figs 1.7 and 1.8: Hysteroscopic view—Secretory phase (*Courtesy*: Dr Luis Alonso Pacheco)

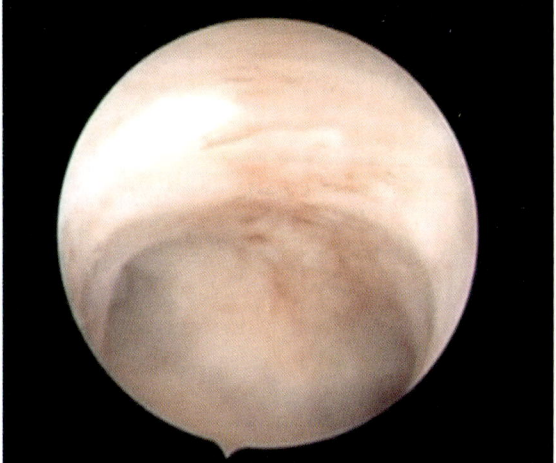

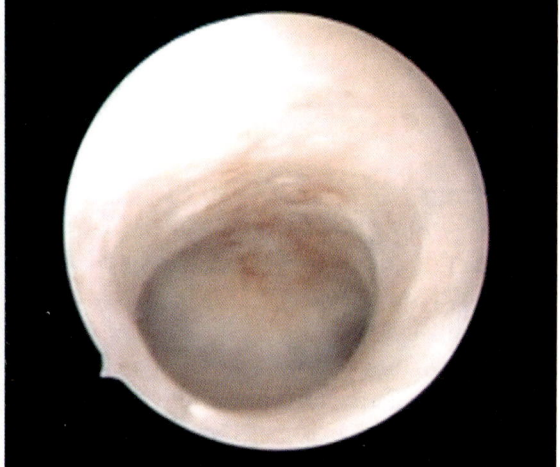

Figs 1.9 and 1.10: Postmenopausal endometrium at different levels of uterine cavity

- These patients having low endo-genous estrogen.
- Hysteroscopic evaluation demonstrates thin endometrium with little vascularity resembling a menopausal uterus.

b. Anovulatory patients of polycystic ovarian syndrome. Most of the patients have hyperestrogenism demonstrating variable presentation of thin to very thick endometrium depending on proximity and adequacy of the most recent bleed. Hysteroscopically, a diverse picture may be seen.

   Since thick endometrium with significant glandular elements and vascularity may be appreciated, it is difficult to differentiate excessive proliferative endometrium from hyperplasia. Also polyps and other intrauterine abnormalities may be hidden by endometrial proliferation. So progesterone withdrawal prior to hysteroscopic evaluation is necessary to form a fair judgment of uterine cavity.

2. Inadequate endogenous hormonal response seen in patients with dysfunctional uterine bleeding.
   a. Inadequate hormonal levels
   b. Inadequate endometrial response to hormones
   On hysteroscopy, endometrium is increased in size, is soft and velvety.

3. Exogenous hormonal agents, e.g. oral contraceptive hormones, hormone replacement therapy, hormonal agents used in prevention of breast cancer like tamoxifen.
   - Patients exposed to tamoxifen have been described as having a higher incidence of endometrial polyps and endometrial thickening.

4. Lesions arising from endometrium: By hysteroscopic examination, majority of the lesions that affect the endometrial cavity or the submucosal myometrium can be detected.
   - Epithelial endometrial lesions, e.g. endometrial hyperplasia, endometrial polyps

- Endometrial stromal tumors
- Mixed endometrial stromal tumors, e.g. adenofibroma
- Lesions arising from myometrium
- Undifferentiated uterine sarcoma
- Endometrial metastasis from extrauterine tumors
- Gestation-related lesions, e.g. placental site nodule and plaque.

But to confirm all lesions of the endometrial cavity, biopsy is essential.

Problems in Hysteroscopic Biopsy

1. Interpretation of hysteroscopic specimen is difficult when lesion is not present in the sample, specially when lesion is in the stroma or in the myometrium. Also in postmenopausal state with very small superficial pieces.
2. As less tissue is obtained, greater is the difficulty in interpretation of samples and less is the degree of reassurance that there is no pathology present in the uterine cavity.
3. In hysteroscopic specimens, it is frequent to see usual artifacts like dissociation and telescoping artifacts due to trauma.

In dissociation, there is disruption of the stroma and alteration of the relation among glands that lie closer together than normal. This false crowding can give appearance of atypical hyperplasia or carcinoma.

Telescoping artifact consists of gland within gland images because of intussusceptions.

Pearls from the History

Entry of hysteroscopy in Ob-Gy field is like a blessings from God. But one should not forget the sleepless nights and lifetime efforts of many known and unknown scientists.

It was the Bozzini, practicing obstetrician and gynecologist, who published the first extensive medical report on his light conductor in 1806. Bozzini's original instrument was used on patients with diseases of the rectum and the uterus.

De'sormeaux in 1865 produced the first hysteroscope.

Pantaleoni in July 1869 accomplished the first hysteroscopy using the instrument of De'sormeaux. He isolated and cauterized a uterine polyp with silver nitrate.

Nitze in 1879 drew and produced an endoscope using the modern technology.

In 1893, Morris used a thin silver-plated tube of brass to see the uterine cavity. Five years later, Duplay and Clado wrote a book with 28 illustrations on hysteroscopy.

In 1908, Charles David wrote his thesis on diagnosis and treatment of intrauterine disease with the aid of hysteroscope.

The 20th century has the privilege of seeing the two important revolutionary landmarks in hysteroscopy, i.e. distension of uterine cavity by CO_2 or water and cold light source for visualization of uterine cavity. Rubin in 1925 recommended CO_2 to insufflate uterus, whereas Schroeder in 1934 had developed 180° hysteroscope and is remembered for his important contribution in determination of intrauterine pressure. In a series of papers published between 1934 and 1942, the French Gynecologist, R Segond, described an operative hysteroscope with an outer diameter of 10 mm with a fixed optic and improved control over, in and outflow of uterine irrigant. Volumiere applied cold light fiber optics and Marleschki (1965) introduced the early form of the contact hysteroscope.

In 1952, a British physicist Sir Professor H H Hopkins and Dr Karl Storz worked together on cold light and rod lens system.

In 1964, Mohiri et al used the first fibre hysteroscope to record fetal images in pregnancy.

Later on, several methods were tried to distend the uterine cavity. In 1963, Silander used transparent balloon with endoscope to distend the uterine cavity. Edstrom and Fernstrom used 35% dextran (high molecular weight fluid from beet sugar) for better visualization of the uterine cavity. In 1970, hysteroendomat was introduced by Gallinat and Lindemann. Lindemann mentioned safety of CO_2 as a distension medium. Later on, the contact hysteroscope (Barbot 1980), and microcolpohysteroscope (Hamou, 1980) evolved one by one.

Due to advancement in technology after 1950, hysteroscopy was started being used for therapeutic purposes. In 1956, Norment performed hysteroscopic removal of submucous fibroid. After that Newwirth and Amin (1976) also tried it. In 1981, Goldrath et al performed first Laser Ablation. Electrodiathermy was used by Decherny and Polan (1983). TCRE using electrical energy was first performed by Decherney and Polan in 1983. Vancialle (1987) described the use of roller ball to perform destruction of endometrium.

So hysteroscopic view of uterus has changed from curiosity to a therapeutic modality. For diagnostic hysteroscopy, we use 4 mm diameter 30° telescope. Stefano Bettocchi and Selvaggi in 1995 developed small diameter instruments with diameter ranging from 1 to 2.9 mm with the help of Karl Storz technology. These telescopes are used for office hysteroscopy with no touch vaginoscopy as well as for easier entry into the cervical canal without any anesthesia. Along with diagnosis, it also permits many operative procedures. Introduction of Versapoint generator (under water bipolar cautery) which can be used in normal saline distension media lead to what is called Modern Operative Office Hysteroscopy.

Nutshell: Hysteroscopy has continued to grow and glow to shine amidst all diagnostic and therapeutic modalities.

Thus hysteroscopy has indeed become a boon for the female patient. And hysteroscope fits completely in the philosophy of uterus or Hustera.

Instruments for Hysteroscopy on My Trolley

PG Paul, George Paul, Geetha R, Sumeetkaur Mehta, Akila B

Hysteroscopy is a truly minimally invasive procedure compared to laparoscopy. Hysteroscopy has become the gold standard in gynecological practice. However, the main obstacles for the popularity of hysteroscopy compared to laparoscopy were difficulties in proper distension of the uterine cavity, lack of smaller calibre and continuous flow hysteroscopes and proper training. Currently, we have good and safe distension equipment with consensus on physiological distension media. We also have a variety of mini-hysteroscopes and resectoscopes available. Safe energy sources for hysteroscopic surgery have also been developed. This chapter aims to describe the basic instrumentation for hysteroscopy and how to choose the right equipment for your type, practice and skill.

HYSTEROSCOPES

There is no distinction between diagnostic and operative hysteroscopy in modern practice. The surgeon should be able to do minor procedures without changing the hysteroscope. Most models have an outer sheath and a separate connecting bridge with ports to insert operative instruments. Some models have an integrated sheath. This model does not need an assembly of the sheath and bridge. Newer hysteroscopes have isolated dual ports for continuous flow of distension media.

Continuous flow with separate inflow and outflow allows the flow of clear fluid in front of telescope providing good vision and drainage of blood-stained fluid through the outflow channel. Both channels have stopcocks which can control the flow of distending media. We keep the inflow completely open, and outflow is controlled to maintain intrauterine pressure and clarity of the media. The inflow and outflow are usually marked with an arrow for identifying where to connect the distension fluid and suction (Fig. 2.1).

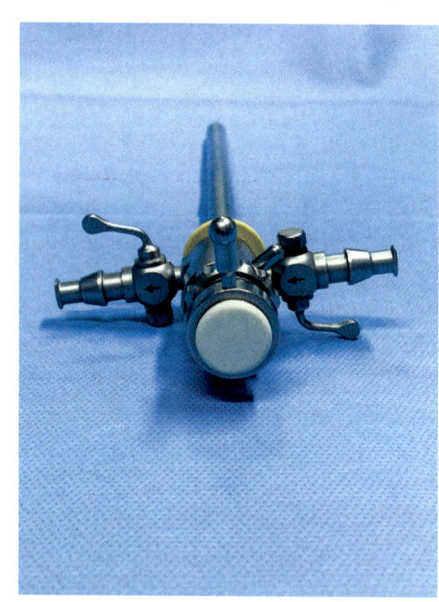

Fig. 2.1: Inflow and outflow channel of resectoscope

The outer diameter (OD) of hysteroscope indicates the width of the sheath. Hysteroscope size ranges from 3–10 mm; the OD of a mini-hysteroscope ranges from 3–5 mm, while the OD of an operative sheath ranges from 5–10 mm. Rigid scopes with an OD exceeding 5 mm usually require some degree of cervical dilation which can cause pain during office hysteroscopy. The working length measures the distance between the distal lens to the proximal eyepiece and ranges from 160–302 mm. Longer working lengths permit the surgeon to operate in the morbidly obese patient. Longer working lengths do not cause differences in picture quality. The depth of field of the scope is usually 2–3 cm and can achieve a good magnification when close to the tissue. Hysteroscopes are available in a variety of viewing angles: 0°, 12°, 15°, 25°, 30°, and 70°. Zero degree scopes provide a wide-angle view. Angled scopes allow for clear views of the cornua and ostia without excessive operator movement. We use 30° scopes for diagnostic procedures and to visualize the ostia, the light cord is rotated to 3 and 9 o'clock positions while the scope is maintained in the midline. For resectoscopic surgeries, 12° and 30° scopes are used.

The 5 mm rigid Bettocchi hysteroscope (Karl Storz) uses a 2.9 mm telescope and gives good image quality. Its oval shape helps in an atraumatic insertion into the cervical canal. The operative channel allows the use of 5 Fr operating instruments (Fig. 2.2). We prefer to use this model for our diagnostic as well as minor operative hysteroscopy. They have a smaller 4 mm model hysteroscope with 2 mm telescope which is quite fragile. In smaller hysteroscopes, there is sharing of the inflow channel with operating channel, so when operating instruments are inserted, the fluid inflow may be compromised reducing the distension. The usual silicone seal on the operative channel causes a jet of fluid leak during instrument introduction and removal. We prefer to use a specially designed seal (Endoscopic seal, OBP, USA) which does not allow fluid leakage even when the stopcock is open (Fig. 2.3).

Versascope (Johnson and Johnson) is a thin 3.2 mm semi-rigid mini-hysteroscope with a disposable sheath and 1.9 mm fiberoptic. It has 5/7 Fr operative channel.

Flexible Hysteroscopes

Flexible hysteroscopes are available in diagnostic and operative models and can have an OD as small as 2.7–4 mm. They are 0°

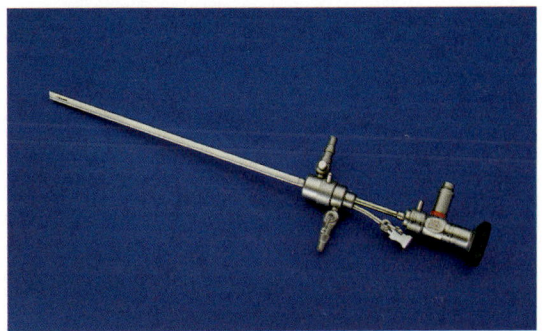

Fig. 2.2: 5 mm Bettocchi® hysteroscope ©Karl Storz Se and Co.KG, Germany

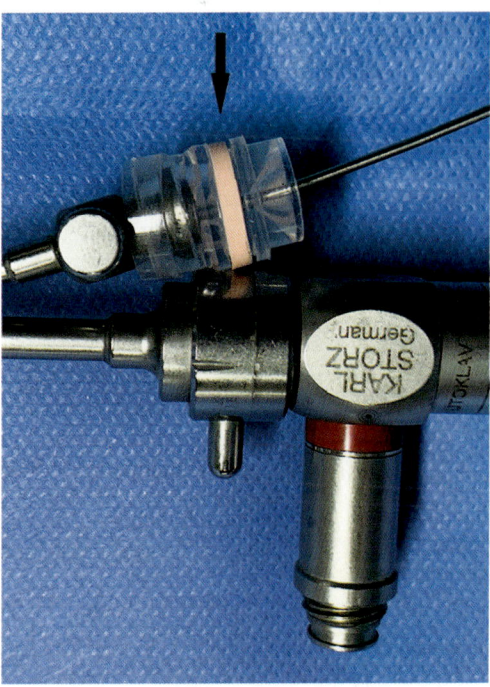

Fig. 2.3: Endoscopic seal (OBP, USA)

fiberscopes, and the tip can bend up to 110°, allowing easy uterine entry with minimal discomfort. It can be easily negotiated through any tortuous cervical canal, but the optical quality is poor compared to rigid scopes.

Digital Hysteroscopes

Disposable and limited use cordless hysteroscopes are now available in the market. They use chip-on-the-tip technology to overcome the poor image in the older fibre scopes. A complementary metal-oxide-semiconductor (CMOS) chip is mounted on the tip of a semirigid cannula which directly takes the images. LED attached to the tip provides the light for the sensors. Endosee (Cooper Surgical, USA) is an all-in-one, hand-held, portable, cordless system for office hysteroscopy and endometrial biopsy. The pictures are less crisp than the rigid scopes. They have a fixed focus, and panoramic view is not ideal.

OPERATIVE INSTRUMENTS AND CATHETERS

Rigid, semi-rigid and flexible instruments are available for hysteroscopic surgery (Fig. 2.4). The size varies from 5–7 Fr and surgeon may select the instrument depending on the type of surgery to be performed. Graspers are used for removing polyps, biopsy forceps for biopsy, scissors for incising septum and adhesions. These instruments are very fragile and can get damaged while in use, so spare sterile instruments must be ready.

Monopolar and bipolar electrodes are available for incising septum or adhesions.

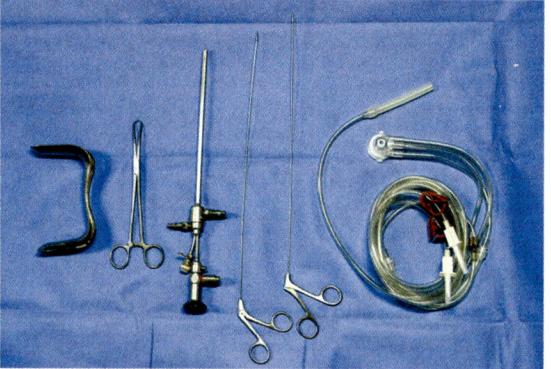

Fig. 2.5: Diagnostic/operative trolley—Sims' speculum, tenaculum, operative hysteroscope, scissors, grasper and Hamou Endomat tubing (Karl Storz)

Special catheters are used for tubal cannulation or tubal sterilization. Novy's catheter or similar designs are used for tubal cannulation.

Our instrument trolley setup for diagnostic/operative hysteroscopy (Fig. 2.5).

RESECTOSCOPES

Gynecological resectoscopes are adapted from urologic resectoscopes, and the OD ranges from 7–9 mm. It has a continuous flow outer sheath, inner sheath with insulated ceramic tip and working element for one-handed operation with spring action (Figs 2.6 and 2.7). The perforations on the outer sheath are larger in gynecological resectoscopes to prevent the holes from getting blocked with debris or chips. The outer sheath has an inflow and outflow channel for distending media. A 4 mm

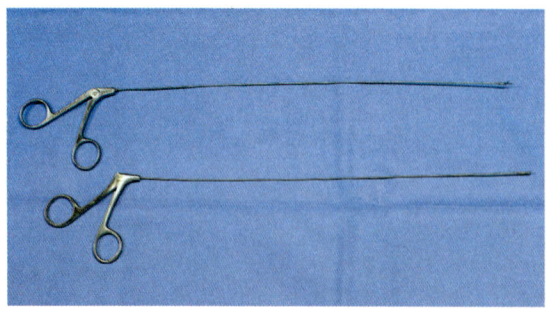

Fig. 2.4: Grasper and scissors

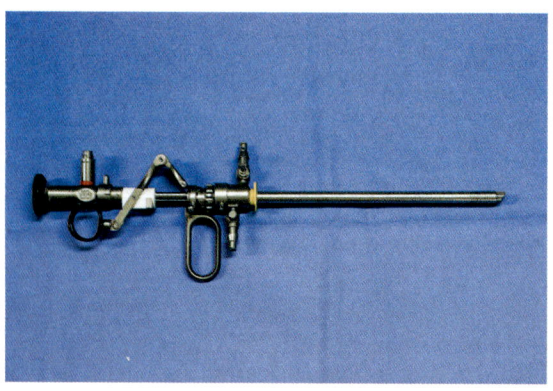

Fig. 2.6: Bipolar resectoscope 26 Fr (Karl Storz)

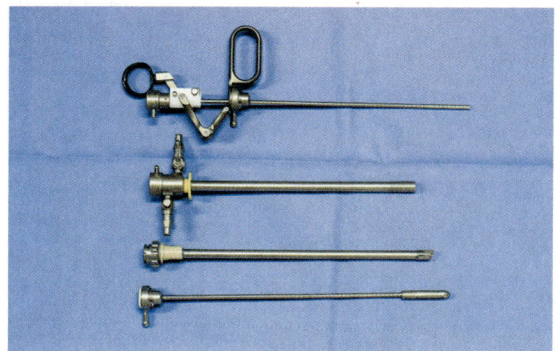

Fig. 2.7: Bipolar resectoscope 26 Fr (Disassembled)

telescope with 12° or 30° is used for visualization. The electrodes are fitted on the working element. Two types of working elements are available—passive and active handles. Passive handle where the electrodes don't protrude out of the sheath when assembled is used in gynecological procedures to prevent inadvertent injury to uterine fundus during introduction or surgery.

When resectoscope is assembled and connected, there are five cables/tubes which interfere with fine movements of resectoscopic surgery. When the handle of the working element is rotated during resection, they can get entangled. So it is very important to organize the cables and tubes for smooth, safe surgery. Most of the resectoscopes have rotatable sheath which avoids the rotation of irrigation/suction tubes during handle rotation (Fig. 2.8).

The working elements also differ in design depending on whether monopolar or bipolar energy being used. If monopolar energy is used, the patient should be grounded, and a non-electrolyte medium like 1.5% glycine should be used as the distending medium. The newer resectoscopes use bipolar energy where saline distending media can be used. It is safer as it causes less fluid, electrolyte imbalance and monopolar return electrode related burns. But it causes more gas-bubble which can hamper the vision as well as a potential gas embolism. Even though saline intravasation does not cause electrolyte changes, fluid intake output should be strictly monitored and never exceeds the upper limit of 2500 mL (normal saline).

Assembling and locking of the resectoscope components need experience. Each model is different and to be learned and practised before the surgery. Another usual error is connecting the irrigation suction on the wrong stopcocks causing poor distension (Figs 2.9 and 2.10). The port close to the camera is usually the irrigation port, an easy way to identify the irrigation port when an arrow mark is not visible (see Fig. 2.1).

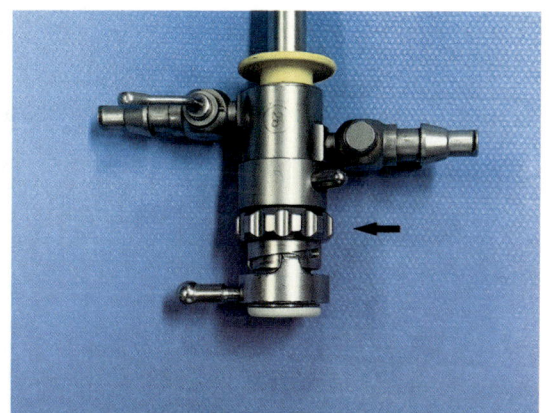

Fig. 2.8: Resectoscope with rotatable sheath (Karl Storz)

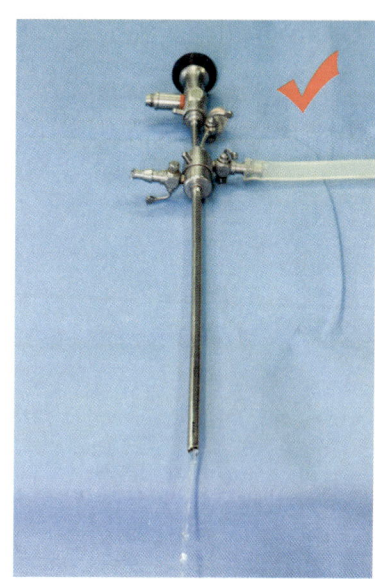

Fig. 2.9: Continuous flow hysteroscope: Correct inflow connection showing flow from the tip of instrument

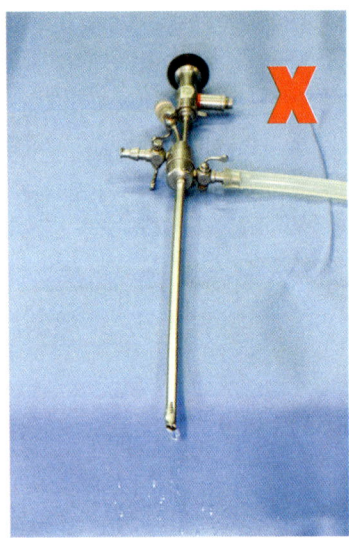

Fig. 2.10: Continuous flow hysteroscope: Incorrect inflow connection showing flow from the perforations on the outer sheath

Different designs of electrode are available such as loop, Collins knife and ball electrodes for both monopolar and bipolar electrosurgery (Fig. 2.11). Loop is used for myoma, polyp and endometrial resection. Ball electrode is used for endometrial ablation. Collins knife electrode is useful for septum incision and adhesiolysis.

Normally, for the introduction of a 26 Fr (circumference) resectoscope, cervix has to be dilated up to 9 mm. To calculate the dilatation required, use the formula:

Diameter (mm) = circumference (e.g. –26Fr)/ π(3.14)

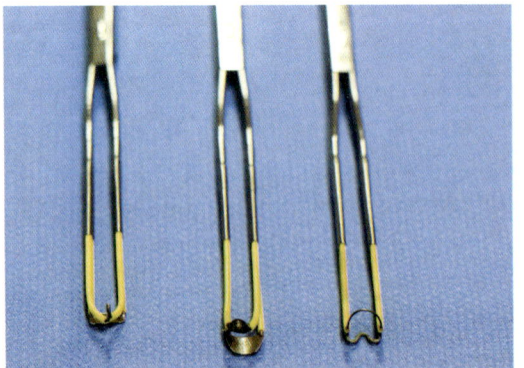

Fig. 2.11: Electrodes—Collins knife, ball and loop electrode

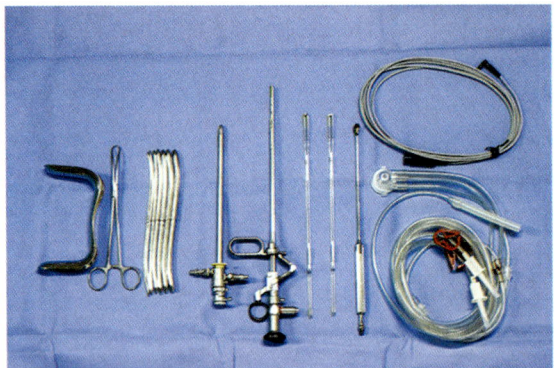

Fig. 2.12: Resectoscope trolley—Sims' speculum, tenaculum, Hegar dilators (0.5 mm gradation), outer sheath, working element with telescope, bipolar electrodes, flushing curette, electrosurgery cable and Hamou Endomat tubing (Karl Storz)

Newer resectoscopes are available in smaller sizes (15–22 Fr) with bipolar electrodes. The advantage of smaller resectoscope is avoidance of difficult cervical dilatation, and smaller resected tissues produce less visibility problems. We use 16.5/22 Fr resectoscopes for the thick septum, adhesiolysis and submucous myomas. The 26 Fr resectoscope is used for endometrial ablations and larger myomas.

We find the old flushing curette useful for removing the resected tissues from the uterine cavity. It is connected to the irrigation, which distends the cavity and the floating tissues can then be easily removed. Our instrument trolley set-up for resectoscopic surgery (Fig. 2.12).

HYSTEROSCOPIC MORCELLATORS

Hysteroscopic morcellators avoid the use of electrosurgery and also remove resected tissue fragments maintaining a clear view during surgery. They are electromechanical morcellators that function through rotating cutting blades. Hemostasis depends on the myometrial contractions.

Many hysteroscopic morcellators are available in the market. Truclear (Medtronic, USA), MyoSure (Hologic, USA) and Intrauterine BIGATTI Shaver (Karl Storz, Germany)

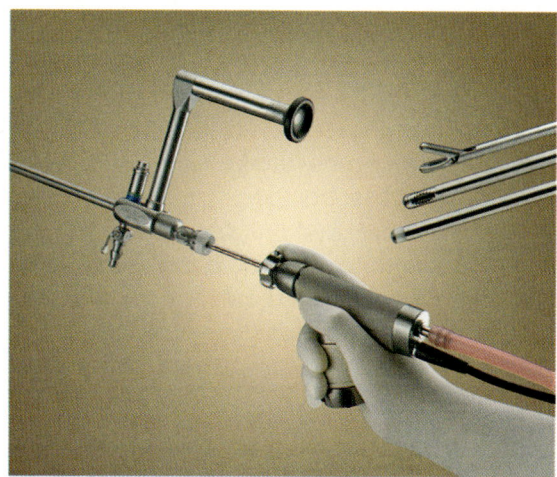

Fig. 2.13: Hysteroscopic morcellator—Bigatti Shaver ©Karl Storz Se & Co.KG, Germany

are the popular models (Fig. 2.13). The outer sheath diameter is 6–9 mm with a 0° telescope and parallel eyepiece. The morcellator blade size is 3–4 mm which are either rotating or reciprocating type. All these devices work with a physiologic saline solution as distension media.

It is useful for polyps and smaller (type 0, 1) myomas. Advantages are, they don't use electrosurgery and need less skill than resectoscopic surgery. Some studies claim a shorter operating time. The disadvantages are the higher cost and not suitable for larger myomas and type 2 myomas.

DISTENSION MEDIA

Fluid media is now the choice of distension media for hysteroscopy. The main advantage of fluid over gas is its ability to flush blood and tissue debris out of the view. Fluid media can be functionally categorized into two groups—electrolyte and non-electrolyte solutions. We prefer normal saline for diagnostic hysteroscopy as it can be used even for bipolar electrosurgery if required. Another advantage is decreased concern for electrolyte imbalance from fluid intravasation. Disadvantages are its miscibility with blood and inability to use monopolar electrosurgery.

DISTENSION SYSTEMS

Good distension of the uterine cavity is important for proper visualisation and safe hysteroscopy. Various types of distension media delivery systems are gravity based, pressure bags and automated pumps. The optimum intrauterine pressure is just below the patient's mean arterial pressure. Higher intrauterine pressure can lead to intravasation of fluid and fluid overload.

Gravity is the simplest method of instilling fluid under constant hydrostatic pressure. The pressure is approximately 70 to 80 mm Hg when the bag is 1 m above the uterus which is not sufficient in most situations. Pressure cuff around the bag filled with the distending media is better than the gravity system but does not allow precise control of the pressure. Modern infusion pumps monitor and maintain a preset intrauterine pressure (Fig. 2.14). These pressure-sensitive pumps reduce the flow rate when the preset level is reached. Such pumps are essential for prolonged operative interventions to avoid fluid overload. These pumps are peristaltic pumps and do not push air into the tubing when the fluid bottle is empty. But if the plastic fluid bottles are punctured, air can enter into the tubing causing a fatal air embolism.

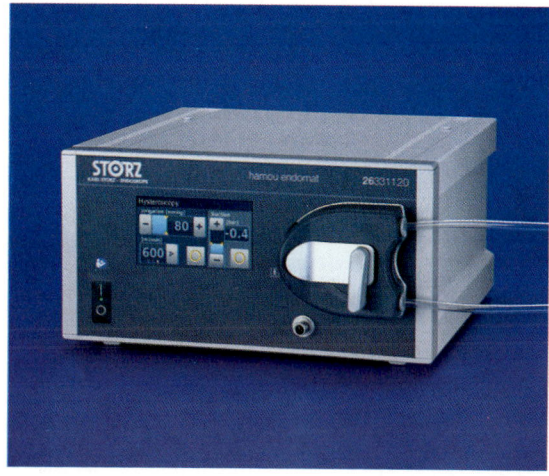

Fig. 2.14: Hamou Endomat ©Karl Storz Se & Co.KG, Germany

Fluid deficit measurement is an important step to avoid fluid overload during operative hysteroscopy. We keep a dedicated staff to manually measure the deficit, and when it reaches 1000 mL, surgeon and anesthesiologist are informed. The procedure is stopped when it exceeds the limit of 1500 mL for Glycine and 2500 mL for normal saline.

Automated fluid management system provides real-time information about the fluid deficit and can also actively manage intrauterine pressure, but it is expensive.

ELECTROSURGERY

Monopolar and bipolar hysteroscopic surgery requires specific instrumentation.

Different types: Needle, loop, Collins knife and ball electrodes are available for both types of electrosurgery. Simple procedures can be performed with electrodes passed through an operating channel of a hysteroscope. Advanced procedures like myoma resection, endometrial ablation requires loop and ball electrode fitted on a resectoscope.

You need to use an electrosurgery generator compatible with the hysteroscope/resectoscope. Selection of the appropriate setting is critical. Modern electrosurgery generators will have dedicated programs which can be easily selected. A lower setting is initially selected and gradually increased to an optimum level, rather than going in the reverse order. If you see a big spark or red glow on the loop, assume the setting is high and reduce it to an appropriate level.

The electrodes should be regularly inspected for insulation damage. The loop electrode should be checked for wear and tear, and periodically replaced.

CAMERA EQUIPMENT

Endoscopic cameras attached to the hysteroscope transmit images to a video monitor. Electronic displays allow the operating room personnel to watch the procedure and are convenient for intraoperative teaching. Images and video clips can be simultaneously recorded on the camera itself or a dedicated video recorder for future reference.

Good light sources and fiberoptic cables are essential for a good image as we use small calibre hysteroscope.

Many compact systems are available where camera, monitor, light source and documentation are all integrated into one unit. This mobile unit is useful for surgeons performing large volume hysteroscopy in different hospitals.

CARE AND MAINTENANCE

Hysteroscope needs delicate handling during the procedure and afterwards. Intraoperatively, the camera should be well supported to avoid stress on the hysteroscope. Care should be taken to avoid using force during introduction and manipulation in distorted uterus to prevent bending of small calibre hysteroscopes. Hysteroscopes should not be kept on the trolley without protective sheath as these telescopes are not as sturdy as laparoscopes. If these telescopes are used for laparoscopy, it should be used with the outer sheath. The common cause for damage is inadvertent fall of speculum and dilators on the telescope.

After disassembling hysteroscopic instruments, they are cleaned under running water, followed by ultrasonic cleaning in enzymatic detergent. It is again rinsed in running water, dried with compressed air and lubricated. Telescopes should never be put in ultrasonic cleaners.

Hysteroscopes and tubings are ideally sterilized by Plasma or Ethylene Oxide sterilizers. But glutaraldehyde or peracetic acid can be used for disinfection except for tubing which has to be sterilized.

SUMMARY

Selection of appropriate instruments for your hysteroscopy practice is important. If you have less workload, sharing of the same telescope for diagnostic and operative surgery can save the cost. But for resectoscopic surgery, make sure the diameter and degree of scope are compatible with the resectoscope. If possible, all hysteroscopes should be of the same brand for compatibility. Always keep spare tubing, cables, operative instruments and electrodes for uninterrupted surgery. It is worth investing on a peristaltic pump for uterine distension as far as safety is concerned. Use an electrosurgery unit compatible with your electrode and resectoscope. Proper maintenance of hysteroscope will avoid unexpected breakdowns.

Camera, Light Source and Distension Media

Milind Telang, Riddhi Desai

Hysteroscopy, as any endoscopy, is a technology driven modality. From the first hysteroscopic attempt by Pantaleoni in 1869, technological advances in the last one and a half century have revolutionized hysteroscopic surgeries.

The most revolutionary of all the techno-logy, has been the invention of fiber optics. With the advent of fiber optics, the way we looked inside the uterus changed. With these, we could bend light using the principle of total internal reflection. These cables allowed for efficient light coupling, thus precise illumina-tion of the anatomy being observed. They enabled carrying of light from an external light source to inside the body cavity and carrying the generated image to the exterior imaging system. All our modern-day equipment use fiberoptics.

With the surge in technological advances, it becomes difficult for beginners and professionals alike to keep pace with it. In this chapter, the authors describe important points to consider while buying endo-camera and light source for hysteroscopy and also discuss important aspects of distension media.

ENDO-CAMERA

The camera is the most important equipment in doing any endoscopic surgery since it acts as the eyes of the surgeon. For proper diagnosis and effective treatment, the quality of view plays a vital part.

There are various camera systems available in the market. Some technical parameters should be kept in mind as the quality of image depends on them.

- Resolution—given by number of vertical lines or pixels. Pixel stands for picture element and is the smallest element of a light-sensitive device. Higher the number of pixels/lines more enhanced the image.
- Aspect ratio: Comparison of horizontal lines to vertical lines. Higher aspect ratio gives better viewing
- Sensitivity (Lux): Minimum quantity of light required to capture the image. Lux is inversely proportional to the sensiti-vity.
- The temporal resolution: Quantity of captured images expressed as frames per second (fps).
- Quality of the reproduction of video/ images.
- Signal-to-noise ratio: A higher ratio indicates that variations in image quality under extreme situations, e.g. hemorrhages or other reasons for loss of light intensity are reduced to a minimum.

- Zoom is the function of image magnification before displaying it on the monitor, which is indispensable when working with miniature scopes.

Thus, an optimal video camera should work with lowest Lux number, while having high resolution in lines/pixels and aspect ratio, high fps, powerful zoom and high S/N ratio.

The camera system consists of the following parts:

Camera Head (Fig. 3.1)

The camera head is the part which is attached to the telescope. Its function is capturing of the illuminated image and transmitting them to the camera control unit (CCU). It consists of image sensors and lenses. Usually, there are additional buttons which allow features like zoom, focusing, white balancing, brightness, etc.

Image Sensor

Image sensors in the camera head convert light signals into electric signals. The image sensor employed by most cameras is a charge coupled device (CCD) also called as 'CHIP'. They create high-quality, low-noise images but consume more power. There are two types of CCDs— single chip and three chip sensors.

Single Chip

The sensors on a CCD chip can only pick-up brightness but not color. In order to produce a color picture with a single chip camera, the pixels of the CCD have to be shared between the 3 primary colors (red, green and blue). 50% of the pixels are used for green, 25% for blue and 25% for red. The camera electronics calculate the missing pixels and produce a colour picture.

Three-Chip

Three-chip camera uses three separate CCDs. One for each red, green and blue. The camera electronics combine 1 pixel from each CCD to a color pixel. As a result, the full resolution is visible in a color picture, therefore, giving a more precise and life-like picture quality than single chip.

Some cameras use complementary metal oxide semiconductor (CMOS) technology instead. They are generally more susceptible to noise and consume less power.

Camera Control Unit (CCU)

It is the main unit where the image is processed after it is digitized. The final image for display is enhanced here. Some CCUs allow filtering, noise reduction, color adjustment, image enhancement, static image capture, video recording, etc. The enhanced video is then transmitted to an external monitor. High definition, medical grade, flat-panel monitors are commonly used and readily available (Fig. 3.2).

High Definition

Modern high definition (HD) cameras offer a very high resolution and almost natural color reproduction and thus are the preferred choice. HD cameras have a high aspect ratio

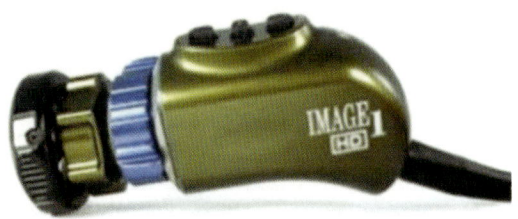

Fig. 3.1: Camera head (Karl Storz)

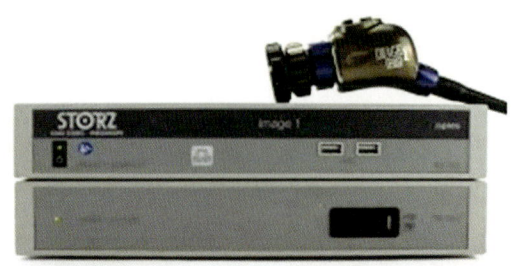

Fig. 3.2: Karl Storz Endo camera CCU with camera head

of 16:9 (most of the cameras have 1280 horizontal lines vs 720 vertical lines or 1920 horizontal lines vs 1080 vertical lines) as compared to the low 4:3 aspect ratio (640 horizontal vs 480 vertical line) of Standard definition (SD) cameras. HD cameras have a high fps. The highest standard readily available is 1080 p at 60 fps. Thus, an HD system offers a superior viewing experience for surgeons.

Light Source

The modern day light delivery system consists of a cold light source and a light cable. A minimum of 175 watts is necessary for a satisfactory vision for office hysteroscopy, but if video recording is desired then 300-watt cold light source is better.

Ideal light source:
- Bright enough to illuminate
- Produces less heat
- Less glare
- Economical

Light is produced outside the endoscope in a cold light source. Light is generated by lamps and kept cool by multiple fans. Light source consists of the following:

1. Lamp
2. Heat filter
3. Condensing lens
4. Intensity control circuit or the shutter

Lamp

Choice of lamp or bulb is the most important part as the quality of light depends on the lamp used. The color temperature of white light is between warm white to cool, which is measured in Kelvins. It ranges from 2700 K to 6500 K. Different bulbs give different kinds of light (Table 3.1).

1. Halogen
2. Xenon
3. LED

Xenon light source and LED light sources (Fig. 3.3) are more popular light sources and the choice depends on the budget and camera system one has. High-end camera systems would require higher intensity and illumination. A proper white balancing, against a white object, before start of the operation is a must for obtaining a natural color, since, white light is composed of the equal proportion of red, blue and green color and at the time of white balancing the camera sets its digital coding for these primary colors to equal proportion assuming that the target is white.

Light Cable

It is a fiberoptic cable connected to the hysteroscope to provide illumination. It transmits light from the light source to the tip of the telescope. The diameter of these cables varies

Table 3.1: Different light sources used in hysteroscopy

	Halogen	Xenon	LED
Watts	200	300	150–175
Material	Tungsten	Silica quartz	Semiconductors mainly gallium
Light	White light with yellowish tint	More natural compared to halogen. White light with bluish tint	White
Color temperature	5000–5600 K	6000–6400 K	Up to 6500 K
Heat generated	High	High	Less
Life (hours)	1000–2000	2000	30,000
Cost	Inexpensive, good for low budget setup	Expensive	Economical and energy efficient

from 3.5 to 5 mm and minimum working length of 180–300 cm. For standard hysteroscopic procedures, cold light cables with a diameter of 5 mm and a length of 180 cm is sufficient.

Two types of light cables are available (Fig. 3.4):
1. Fiberoptic cable
2. Liquid crystal gel cable

Optic cables: These cables are made up of a bundle of optical fiber glass thread. They work on the phenomenon of total internal reflection. The light enters at one extremity and passes in zig zag manner. They have a very high quality of optical transmission, but are fragile and tend to break with wear and tear. Even though fragile, we use optical fiber cables more routinely as they are flexible and thus makes them much easier to maintain.

Gel cables: These cables are made up of a sheath that is filled with a clear optical gel (liquid crystal). They are capable of transmitting 30% more light than optic fibers. They

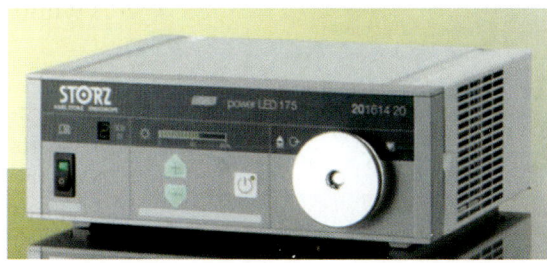

Fig. 3.3: LED light source (Karl Storz)

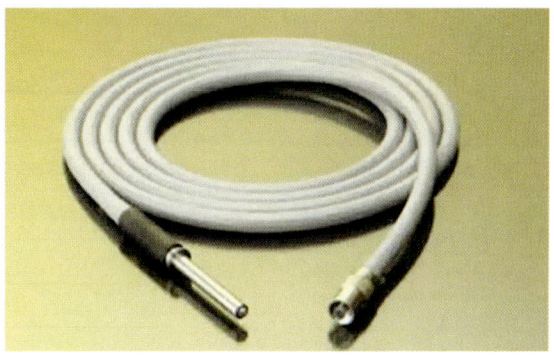

Fig. 3.4: Light cable

are very fragile as the quartz crystals in them can easily break. To make them more rigid, these cables are encased in a metal sheath. This makes them difficult to maintain.

Points to remember while buying camera system and light source:
1. Budget and the type of work done by surgeon dictates the buying process
2. Invest in 3-chip or high definition (HD) camera systems if the same set up is going to be used for hysteroscopy as well as laparoscopy.
3. Xenon or LED light sources are preferable for high definition systems.
4. Choose companies that offer good on-site maintenance and servicing of equipment.
5. Usually choose all components of one company as will make life easier in the OR.

Distension Media

The endometrial cavity is virtual cavity and needs to be separated from each other to visualize the cavity fully. A pressure of approximately 45–70 mm Hg is needed to distend the uterine musculature. Always plan hysteroscopy in proliferative phase as then the pressure required to distend will be minimal.

Various distension media are available and their advantages and disadvantages are summarized in Table 3.2.
1. Gas: CO_2
2. Liquids:
   - Low density—electrolyte—normal saline, lactated Ringer's, dextrose
   - Non-electrolyte—glycine, mannitol, sorbitol
   - High density—dextran 70 (Hyskon)

Points to remember while choosing the distention media for the procedure: The choice of distention media depends on the type of procedure (diagnostic/operative/office) and the instrumentation that will be used for the procedure.

Table 3.2: Types of distension media in hysteroscopy

	Gas	Liquids		
		Electrolyte	Non-electrolyte	High density
Example	CO_2	Normal saline, lactated Ringer's, dextrose	Glycine, mannitol, sorbitol	Dextran 70 (Hyskon)
Viscocity		Low viscosity	Low viscosity	High viscosity, molecular weight 70,000 MW
Pressure	80–100 mm Hg with a flow rate of 60–80 mL/min, maintained by the hysteroflator	40–60 mm Hg	40–60 mm Hg	50 mL is infused with a syringe from the sheath of hystero-scope. 100 mL is enough to achieve a good uterine disten-sion
Advantages	1. Cheap 2. Good conductor of light, thus gives good vision	1. Cheap 2. Easily available 3. Isoosmolar and metabolically inert 4. Good conductor of electricity, thus bipolar energy source can be used 5. Gives good vision	1. Cheap 2. Does not need a separate disten-tion system, when the plastic con-tainer is elevated to a height of 80 cms, gravity can help distend the uterus. 3. Not a good conductor of electricity. There are no electrolytes to disperse the current, thus it is the best choice for operative surgery with the use of monopolar current.	1. As it is highly viscous, it does not mix with blood or spills in the peritoneal cavity. 2. It has a good refractive index and thus gives a good vision.
Disadvantages	1. Operative hystero-scopy is difficult due to blood and fumes	1. Mixes easily with blood thus obscuring vision 2. Continuous moni-toring of inflow and out flow is necessary	1. Mixes easily with blood thus obscuring vision 2. Continuous moni-toring of inflow and out flow is necessary	1. Expensive 2. Not readily available 3. 'Caramelizes' on the scope and instruments if not immediately washed with warm water.
Risks	Risk of gas embolism can be minimized by low working pressure and faster operative time.	Volume overload can occur. This can lead to left heart failure and pulmo-nary edema. This can be prevented by continuous inflow-outflow monitoring.	Glycine is hypo osmolar, it gets metabolized into ammonia and thus causes hyponatremia. It can also cause alteration of nerve impulses and membrane potentials thus causing muscle dysfunction.	Anaphylactic reactions, coagula-pathies, pulmonary edema and occasional report of death.

The AAGL[1] and the BSGE/ESGE[2] guidelines on choice of distention media are summarized below (AAGL Level C evidence, BSGE/ESGE Grade D recommendation).

- The guidelines recommend, CO_2 only for diagnostic hysteroscopy. Fluid media are ideal for operative hysteroscopy.
- Isotonic electrolyte-containing distension media, such as normal saline, to be used for diagnostic as well as operative hysteroscopy where bipolar energy source is used because they are less likely to cause hyponatremia, if fluid overload occurs.
- Hypotonic, electrolyte-free distension media, such as glycine and sorbitol, should only be used with monopolar electrosurgical instruments.

BSGE/ESGE guidelines describe the ideal distending medium as:

- Allows clear visualization of the uterine cavity
- Isotonic
- Nontoxic
- Hypoallergenic
- Non-hemolytic
- Be rapidly cleared by the body
- Readily available
- Inexpensive

Normal saline satisfies all these criteria and for this reason has become the fluid distension medium of choice for both diagnostic as well as operative procedures. Normal saline is preferred for 'vaginoscopic approach'. In office hysteroscopy, normal saline as distension media is associated with increased compliance and better cost benefit ratio. With the advent of miniature hysteroscopes, bipolar miniature resectoscopes like the Gubbini and Betocchi systems and also with the availability of various hysteroscopic morcellators (Tru clear, Bigatti shaver) the use of normal saline is on the rise. Ideally the use of automated, microprocessor-controlled irrigation and suction unit for distention is recommended.

Bibliography

1. AAGL Practice Report: Practice Guidelines for the Management of Hysteroscopic Distending Media? (Replaces Hysteroscopic Fluid Monitoring Guidelines. J Am AssocGynecol Laparosc. 2000;7:167–168.) J Am AssocGynecol Laparosc. (2013) 20, 137–148.
2. Umranikar S, Clark T,SaridoganE et al. BSGE/ESGE guideline on management of fluid distension media in operative hysteroscopy. GynecolSurgDOI 10.1007/s10397-016-0983-z.

Which Energy Source?
Monopolar or Bipolar

Rajesh V Darade, Priyanka Pramod Sawadkar

INTRODUCTION

Electrosurgery is the most common energy source used in hysteroscopic surgery. Two forms of energy are used monopolar and bipolar.

PRINCIPLES OF ELECTROSURGERY

Electricity is flow of electron through a conducting medium. Depending on the direction of the current flow we call it direct or alternating current. When current flows continuously from one pole to other pole of an electric circuit, it is called direct current (DC). When current flows changes its direction it is called alternating current (AC). Household electricity is an alternating current and it changes its direction 50 times per second which is called frequency of current (50 HZ). This low frequency current cannot be used for electrosurgery. When it passes through our body it will stimulate our nerves and cause heart block and cardiac arrest. The nerve stimulation and, therefore, paralysis can be avoided by applying for a fraction of time shorter than required to lower the threshold potential. This can be achieved by increasing the frequency of current to a level of 100 kHz (100000 cycles per second). All modern electrosurgical units produce an electric current of 500 kHZ to 2 MHz (radio frequency).

When a high frequency current is applied to the body tissue, certain biochemical effects occur. Cells contain water, electrolytes and non-electrolyte particles. When a flow of electron are applied to the cells, the positive charged particles (sodium and potassium ions) move towards it and negative charged moves away from it. During the fast flow of these charged particles, it collides with each other or with other uncharged molecules producing friction and, therefore, heat. The temperature rises in the cell. If the tissue is heated very slow and temperature raises above 60°C the protein gets denatured by losing its structure an effect called coagulation. If the temperature rise is quick by applying more energy, temperature rises quickly to 100°C. The cellular water turns into steam and which results in cell rupture a process called vaporization. In electrosurgery, our aim is to produce a combination of above tissue effects. The tissue effect from the heat depends directly on the temperature inside the tissue and the time required to reach that temperature. Clinicians use electrosurgery to cutting the tissue or coagulating it.

Electrosurgery requires a circuit for the passage of electrons that includes two electrodes, the patient, the electrosurgical generator or unit (ESU) and the connecting wires. In monopolar circuit, current flows through the active electrode to the tissue, pass through body and returns to the generator through the patient plate. Monopolar instrument is so designed that the entire patient is involved in the circuit and circumstance that provides a greater opportunity for current to be diverted to undesirable location. In bipolar circuit, current flow is limited between the closely placed electrodes and less chance for current diversion. So the surgeon has to be more knowledgeable about electrosurgery when using monopolar energy to avoid complications.

ELECTROSURGERY IN HYSTEROSCOPY

In fluid medium electrosurgery presents several challenges in establishing and maintaining the tissue effects. Because electrolyte containing distention media such as saline are effective conductors, they disperse the current from the active electrode of a monopolar instrument, preventing the creation of the zone of high current density necessary to achieve the desired electrosurgical tissue effect. So it is necessary to use electrolyte-free distension media, such as sorbitol, glycine, or mannitol for monopolar electrosurgery. Bipolar resectoscopic instruments are generally designed with a distal active electrode and a more proximal dispersive electrode, a configuration that is necessary for the completion of a circuit in an electrolyte-rich medium like normal saline. Distance between the two electrodes is greatly decreased in bipolar system so as to reduce the impedance, and a steam envelope forms around these electrodes completing the circuit when unit is activated. When the activated bipolar electrode is not in contact with tissue, the electrolytes solution in the uterus dissipates it. When the loop is sufficiently close to tissue, the high bipolar voltage spike are between the electrode converts the conductive sodium chloride solution into a non-equilibrium vapour layer once formed, this plasma effect

can be maintained at lower voltages. With tissue contact, there is disintegration of tissue via molecular dissociation. The cell membranes rupture producing visible cutting. Clinically, there is precise tissue effect with minimal collateral damage, as the charged ions have an estimated penetration depth in tissue of only 50–100 micrometer (0.5–1 milimeter). The depth of coagulation is determined principally by the electrode configuration and by the system design, as well as by the technique used by the operator (time and pressure of contact).

Monopolar and bipolar instruments, when used to vaporize tissue, produce the same vapor cloud that, in fluid media, manifests as bubbles that largely consist of hydrogen, CO and CO_2, each of which is highly soluble in blood. Although they usually enter the systemic circulation and rapidly dissolve in blood and do not produce gas embolism.

MONOPOLAR RESECTOSCOPE

Monopolar hysteroscopic surgery requires specific instrumentation. Simple procedures can be performed with unipolar electrodes passed through an operating channel of a hysteroscope. Major hysteroscopic procedures are performed with resectoscope. It was originally designed for transurethral resection of prostate. In gynecological surgery, a modified resectoscope with larger perforations on the sheath is used. It has a continuous flow outer sheath, inner sheath with insulated ceramic tip, working element for one handed operation with spring action. The size of whole assembly is 26 F, i.e circumference is 26 mm. A 4 mm telescope is used for visualization. Smaller resectoscopes are also available. Different types of electrodes are available and are chosen depending on the type of surgery to be performed. Electrode is fitted on the working element and connected to the surgery unit. A peristaltic pump with pressure and volume control designed for hysteroscopic surgery is not suitable and can be dangerous.

After the resectoscope assembled properly inflow is connected to irrigation pump and any residual air bubbles evacuated. Irrigation pressure of 100–110 mm Hg and flow rate of 200–400 mL/min is set. Outflow is connected to the suction pump and is usually kept in closed position. A setting of 80–90 watts pure cutting current is selected on the electrosurgery generator. Coagulation current is set at 50–60 watts. Cervix is dilated depending on the size of resectoscope so that it can be introduced without much resistance. Irrigation pump is started and a good visualization of the cavity is achieved by minimally opening the outflow stopcock.

Advantages of Monopolar Resectoscopic Surgery

1. More efficient and cost effective than bipolar resectoscopes.
2. Working of monopolar resectoscope is easy.

Disadvantages of Monopolar Resectoscopic Surgery

1. Fluid overload, glycine toxicity, electrolyte imbalance and dreadful complications like TURP syndrome and cerebral edema are common.
2. Tissue damage and charring of tissue is more with monopolar.
3. Electrosurgical complications are more as energy passes through other body tissues.
4. Complication like perforation, damage to surrounding tissues with energy is more common.

BIPOLAR RESECTOSCOPE

Bipolar hysteroscopic surgery requires specific instruments like dedicated bipolar electro-surgical generator. The working element of a bipolar resectoscope will have two components, thin loop act as an active electrode and the broad "C" shaped non-insulated part act as return electrodes are available for bipolar electrosurgery. Different designs like loop, Collin's knife and surgery ball electrodes are available for bipolar electrosurgery. The working element is then connected to the dedicated bipolar ESU. No patient return electrode is needed for bipolar electrosurgery.

Advantages of Bipolar Resectoscopic Surgery

1. Tissue damage is less with bipolar electro-surgery as the tissue temperature achieved is less compared with monopolar.
2. Less stickiness of electrodes in bipolar electrosurgery due to its plasma effect.
3. Has more coagulating effect, therefore, achieving better hemostasis during surgery.
4. Electrosurgical complications are less as the patient is not a part of the circuit.
5. Fluid overload can be easily treated with diuretics alone.
6. Excellent dissection and coagulation at low settings.

Disadvantages of Bipolar Resectoscopic Surgery

1. It is costlier because of the need for specific instrumentation due to difference in the electric circuit design.
2. Bipolar resectoscopic loops have to be changed frequently.
3. Bipolar resection is slower than monopolar (Table 4.1).

ELECTROSURGICAL COMPLICATIONS IN HYSTEROSCOPIC SURGERY

Electrosurgical complications are possible with improper use of both monopolar and bipolar hysteroscope.

Perforation of uterus may sometimes occur with an activated electrode that can subse-quently injure bowel, bladder or other intraperitoneal structures including blood vessels. Such injuries need to be explored with laparoscope immediately.

Current diversion can occur during the improper use of monopolar resectoscope causing burns to cervix, vagina or vulva. Electrode insulation damage can also lead to same.

Current diversion can also be seen if there is loss of contact between the external sheath

Table 4.1: Difference between monopolar and bipolar resectoscopic surgeries

Character	Monopolar	Bipolar
Distention media	Mostly 1.5% glycine. Others are glucose, dextran, mannitol, sorbitol	Mostly 0.9 % saline. Others are ringer lactate, dextrose 5 %, 50% saline
Flow of energy	Electrosurgical unit, active electrode, whole patient, neutral plate, electrosurgical unit	Electrosurgical unit, active electrode, patient tissue, return electrode, electrosurgical unit
Mechanism of working	Continuous sinusoidal wave without cooling-off period. Causes rapid heating with cell explosion	Gives low energy to tissue
Complications	Greater chances of current diversion and fluid overload Dreadful complications like TURP syndrome, cerebral edema are more common	Less common

and the cervix, the current can be diverted to another path, which could result in a zone of high current density on the vagina or vulva causing burns.

GUIDELINES TO REDUCE COMPLICATIONS

The following principles serve to reduce the risk of electrosurgical injuries.

1. Every manipulation should be soft, precise and quick with use of minimal power and electrode under optical control with complete visibility of optical field.
2. The foot pedals controlling the electrode should not be placed in a location that facilitates inadvertent activation by surgeon or assistants.
3. The dispersive electrode should be securely affixed to the patient, usually on the thigh or buttocks, in a location that is not scarred or unhealthy. Most microprocessor controlled generators posses an impedance-based safety mechanism to ensure that the dispersive electrode is attached to the generator and to detect inadequate attachment to the patient.
4. Advancement of an activated electrode should be under vision.
5. The use of electrode with damaged insulation should be avoided. Check for insulation damage before surgery.

6. It is probably safer to use low-voltage ("cutting") current to avoid current diversion complication. Coagulation current should be sparingly used.
7. Cervix should not be over dilated as it can cause loss of close contact between the cervix and sheath to prevent current diversion. During resection simultaneous withdrawal of whole resectoscope with the electrode can also lead to similar situation.
8. The electrode should be activated only when near to, or in contact with the target tissue and the temptation to over desiccate tissue should be avoided. One sign of current diversion is the absence or reduction of the electrosurgical effect. The power setting should not be increased for absence of tissue effect and it may be a sign of current diversion.
9. A metal speculum in vagina during resection can conduct current from sheath to vulva and vagina causing thermal injury. So no metallic object should be kept vaginal during activation.

SUMMARY

Hysteroscopic surgery needs energy sources like any other surgery and monopolar electrosurgery is the most commonly used one.

Monopolar resectoscopic surgery is faster and cheaper compared bipolar techniques. But improper use can result in complications and surgeon has to be more knowledgeable and need to adhere to the safety guidelines. No difference have been found between women operated with monopolar resectoscope or bipolar and are at no higher risk of adverse obstetric outcome at term and during labour compared to general population. Vaginal delivery seems to be safe and hysteroscopic metroplasty in experienced hands seems not to be harmful for mother or their newborns no matter if monopolar or bipolar resectoscope has been used. Compared with monopolar systems, there are several design and construction issues that make bipolar resectoscopes less efficient than monopolar versions. Hysteroscopic surgery with bipolar energy can overcome most of the complications associated with current diversion. Fluid overload treatment is simpler with bipolar electrosurgery, but should be avoided by adhering to the fluid management safety protocols. Therefore, when available bipolar system should be preferred.

Bibliography

1. Berge A, Sandvik L, Langebrekke A, Istre O - RCT-monopolar *vs* bipolar.
2. HueberPA, Al-Asker A, Zorn KC. Monopolar vs bipolar TRUP. Can UrolAssoc J 2011;5 (6): 390–91.
3. Munro MG. Mechanisms of thermal injury to the lower genital tract with radiofrequency resectoscopic surgery. J Minim Invasive Gyanacology.
4. RazBahar, MD, Michal Shimonovitz, B med Sc, Avi: Benshushan journal of minimally invasive Gynacology, volume 2-0, issue 3, PP 376–80.

Office Hysteroscopy

Genesis of Office Hysteroscopy

Rahul Manchanda, Nidhi Chandil, Esha Sharma

Pantaleoni first performed hysteroscopy in 1869, but it was not until the early 1970s that hysteroscopy became part of the gynecologist's armamentarium.

During the 1970s and 1980s, 'traditional technique' of hysteroscopy was routinely performed. This approach involved the use of a speculum and cervical forceps while viewing and examining the cervix under distension using CO_2 as the preferred gaseous medium. Owing to the large diameter of the hysteroscope, preparatory cervical dilatation was mandatory, using local or general anesthesia, followed by hospitalization during recovery (inpatient hysteroscopy) (Figs 5.1 and 5.2).[1]

In the early 1990s, advances in technology and techniques made hysteroscopy less painful and invasive. At the same time, the number of ambulatory procedures (office hysteroscopy) was seen to rise, which may also be attributed to the fact that office hysteroscopy has the inherent benefit of obviating the need for anesthesia and dilatation of the cervical canal.[2-4] The standard rigid hysteroscopes used for decades had a diameter >5 mm and so cervical dilatation and

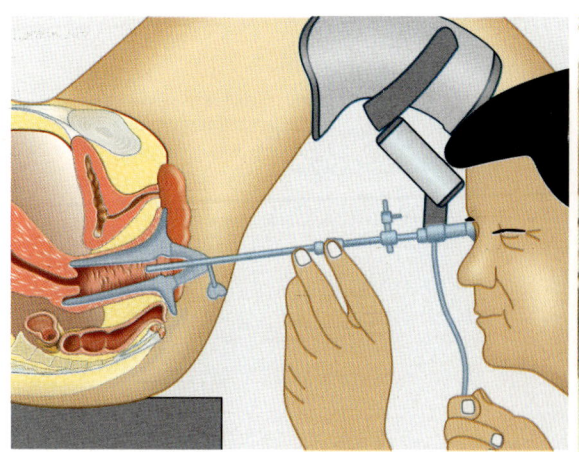

Fig. 5.1: Initial days of hysteroscopy

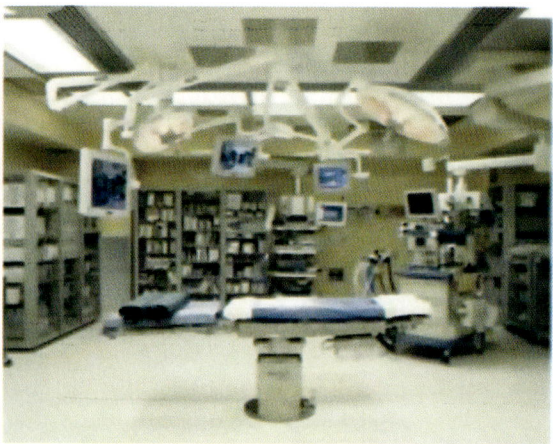

Fig. 5.2: Current set up of hysteroscopy

local or general anesthesia was required. The miniaturization of the instruments effectively reduces the difficulties both for the operator and for the patient, allowing even less skilled gynecologists to perform office hysteroscopy.[5] Moreover, it has been demonstrated that a smaller hysteroscope size make its introduction easier and less painful compared with conventional ones (Figs 5.3 and 5.4).[6, 7]

Office-based hysteroscopy allows us to visualize the uterine cavity for diagnostic or therapeutic purposes. Office procedures have lower complications and faster recovery and are easier to schedule, quicker, and more cost-effective.[8,9] The entire procedure takes less than 15 minutes.

These new scopes enable diagnostic and operative hysteroscopy to be performed simultaneously, in the office setting, without cervical dilatation and consequently without anesthesia or analgesia (**Bettocchi and Selvaggi, 1997**). Hysteroscopy not only allows for providing tissue, but permits the gynecologist to choose selected areas for directed biopsy and identify polyps and submucous fibroids. The latter are routinely missed by blind procedures such as a D&C.

Indication of Office Hysteroscopy

Diagnostic

- To evaluate patients with abnormal uterine bleeding resistant to medical management
- Filling defects identified by ultrasound or hysterosalpingography can be confirmed or mapped by hysteroscopic visualization.
- Routine hysteroscopy in infertility workup.
- Localization and removal of embedded intrauterine devices (IUDs) or IUD remnants.
- Post-myomectomy
- Post-uterine surgery or complication

Operative

- Myomectomy
- Uterine septoplasty
- Polypectomy
- Endometrial ablation
- Sterilization
- Retrival of IUCD

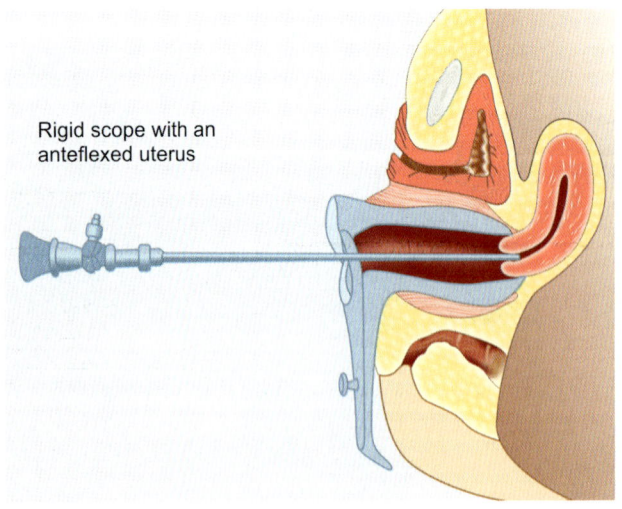

Rigid scope with an anteflexed uterus

Fig. 5.3: Rigid hysteroscope

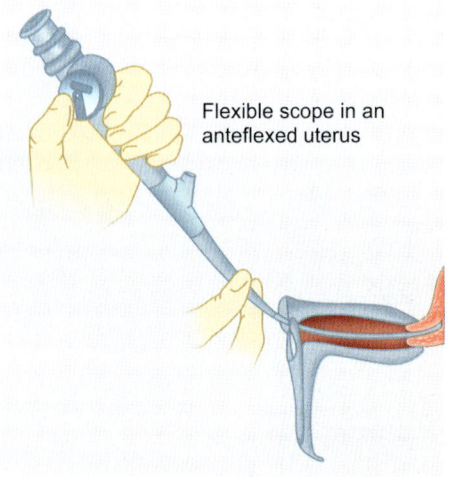

Flexible scope in an anteflexed uterus

Fig. 5.4: Flexible hysteroscope

Instruments of Office Hysteroscopy

Bettocchi's office hysteroscope (Karl Storz, Canada) (Fig. 5.5)

- 2.9 mm scope with 1.8 mm working channel (5 Fr)
- 4.3 mm diagnostic
- 5 mm operative

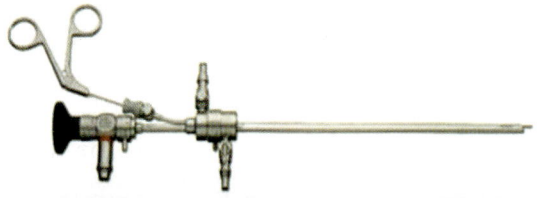

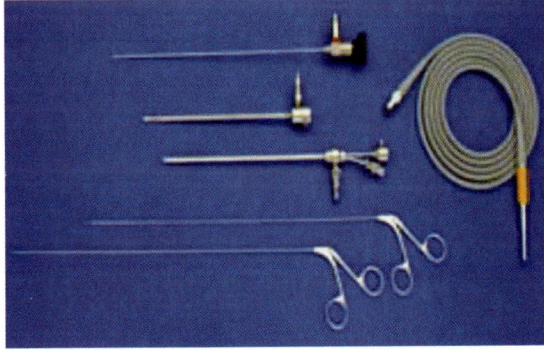

Fig. 5.5: Bittocchi's office hysteroscope

Other Instruments (Fig. 5.6)

- ➤ Ovum forceps
- ➤ Polyp forceps
- ➤ Ring forceps
- ➤ Myoma (Corson) grasper
- ➤ Suction curette
- ➤ Sharp curette
- ➤ Cutting loop

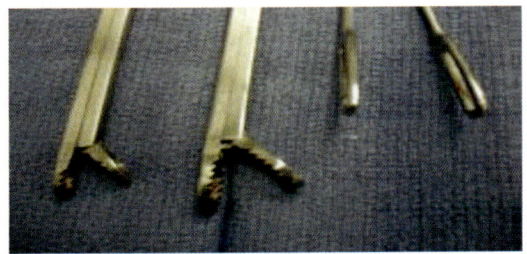

Fig. 5.6: Hysteroscopy instrument

Gynecare versapoint—bipolar electrode utilizing saline, used in myomectomy, polypectomy, adhesiolysis and septal resection (Fig. 5.7).

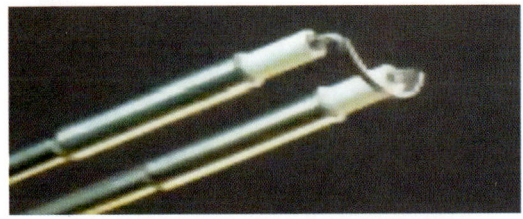

Bipolar loop resecting

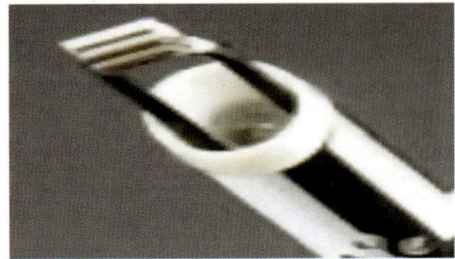

0° vaporizing

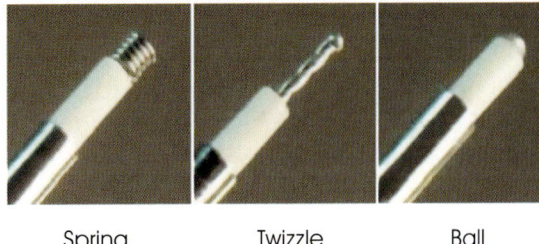

Spring   Twizzle   Ball

Fig. 5.7: Gynecare versapoint

Hysteromat and fluid delivery system: Closed systems should be used as they allow more accurate measurement of the fluid input and output (Fig. 5.8).

Preop Prerequisite

- Hysteroscopy should be performed during early proliferative phase or with endometrial thinning.
- Informed consent of the procedure, its alternative, and complication related to procedure, should be taken prior to surgery.
- Surgeon should be familiar with the instrument and procedure.

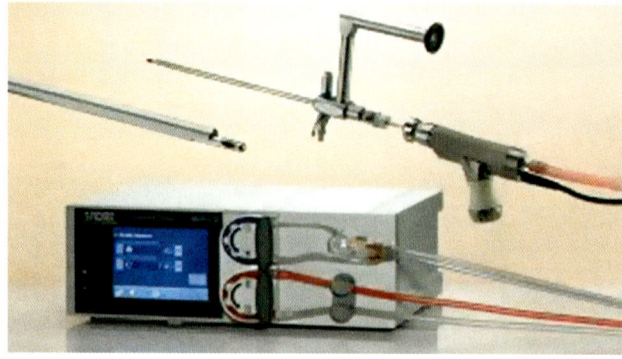 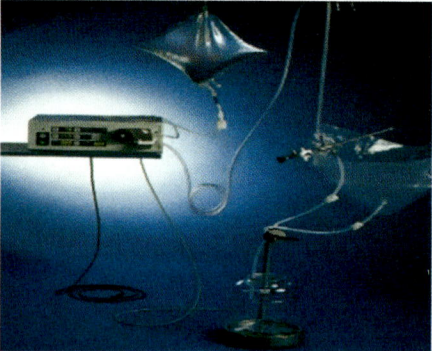

Fig. 5.8: Hysteromat with fluid delivery system

OFFICE SETUP

Hysteroscopy can be performed in a routine office exam room, although a room dedicated to procedures will facilitate its use. A video camera and monitor to display the findings to the patient is a very nice addition.

The establishment of an office hysteroscopy unit is described in Table 5.1 and Fig. 5.9.

1. *Position of patient*
   ➤ Patient is placed in dorsal lithotomy position (Fig. 5.10). Table should be flat. Do not use Trendlenburg tilt.
   ➤ Legs should be positioned in Allen Stirrup's or Candy cane
   ➤ Collect fluids with drapes/pouches.
2. *Distension media*: Historically, office hysteroscopy has been performed using carbon dioxide. Fluid distention systems, such as the Disten-U-Flo, make use of low viscosity fluids and continuous flow hysteroscopes, alleviating the expense of a CO_2 insufflating unit and remaining functional in the presence of bleeding.

Isotonic electrolyte-containing distension media such as normal saline should be used

Table 5.1: Minimal equipment for office hystero-scopy·

- 30° for oblique telescope and 5.5 mm continuous flow diagnostic hysteroscopic sheath
- Light source and light cable
- Disten-U-Flo system or CO_2 insufflator biopsy forceps
- Continuous suction aspiration equipment·
- Cervical speculum
- Cervical tenaculum
- Ring forceps and prep bowl
- Finger grip control syringe with needle extender and #21 needle·
- 1% Lidocaine without epinephrine
- Small cervical dilator
- Sterile drape under the buttocks

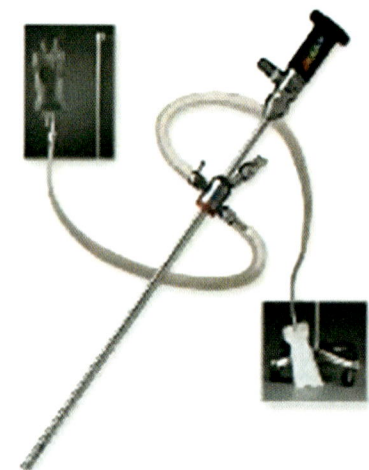

Fig. 5.9: Disten-U-Flo fluid management system with CIRCON ACMI GY5-CFH continuous flow hysteroscope

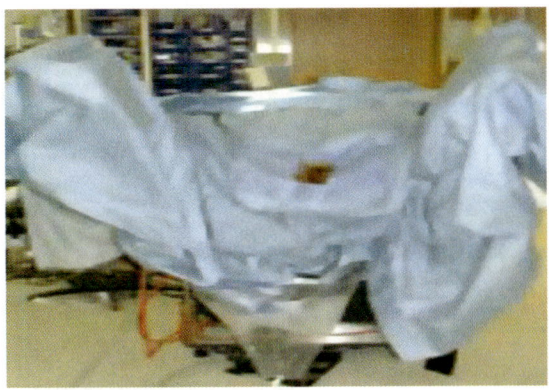

Fig. 5.10: Lithotomy position

with mechanical instrumentation and bipolar electrosurgery because they are less likely to cause hyponatremia, if fluid overload occurs.

Hypotonic, electrolyte-free distension media, such as glycine and sorbitol, should only be used with monopolar electrosurgical instruments.

3. *Operative considerations*
   - Dilatation is not required with 2.9 mm office hysteroscope, alleviate need for local or general anesthesia.
   - A paracervical and intracervical block administered, if necessary.
   - Vaginoscopic method: In 1997, Bettocchi et al [2] developed the 'vaginoscopic approach' or 'no-touch technique' for the atramautic insertion of the hysteroscope into the external uterine orifice, without the aid of the speculum or the tenaculum, introducing the scope directly into the vaginal canal. This vaginoscopic method results less pain as speculam insertion is most painful step during hysteroscopy (Fig. 5.11).

   - The best view of the entire uterine cavity is obtained when the hysteroscope is placed at the junction of the lower uterine segment and upper cervical canal. The hysteroscope can then be advanced into the cavity for a closer view.

   - Visualize all landmarks including external uterine ostium, cervical canal, internal os, endometrial cavity with all 4 walls (anterior, posterior, right and left lateral walls), fundus and both ostia.

   - Hysteroscope should be placed into the lower vagina and, with the introduction of the distension medium at a pressure of 30–40 mm Hg (the same pressure used for the distension of the uterine cavity), progressively distend the vaginal cavity, without causing pain (Figs 5.12 and 5.13).

   - *A fluid deficit of more than 1000 mL should be used as threshold to define fluid overload when using hypotonic solutions in healthy women of reproductive age.*

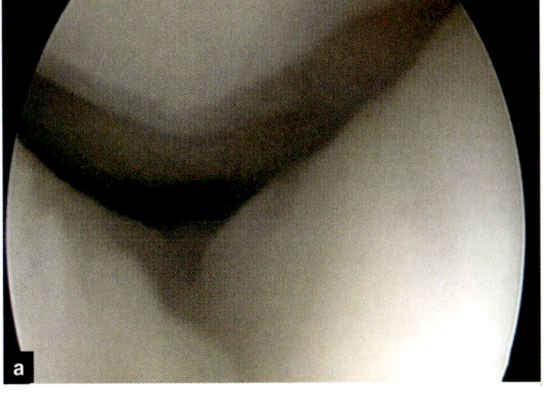
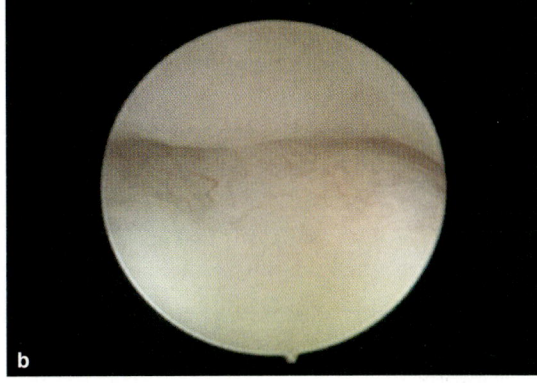

Fig. 5.11: Vaginoscopic view of (a) vagina and (b) external uterine ostium

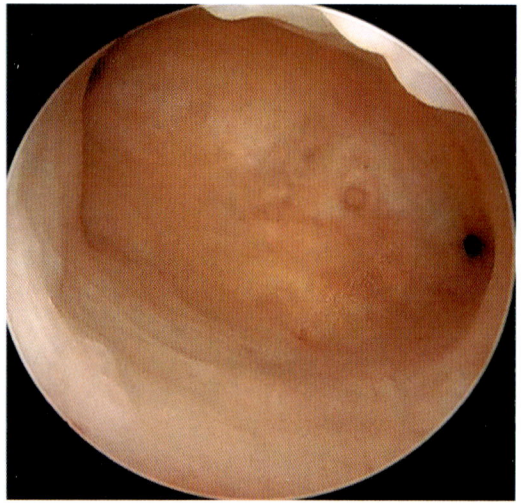

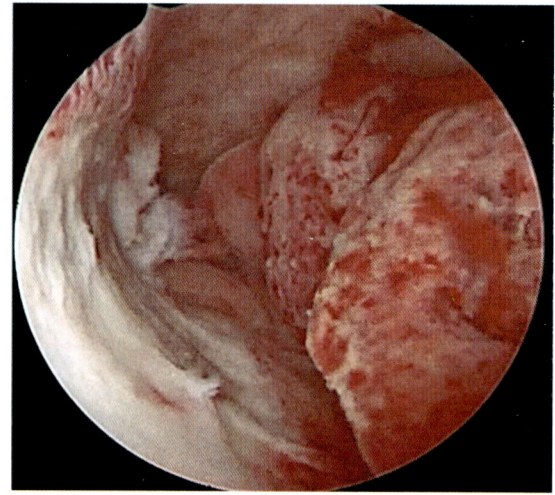

Fig. 5.12: Hysteroscopic view of urerine cavity with both ostia

5.13: Multiple polyp inside the cavity

A fluid deficit of 2500 mL should be used as threshold to define fluid overload when using isotonic solutions in healthy women of reproductive age. Procedure should be abandoned once the threshold is achieved.

General Principles of Operative Hysteroscopic Myomectomy

- Attempt should be made to resect type 0 and 1 fibroids only.
- Electrode should be advanced toward the surgeon only.
- Restrict resection to endometrial surfaces, if deep intramural lesion noted—be patient!! Often once the pseudocapsule is breached, the uterus will contract and expel the myoma into the field.
- Beware of progressive myometrial eversion, end resection at capsular level.
- Deflate the endometrium and uterine massage should be done, once the resection is complete.
- Reinspect endometrial cavity 2–3 minutes after removing hysteroscope.
- Sharp curettage can be performed, if copious endometrial debris, blood, or copious resected myoma or polyp present inside the cavity.

- Consider estrogen therapy to aid in re-epithelialization of endometrium in patients desiring fertility.

PROBLEMS ASSOCIATED WITH OFFICE HYSTEROSCOPY

The procedure is generally well-tolerated in the office setting, but the most common cause for discontinuation of office hysteroscopy is pain. Women who undergo outpatient hysteroscopy complain of discomfort primarily during cervical manipulation and cervical dilation, uterine distension, uterine contractions (caused by endometrial biopsy, polypectomy, or ablation), and tubal manipulation (transcervical sterilization).

Less pain with:

- Mini-hysteroscope 2.9 mm instrument
- Vaginoscopic method—no speculam, no tenaculam, no cervical dilatation.
- Lesser intrauterine pressure (30–40 mm Hg).
- Skilled surgeon
- Surgery in mucosa (polyps, biopsies and lysis of adhesion)

Greater risk of pain:

- Previous cesarean section
- Anxiety
- Menopausal
- Longer procedure (>15 min)

Each of these sensations is managed by the complex innervation of the uterus, cervix, fallopian tubes, and endometrium. The sympathetic nerves of the thoracic and lumbar spine (T10–L1) travel with the superior hypogastric plexus (presacral nerve). They

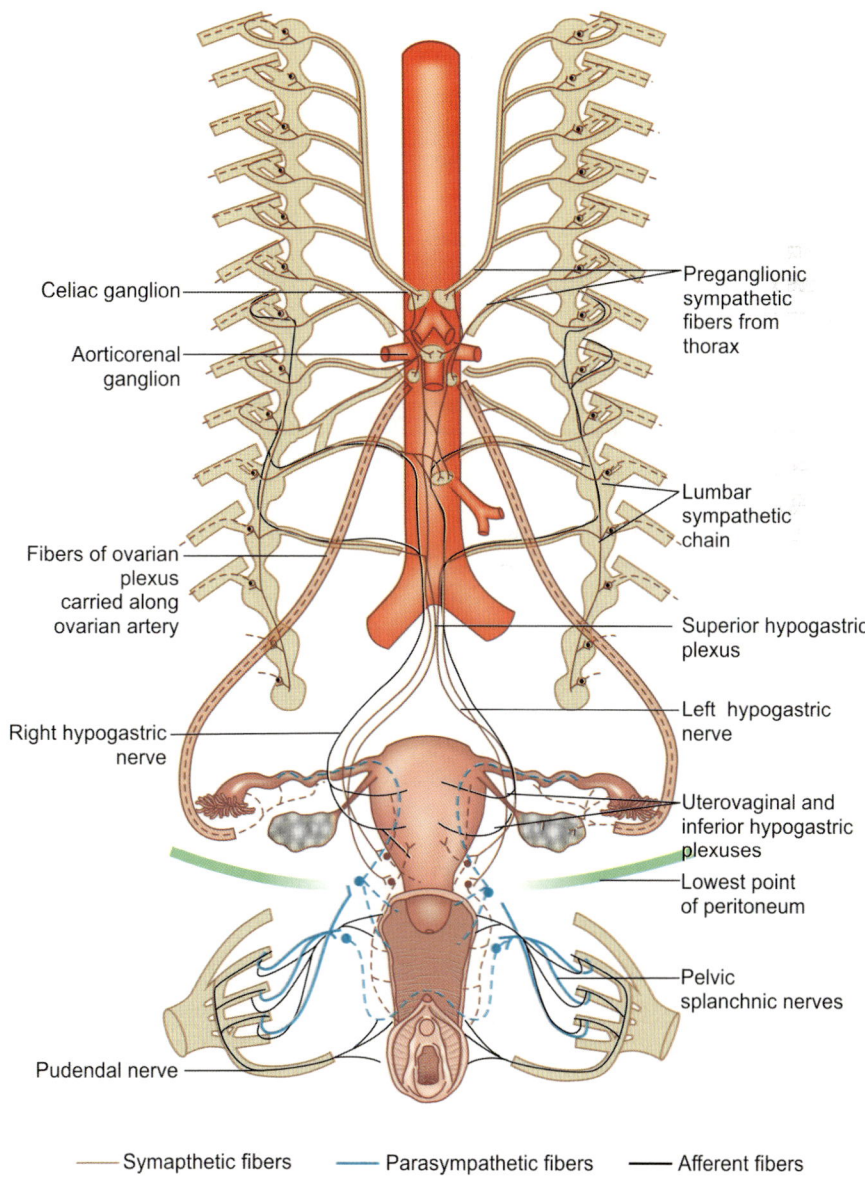

Celiac ganglion

Aorticorenal ganglion

Fibers of ovarian plexus carried along ovarian artery

Right hypogastric nerve

Pudendal nerve

Preganglionic sympathetic fibers from thorax

Lumbar sympathetic chain

Superior hypogastric plexus

Left hypogastric nerve

Uterovaginal and inferior hypogastric plexuses

Lowest point of peritoneum

Pelvic splanchnic nerves

—— Symapthetic fibers   —— Parasympathetic fibers   —— Afferent fibers

Fig. 5.14: Sympathetic and parasympathetic innervations of uterus and adnexa

then divide into the two hypogastric nerves and reach the uterine fundus via the uterosacral ligament. Sympathetic fibers further innervate the uterus via the ovarian plexus. Parasympathetic nerves of sacral origin (S2–S4) form the uterovaginal and inferior hypogastric plexus, innervating mainly the cervix and the lower uterine segment. This is known as Frankenhauser's paracervical nerve plexus. The inferior ovarian nerves arise directly from the hypogastric plexus and innervate the fallopian tubes. The innervation of the endometrium and the myometrium is poorly understood. However, uterine activity has been shown to cause patient pain and discomfort (Fig. 5.14).[10]

Larger diameter hysteroscopes are associated with increased pain during dilation, but the 5 mm hysteroscope may be necessary for certain procedures. It has been shown that longer procedures are more uncomfortable for patients and, therefore, knowledge of the instrument and preparation of the procedure room will optimize chances of success.

Measures to Reduce Pain During Office Hysteroscopy

- Either no speculam or wet speculum should be used, if necessary.[11]
- Cervical dilatation is not required with 2.9 mm office hysteroscope. Local anesthesia with a PCB has been found to decrease pain with introduction of the hysteroscope when cervical dilatation is required.[12]
- Recommendations for maximum dosing state that providers should not exceed 4.5 mg/kg 1% lidocaine without epinephrine or 7 mg/kg 1% lidocaine with epinephrine.
- *Nitrous oxide:* Nitrous oxide may be helpful in reducing pain from hysteroscopy and hysteroscopic sterilization. Nitrous oxide has analgesic, anxiolytic, and amnestic properties, and vasodilates smooth muscle.[13,14]
- *The power of words:* Providers should remember the power of their words and

always use the neutral words. Literature from interventional radiology finds that negative words increase the pain, anxiety, and discomfort that patients experience during outpatient procedures.[15]

- **Soft music** played in the procedure room has been shown to decrease patient anxiety and pain with hysteroscopic procedures.[16]

Office hysteroscopy is advantageous both for the patient and the physician. For the patient, it is little more than an extended office visit, usually providing a prompt diagnosis to a problem. Diagnostic office hysteroscopy is a safe procedure, with a few significant complications, and the patient can resume normal activities immediately. Savings in terms of physician time average one to two hours when compared to a hospital D&C. These savings occur primarily as a result of minimal office preparation, decreased turnover time between procedures, no anesthesia, and no commute between the hospital and office.

References

1. Bettocchi S, Ceci O, Spinelli ML, et al. Office hysteroscopy. Ref Gynecol Obstet. 2010;12:1e9.
2. Bettocchi S, Selvaggi L. A vaginoscopic approach to reduce the pain of office hysteroscopy. J Am Assoc Gynecol Laparosc. 1997;4: 255e258.
3. Paschopoulos M, Paraskevaidis E, Stefanidis K, Kofinas G, Lolis D. Vaginoscopic approach to outpatient hysteroscopy. J Am Assoc Gynecol Laparosc. 1997;4: 465e467.
4. Cicinelli E. Diagnostic mini-hysteroscopy with vaginoscopic approach: rationale and advantages. J Minim Invasive Gynecol. 2005;12:396e400.
5. Campo R, Molinas CR, Rombauts L, et al. Prospective multicentre randomized controlled trial to evaluate factors influencing the success rate of office diagnostic hysteroscopy. Hum Reprod. 2005;20:258e263.
6. Valle RF. Office hysteroscopy. Clin Obstet Gynecol. 1999;42:276e289.
7. Campo R, Van Belle Y, Rombauts L, Brosens I, Gordts S. Office mini-hysteroscopy. Hum Reprod Update. 1999;5:73e81.

8. Loffer FD: "Hysteroscopy with selected endometrial sampling compared with D&C for abnormal uterine bleeding: the value of a negative hysteroscopic view." Obst Gyne 1989, 73:16–20.

9. Isaacson KB editor: Office Hysteroscopy, St. Louis, Mosby-Year Book, 1996.

10. Smith GM, Stubblefield PG, Chirchirillo L, McCarthy M. J. Pain of first-trimester abortion: its quantification and relations with other variables. Am J Obstet Gynecol. 1979;133:489–498.

11. Hill DA, Lamvu G. Effect of lubricating gel on patient comfort during vaginal speculum examination: a randomized controlled trial. Obstet Gynecol. 2012;119(2, Part 1):227–231.

12. Chudnoff S, Einstein M, Levie M. Paracervical block efficacy in office hysteroscopic sterilization: a randomized controlled trial. Obstet Gynecol. 2010;115(1): 26–34.

13. Zacny JP, Hurst RJ, Graham L, Janiszewski DJ. Preoperative dental anxiety and mood changes during nitrous oxide inhalation. J Am Dent Assoc. 2002;133(1):82–88.

14. Becker DE, Rosenberg M. Nitrous oxide and the inhalation anesthetics. Anesth Prog. 2008;55(4):124–130; quiz 31-32.

15. Lang EV, Hatsiopoulou TK, Berbaum K, et al. Can words hurt? Patient-provider interactions during invasive procedures. Pain. 2005;114: 303–309.

16. Angioli R, De Cicco Nardone C, Plotti F, et al. Use of music to reduce anxiety during office hysteroscopy: prospective randomized trial. J Minim Invasive Gynecol . 2014;21(3): 454–459.

Office Hysteroscopy and Outpatient Transvaginal Endoscopy in Low Resource/ Minimal Setting

Ichnandy Arief Rachman, Ditha Loho

BACKGROUND

Transvaginal endoscopy (TVE) has been recognized as an alternative procedure of standard laparoscopy performed in the treatment of infertility patients whose cause is unknown. TVE is a modification of culdoscopy used to evaluate the posterior uterus, lateral pelvic wall and adnexa. This procedure is considered a part of the natural orifice transluminal endoscopic surgery (NOTES) procedure so it does not cause scars on the abdominal area which is very important for most women. Compared to more invasive and more expensive diagnostic laparoscopy. TVE is the diagnostic procedure of choice that can be performed at the office setting for infertility patients without clear pelvic pathology.[1–3]

Hysteroscopy is a form of an inspection of the cervix and intrauterine through the endoscope. Hysteroscopy is now considered as the gold standard for detecting uterine cavity abnormalities in infertility.[4,5] TVE can be done in the office under local anesthesia.[6]

Combined with office hysteroscopy and chromotubation, it can replace hysterosalpingography (HSG) as the first-line diagnostic test for the infertile woman.[2] Studies have shown high patient tolerability with less pain reported postprocedure than with HSG.[2]

As infertility cases are getting higher in most countries, cost for infertility management will be big burden especially in developing countries. This chapter will elaborate and discuss about TVE instrumentation, indication–contraindication, cost and benefit that we can have. Also about the patient selection, preparation and the challenges that we have to encounter to make this procedure as a daily office routines.

Instrumentation for Office Hysteroscopy and Transvaginal Endoscopy

The standard office hysteroscope consists of a 2.9 mm 30° forward—oblique rigid telescope assembled in a single-flow diagnostic sheath for a total instrument diameter of 3.7 mm (Fig. 6.1).[7]

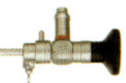

Fig. 6.1: Karl Storz endoscope

As for the transvaginal endoscopy, there are 2 types of instruments currently used, namely 'reusable instruments' developed by Stephan Gordts in collaboration with Karls Storz, Tutlingen, Germany[4] and 'disposable instruments' developed by Antoine Watrelot in collaboration with fertility focus, sommerset, United Kingdom.[8]

"Reusable instruments" by Karl Storz, Tutlingen, Germany is a trocar system consisting of a special dilator needle created to ensure safety and anticipate injury while entering the Douglas pouch.[6] These reusable instruments are more preferable to use in the low resource setting (Fig. 6.2).

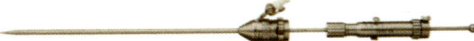

Fig. 6.2: "Special needle dilator trocar system"

The system is comprised of 3 components:[6]

1. *Springload needle* with a diameter of 1.5 mm and length of 30 cm
2. *Dilating sheath* with a diameter of 3.8 mm and length of 30 cm
3. *Outer trocar* with a diameter of 4.4 mm and length of 20 cm (Fig. 6.3)

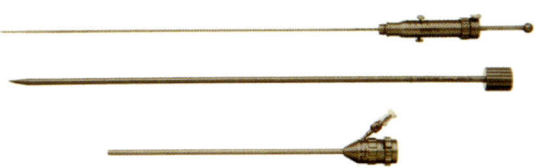

Fig. 6.3: "Springload needle", "dilating sheath", and "outer trocar"

The 'outer trocar' can be replaced with a 5.6 mm diameter *operative outer*.

Trocar with one *working channel* allowing the use of a 5 Fr instrument.[6] The process of replacing the outer sheath with the operative outer sheath is guided with a guidewire (Figs 6.4 and 6.5).[6]

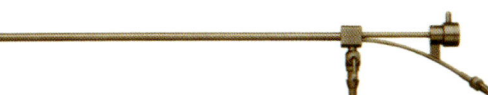

Fig. 6.4: *Operative outer sheath* 6 with a diameter of 6.6 mm, and length of 29 cm

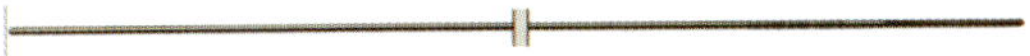

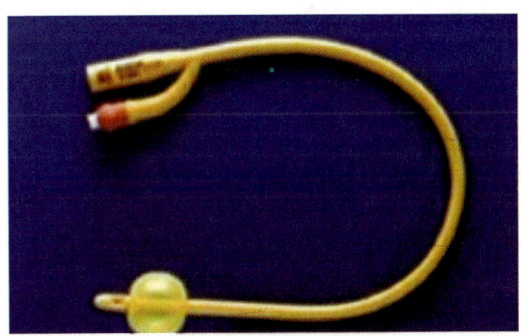

Fig. 6.5: Karl Storz *guidewire,* with a diameter of 2.9 mm, and length of 36 cm

Aside from the aforementioned instruments, other instruments needed to perform the procedure include:[6]

1. A Graves-Weismann speculum or Colin speculum (Fig. 6.6) with one-sided lateral opening.

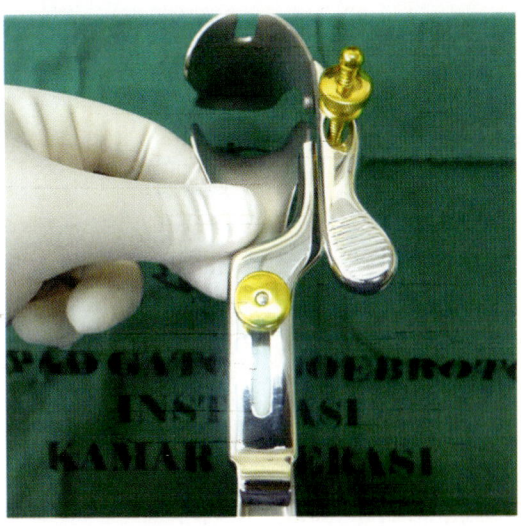

Fig. 6.6: Graves-Weismann speculum

2. No. 8 urinary Foley's catheter to perform chromotubation (Fig. 6.7).

Fig. 6.7: Foley's catheter

3. *Electronic pump* or *pressure bag*
   Electronic pump adjusts the pressure automatically as we set it. But *pressure bag* gives us a sufficient and adequate function compare to the more expensive electronic pump (Figs 6.8 and 6.9).

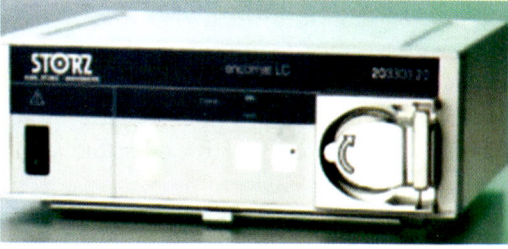

Fig. 6.8: Karl Storz endomat *electronic pump*

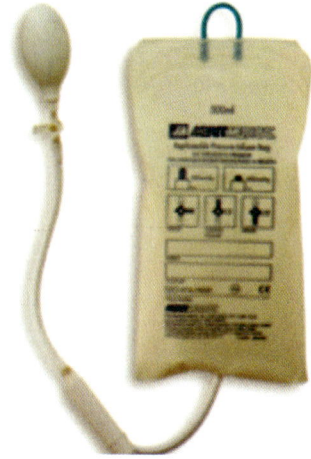

Fig. 6.9: Pressure bag

Disposable instruments is a system comprised of 2 introducers, one to enter the uterine cavity and the other to enter the pelvis. At the end of either 'introducers' is a 2–3 mL balloon to fixate the introducer.[8] These *disposable instruments* are more expensive and not cost effective to be used in a low resource setting (Fig. 6.10).

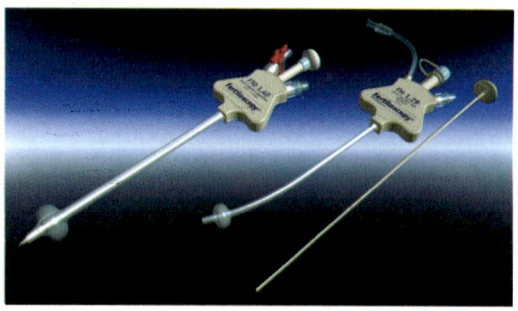

Fig. 6.10: *Disposable instrument*

TROCAR INSERTION TECHNIQUE

The indication for TVE is mainly for infertility patients with an anteflexed uterus and unidentifiable cause, while some relative contraindications for this procedure are retroflexed uterus, history of pelvic surgery, Douglas pouch obstruction, acute pelvic infection.[2,3,6,8,9] The gravest complication that may occur is rectum perforation.[10] TVE is performed **after** a prior office hysteroscopy has been performed.[6,8,9]

The steps in performing TVE are as follows:[6]

a. Application of a Graves-Weismann or Collin speculum with a one-sided lateral opening.

b. Injection of a local anesthesia posterior to the cervix.

c. Elevation of the posterior of cervix to clearly visualize the posterior wall.

d. Application of the *special needle dilator system* approximately 15 mm inferior to the posterior cervical lip (Fig. 6.11a to d).

After the trocar has been correctly inserted, the "spring load needle" is removed, Foley catheter is inserted, and the tenaculum and speculum are removed (Fig. 6.12).[6]

Following removal of speculum, warm saline flow is started, and the endoscope is inserted into the trocar, allowing the evaluation process to be initiated (Fig. 6.13).

INTRAPERITONEAL EVALUATION

TVE exploration is intended for direct observation of the internal genitalia in the most minimally-invasive manner, without compromising the diagnostic accuracy.[11,12] The initial evaluation will be comprised of the posterior uterine wall, and with the former as guidance, we can identify the rectum, bilateral pelvic walls, both tubes, salpingoscopy, and both ovaries.[1,6,9,12] In combination with chromotubation, TVE may replace the need for HSG and diagnostic laparoscopy (Figs 6.14 to 6.18).[1,3,9]

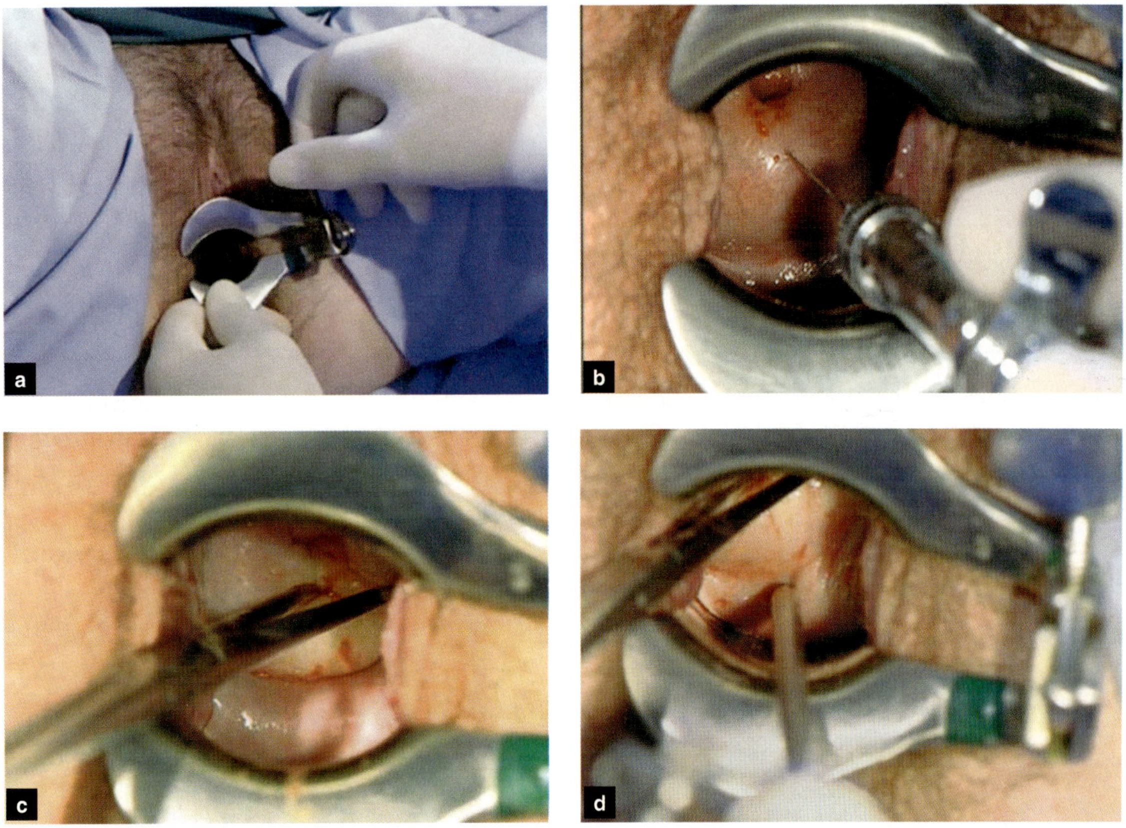

Fig. 6.11: Application technique of *special needle dilator trocar system*

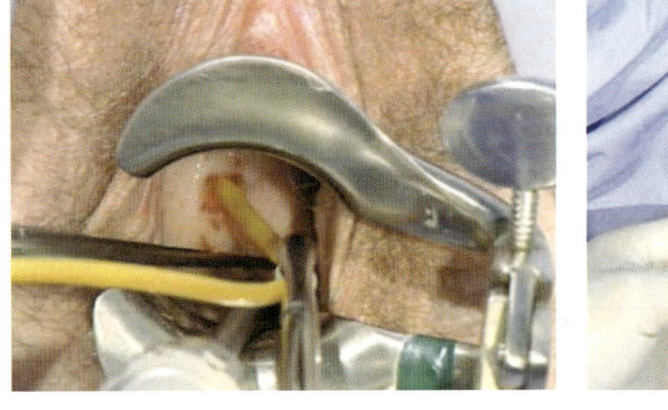
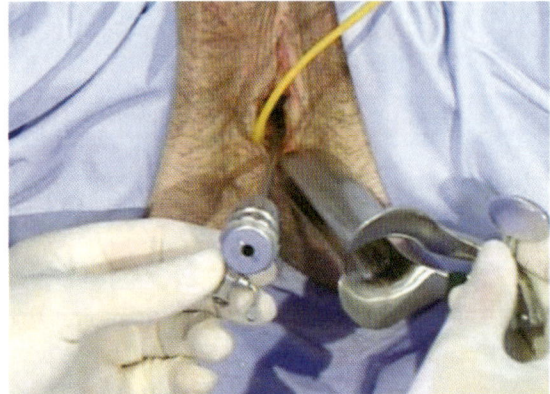

Fig. 6.12: Speculum removal technique

The use of warm saline as distension medium provide the "hydrofloatation" effect, allowing for clear visualization of pathologies such as endometriosis lesions (Fig. 6.16a and b).[1,11,12]

The following figures demonstrate the appearance of pathologies encountered in TVE.

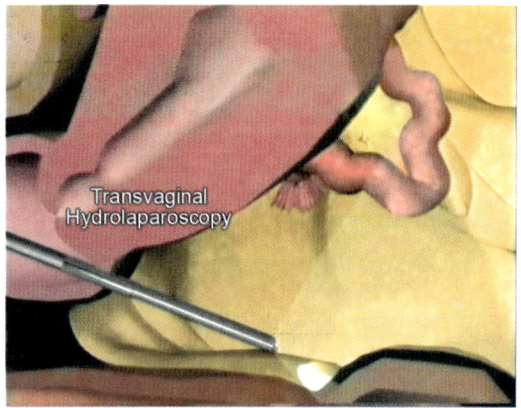

Fig. 6.13: Evaluation process of TVE

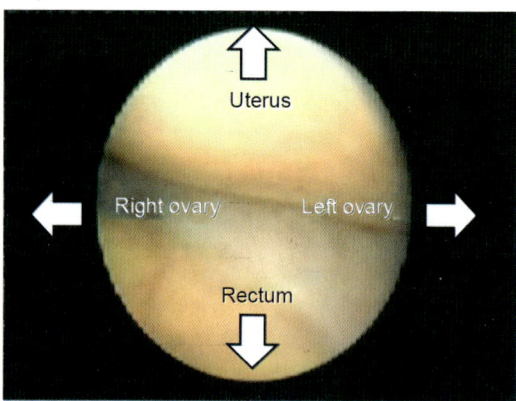

Fig. 6.14: Capture from Karl Storz TVE educational video

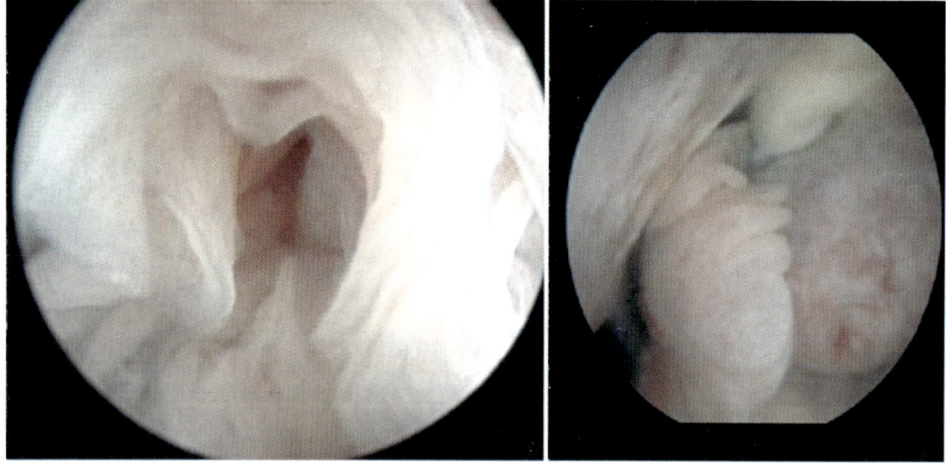

Fig. 6.15: Salpingoscopy and chromotubation

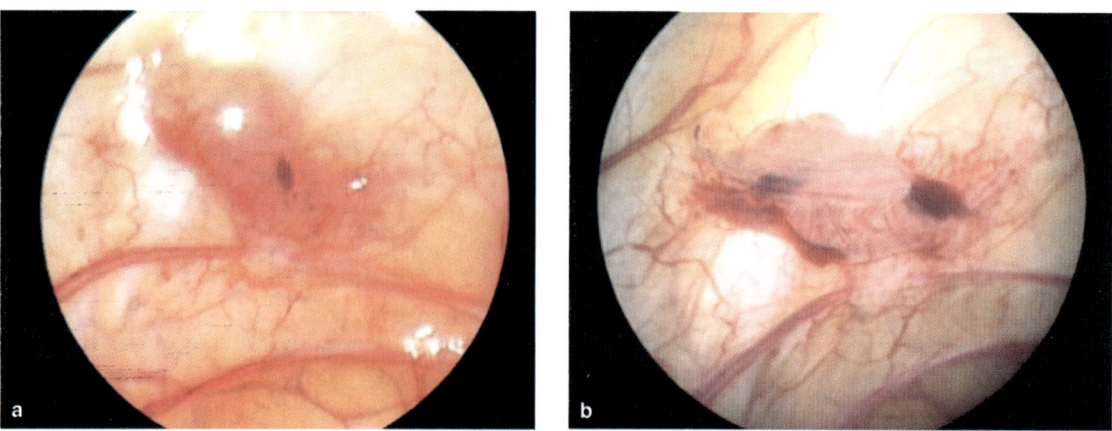

Fig. 6.16: Comparison of endometriosis lesion on (a) laparoscopy and (b) transvaginal endoscopy

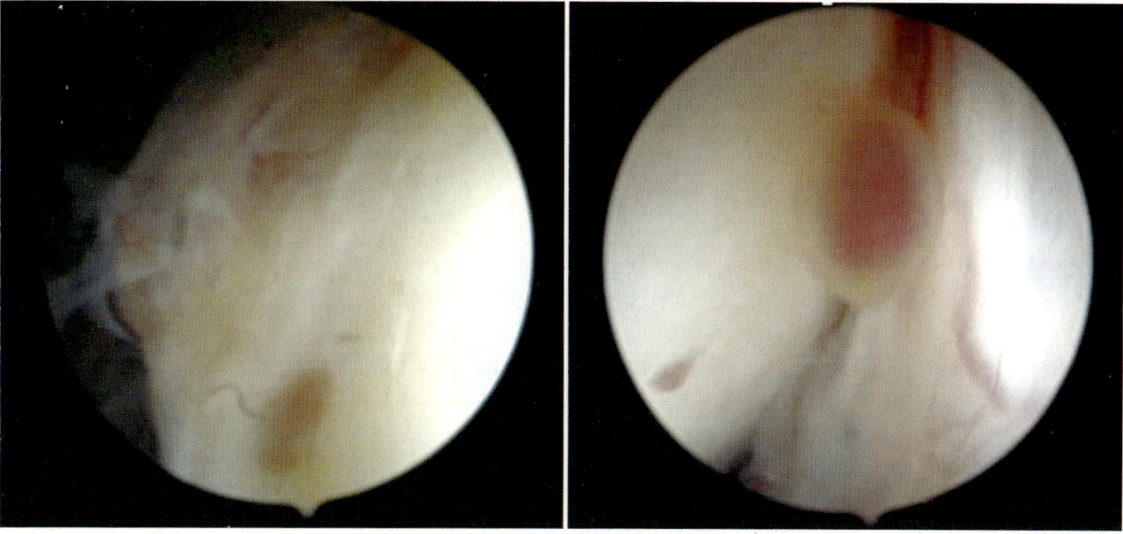

Fig. 6.17: Endometriosis lesion

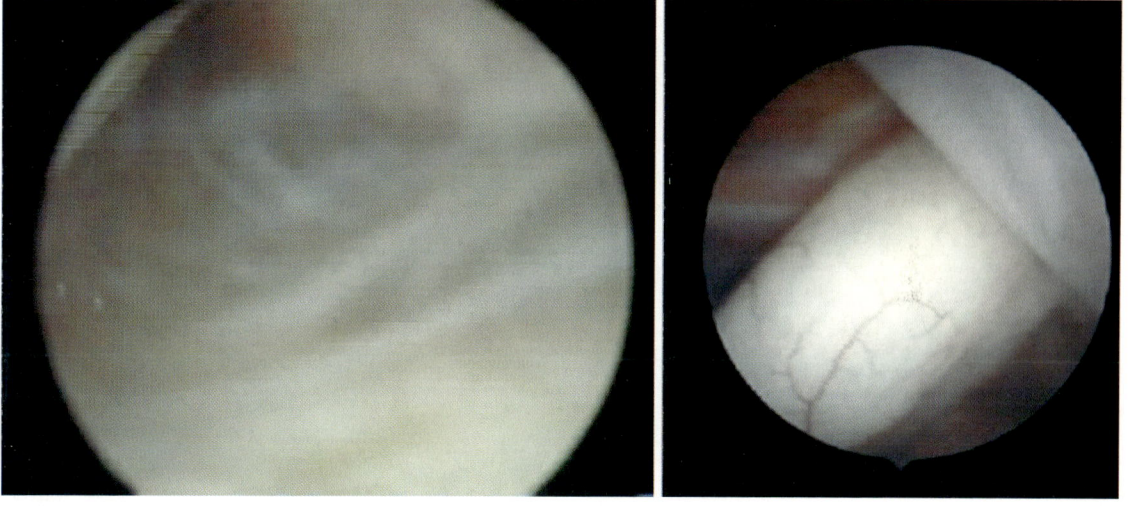

Fig. 6.18: Adhesion and appendicitis

DISCUSSION

In conjunction with hysteroscopy and chromotubation, TVE can substitute HSG as the initial diagnostic procedure in infertility case.[1–3,8,9] Various studies have demonstrated a lower post-procedural pain level in comparison with HSG.[2,3]

With adjoining salpingoscopy, TVE is equally effective as laparoscopy in diagnosing female pelvic pathologies,[2,3,8] with lower cost, shorter procedure duration, and comparable accuracy. Limitations of TVE include limited panoramic view and difficulty of performing the procedure in patients with a retroflexed uterus or adhesions, which may increase the risk of rectum perforation.[9,10]

We do not need to worry about the excess media distension in the peritoneal cavity that use in the hysteroscopy procedure. All of the excess liquid will be taken out during the end of transvaginal endoscopy procedure.

CONCLUSION

TVE is a part of NOTES procedure that may be performed in the outpatient clinic or *office setting*. The procedure is very cost effective, fast, and accurate in the initial investigation of infertility patients and can be performed as a *one day care* procedure. A distinct training method is needed for an endoscopist prior to being certified competent in this procedure.

References

1. Gordts S, Brosen I. Rationale of Transvaginal Laparoscopy in Atlas of Transvaginal Endoscopy. Informa Health Care 2007:4–7.

2. Gordts S, Campo R, Rombauts L, Brosens I. Transvaginal hydrolaparoscopy as an outpatient procedure for infertility investigation. Hum Reprod 1998;13:99–103.

3. De Wilde RL, Brosens L. Rationale of first-line endoscopy-based fertility exploration using transvaginal hydrolaparoscopy and mini hysteroscopy. Hum Reprod 2012;0;1–7.

4. Cholkeri-Singh A, Sasaki KJ. Hysteroscopy for infertile women: a review. J Minim Invasive Gynecol 2015;22:353–62.

5. Salazar CA, Isaacson KB. Office Operative Hysteroscopy: An Update. J Minim Invasive Gynecol 2018;25:199–208.

6. Lundorff P, Gordt S. Transvaginal Endoscopy: Instrumentation and Technique in Atlas of Transvaginal Endoscopy. Informa Health Care 2007:25–32.

7. Campo R, Molina CR. Diagnostic Hysteroscopy in Atlas of Transvaginal Endoscopy. Informa Health Care 2007:9–23.

8. Watrelot A. Fertiloscopy in Atlas of Atlas of Operative Laparoscopy and Hysteroscopy. Informa Health Care 2007:113–32.

9. Shibahara H, Suzuki T, Suzuki M. Diagnostic and Therapeutic Transvaginal Hydrolaparoscopy in Advance Gynelogoic Endoscopic. Intech, 2011.

10. Verhoeven HC, Brosens I. Risks and Complications of Transvaginal Access to the Peritoneal Cavity in Atlas of Transvaginal Endoscopy. Informa Health Care 2007: 41–4.

11. Gordts S, Campo R, Puttemans P, Verhoeven H, Gianaroli L, Brosens J, Brosens I. Investigation of the infertile couple: a one-stop outpatient endoscopy-based approach. Hum Reprod 2002;17:1684–87.

12. Gordts S. Normal Tubo-ovarian Events at Transvaginal Laparoscopy in Atlas of Transvaginal Endoscopy. Informa Health Care 2007:33–39.

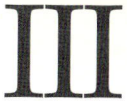

Challenges in Dealing with Submucous Myoma

Uterine Fibroids: Classification and Management

Marie Hanna, Nash S Moawad

INTRODUCTION

Uterine leiomyomas (fibroids) are common tumors arising from the smooth muscle cells of the uterus. It is difficult to report prevalence of fibroids as they are frequently asymptomatic and screening tests are neither routine nor recommended. It is estimated that between 55% and 77% of women have fibroids.[1,2] Submucosal myomas, in particular, account for 5.5 to 16.6% of all uterine myomas[3]. These may be asymptomatic or can be associated with significant symptoms such as abnormal uterine bleeding, pain, dysmenorrhea, pressure symptoms such as bowel or bladder dysfunction, infertility or recurrent pregnancy loss. This chapter will focus on the classification systems of leiomyomas, in addition to current treatment options, with particular attention to hysteroscopic myomectomy of submucosal fibroids.

Classifications

Three classifications will be described in this chapter, namely the Wamsteker/ESGE classification, Lasmar's STEPW classification, and the International Federation of Gynecology and Obstetrics (FIGO) classification. Classification systems were created to facilitate documentation and communication of the fibroid location and size, help with counseling

patients on the surgical risks and expectations, as well as predict surgical difficulty and success rates.

The classification system by Wamsteker et al (Box 7.1) was developed for submucosal fibroids in 1993 in order to predict the degree of difficulty of transcervical hysteroscopic resection based on the degree of intramural penetration. The authors concluded that complete resection was not always possible with submucosal fibroids with deep intramural extension, and that repeat procedures may be required in certain cases[4]. The classification system was later adopted by the European Society of Gynecological Endoscopy (ESGE) (Fig. 7.1).[5] The system classifies submucosal fibroids as type 0, 1 or 2 Type 0 is a pedunculated intra-cavitary fibroid without intramural extension. Type 1 is a sessile fibroid with less than 50% of the fibroid penetrating into the myometrium (Fig. 7.2). If the fibroid's intramural extension is >50%, it is classified as type 2. The extent of intramural extension is determined by visualization of the angle of the fibroid with the endometrium at its attachment, with an acute angle suggesting a type 1 fibroid, while an obtuse angle suggesting a type 2 fibroid.[4]

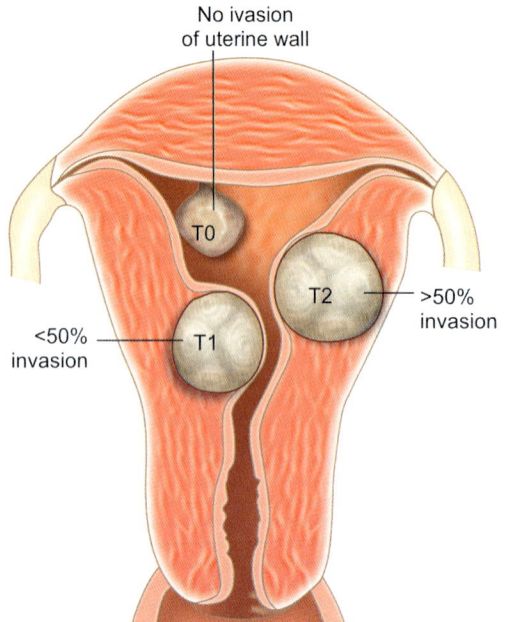

Fig. 7.1: Wamsteker/ESGE Classification of sub-mucosal leiomyomas
*Reprinted/adapted by permission from **Springer Nature**: Hysteroscopy by Haimovich, Tinelli and Alonso, 2018.*

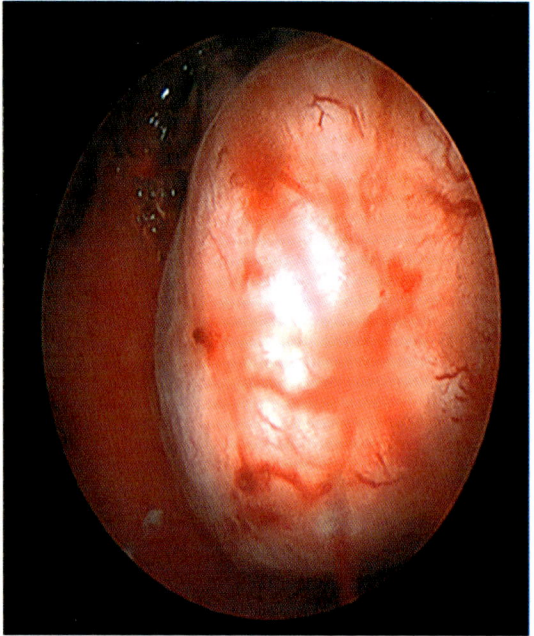

Fig. 7.2: Large type 1 submucosal myoma
*Reprinted/adapted by permission from **Springer Nature**: Uterine Fibroids: A Clinical Casebook by Nash S Moawad, 2018.*

Box 7.1: Classification of submucous myomas

Type 0
• Entirely within endometrial cavity
• No myometrial extension (pedunculated)

Type 1
• <50% myometrial extension (sessile)
• <90° angle of myoma surface to uterine wall

Type 2
• >50% myometrial extension (sessile)
• >90° angle of myoma surface to uterine wall

Modified from Wamsteker et al. Obstet Gynecol. 1993;82:736–740.

*Reprinted/adapted by permission from **Springer Nature**: Uterine Fibroids: A Clinical Casebook by Nash S Moawad, 2018*

Another classification system, developed in 2005 by Lasmar et al (Fig. 7.3), used five parameters to classify submucosal fibroids.[6]

These five parameters included size, topography, extension of the base in relation to the uterine wall, penetration into the myometrium, and whether the fibroid is arising from the lateral wall (STEPW). Lasmar et al showed in a study of 62 hysteroscopic myomectomies, that the STEPW classification had greater correlation with surgical difficulty than the ESGE classification system. A follow-up multicenter study in 2011 with 465 myomectomies again showed greater correlation of the STEPW classification with complete or incomplete removal of the fibroid by hysteroscopic myomectomy, when compared to the ESGE classification (Fig. 7.3).[7]

The International Federation of Gynecology and Obstetrics (FIGO) abnormal uterine bleeding (AUB) classification system (Fig. 7.4) includes the following uterine fibroid subclassification: Submucosal, intramural and subserosal leiomyomas.[8] Types 0, 1 and 2 are

	Size (cm)	Topography	Extension of the base	Penetration	Lateral wall	Total
0	≤2	Low	≤ 1/3	0		
1	2–5	Middle	1/3 – 2/3	≤ 50%	+1	
2	>5	Upper	> 2/3	> 50%		
Score	+	+	+	+	+	

Score	Group	Complexity and therapeutic options
0–4	I	Low complexity hysteroscopic myomectomy.
5–6	II	High complexity hysteroscopic myomectomy. Consider GnRH use? Consider Two-step hysteroscopic myomectomy.
7–9	III	Consider alternatives to the hysteroscopic technique

Fig. 7.3: Lasmar's STEPW classification for submucosal leiomyomas and prediction of surgical difficulty

reminiscent of the Wamsteker (ESGE) classification. Type 0 is intracavity and attached to the endometrium by a stalk, type 1 is <50% intramural involvement, and type 2 is at least 50% intramural extension.

The other types in the FIGO classification system refer to intramural, subserosal and hybrid fibroids. Type 3 is 100% intramural, but is in contact with the endometrium. Type 4 is completely intramural without

SM - Submucosal	0	Pedunculated intracavitary
	1	<50% Intramural
	2	≥50% Intramural
O - Other	3	Contacts endometrium; 100% intramural
	4	Intramural
	5	Subserosal ≥50% intramural
	6	Subserosal <50% intramural
	7	Subserosal pedunculated
	8	Other (specify e.g. cervical, parasitic)
Hybrid leiomymas (impact both endometrium and serosa)	Two numbers are listed separated by a hyphen. By convention, the first refers to the relationship with the endometrium while the second refers to the relationship to the serosa. One example is below	
	2–5	Submucosal and subserosal, each with less then half the diameter in the endometrial and peritoneal cavities, respectively.

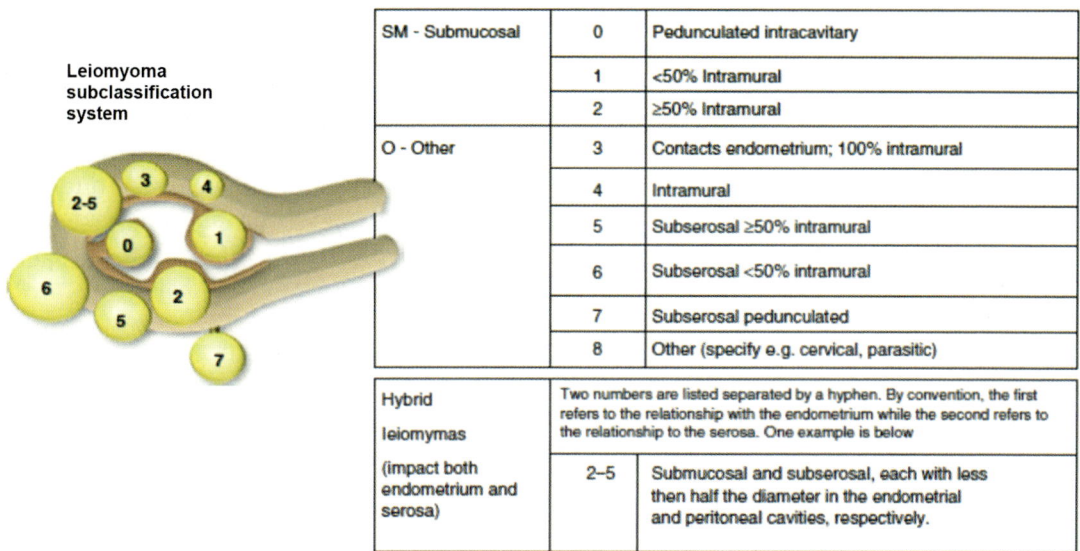

Fig. 7.4: FIGO fibroid subclassification system

Reprinted/adapted by permission from ***Springer Nature:*** *Hysteroscopy by Haimovich, Tinelli and Alonso, 2018.*

extension to the endometrial or serosal surfaces. Types 5–7 are subserosal and mirror of the classification of types 0–2 submucosal fibroids. Type 5 is at least 50% intramural, type 6 is <50% intramural, and type 7 is attached to the serosa by a stalk. Type 8 describes a group of fibroids that has no relationship to the myometrium. For example, they may be cervical lesions or found on the round or broad ligaments or away from the uterus. Hybrid fibroids are indicated by two numbers separated by a hyphen. The first number refers to their relationship with the endometrium, and the second number refers to their relationship with the serosa. A relatively common hybrid fibroid is type 2–5.

Treatment Strategies for Submucosal Fibroids

There are a variety of treatment options for fibroids. Asymptomatic fibroids can be managed expectantly, while symptomatic fibroids can be managed medically, surgically, or with other new technologies. Surgical options include: Ablation, resection (myomectomy), or hysterectomy.

Treatment decisions depend on the fibroid classification, the patient's presenting symptoms, age, desire for future fertility, response to conservative measures, and surgeon's preference and expertise. Surgical treatment aims at removing the symptomatic fibroid(s). Indications for surgical management include lack of response to medical management, recurrent pregnancy loss, infertility and concern for malignancy[9]. Prior to hysteroscopic myomectomy in 1976, abdominal hysterectomy and abdominal myomectomy were the traditional management options for symptomatic submucosal myomas.[5]

In this discussion, we will focus on hysteroscopic excisional procedures of submucosal myomas, as this approach is minimally invasive and allows for direct visualization with identifying and treating intrauterine pathology. Contraindications to hysteroscopic surgery include active pelvic infection, suspected or confirmed malignancy, or pregnancy.[10] Based on a study of women with large symptomatic submucous myomas, hysteroscopic myomectomy should be the treatment of choice in patients with submucosal myomas 6 cm or less in diameter and menorrhagia. If the myoma is greater than 6 cm, hysteroscopic myomectomy can still be considered, but it may require 2 surgical sessions for complete resection (a staged, or 2-stage procedure). Despite the possibility of 2 surgical sessions, some studies suggest that it still offers a shorter hospital stay and more rapid recovery than the laparoscopic approach.[11,12]

Resectoscopic Myomectomy

The first resectoscopic hysteroscopic myomectomy was performed in 1976 by Neurwith and Amin, using a urologic resectoscope and monopolar electrosurgical loop.[13] In 1984, Hallez created a gynecologic resectoscope featuring a smaller diameter, new positioning of the evacuation openings and continuous flow, which allowed better intrauterine visualization. They further improved the technique, and in 1994, reported a 9-year retrospective analysis of 284 patients with submucosal myomas who underwent hysteroscopic myomectomies. They used a pure cutting current (150 W), always starting from the fundus and moving caudad towards the internal cervical os, and concluded that albeit difficult, it is a safe procedure with a low risk of long-term complications.[14]

Traditionally, the resectoscope used monopolar energy attached to a loop wire electrode. The risks involved with monopolar energy included thermal injury, fluid overload, and hyponatremia due to the use of non-conducting, non-physiologic distension media such as mannitol or glycine.[15] Newer resectoscopes use bipolar radiofrequency energy (Fig. 7.5), which has been shown to be as effective as monopolar energy in removing polyps.[16] In addition, bipolar resectoscopes do not require the use of non-ionic distension media, as the current travels between the two electrodes at the tip of the resecting loop, and does not disperse to the surrounding conductive medium. Another technique that has been used to limit intravasation is hydromassage, which stimulates uterine contractions by rapid changes in intrauterine pressure using saline.[12] When using the electrosurgical tools, it is important to move from cephalad to caudad (fundus to os), without forward motion to decrease the risk of uterine perforation.[17]

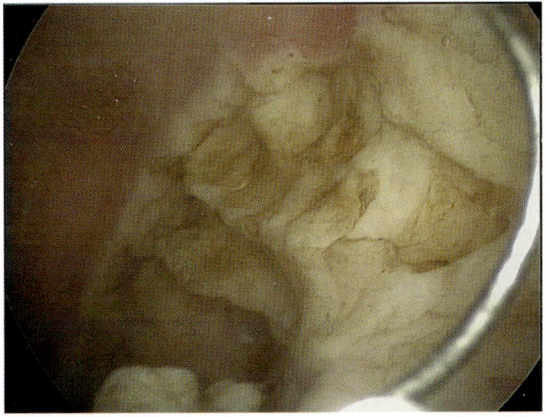

Fig. 7.5: Bipolar loop electrode used for hysteroscopic myomectomy of large type 1 submucosal myoma
*Reprinted/adapted by permission from **Springer Nature**: Uterine Fibroids: A Clinical Casebook by Nash S Moawad; 2018.*

Hysteroscopic Morcellators

In 2005, hysteroscopic morcellation was introduced by Emanuel and Wamsteker as a new technique to remove intrauterine myomas.[18] The intrauterine morcellator (IUM) consists of a set of two metal tubes that fit into each other (Fig. 7.6). The inner tube rotates within the outer tube, and is attached to a vacuum. Both tubes have a cutting window, therefore the lesion can be cut as the inner tube rotates, and the tissue is aspirated through the device into a collecting pouch for histopathologic analysis.[18,19] The IUM is introduced into the uterine cavity with a hysteroscope,

and saline is used for distension and irrigation of the uterine cavity. The goal, with this technique, was to resolve some of the difficulties experienced during traditional resectoscopic surgery such as excessive intravasation of non-conducting, non-physiologic, electrolyte-free distension media, causing hyponatremia, pulmonary edema, heart failure, cerebral edema and death. There is also a risk of internal and external burns when electric current was used, in addition to some studies suggesting resectoscopy to be relatively time-consuming and difficult to learn.[18,20] The morcellator also automatically retrieves the fibroid chips and stores them for submission to microscopic examination.

In two systematic reviews, patients treated with intrauterine morcellation had shorter procedure duration than those treated with electrosurgical resection. There was also an association with smaller fluid deficit and lower odds of incomplete lesion removal.[20,21] Intraoperative and short-term postoperative complications were similar between the morcellation and resectoscopic groups. Long-term outcomes of morcellation were unavailable due to the novelty of the technique. Analysis was limited by heterogeneity of the study design, devices, and treated lesions, in addition to small sample size.[21] Literature has shown successful removal of types 0 and 1 myomas,

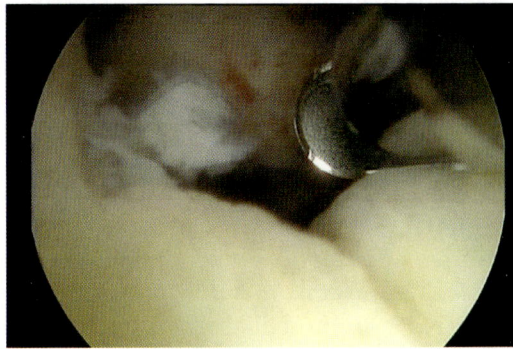

Fig. 7.6: Hysteroscopic morcellators are the most recent advances in hysteroscopic myomectomy
*Reprinted/adapted by permission from **Springer Nature**: Uterine Fibroids: A Clinical Casebook by Nash S Moawad, 2018.*

but has been limited to case studies for removal of type 2 myomas, due to increased intramural extension.[22] These fibroids are typically more amenable to removal with traditional resectoscopic loops, but require special expertise in this technique.

The Cold Loop Technique

A technique more commonly used in Europe is cold loop resectoscopy. First introduced in 1995 by Mazzon, this procedure was proposed with the intention of creating a safe, efficient procedure, in addition to maintaining the integrity of the surrounding endometrium and myometrium.[23] In 2015, Di Spiezio reported a safe one-step combined procedure for hysteroscopic myomectomy.[24] First, an electric loop powered by a 100 W monopolar current in cutting mode was used to excise the intra-cavitary portion of the myoma. This was followed by a cold blade without energy to enucleate the myoma from the myometrium, similar to the blunt dissection technique traditionally used in abdominal and laparoscopic myomectomy. Finally, the myoma is extracted using an angled cutting loop. A retrospective study of 1,434 procedures showed efficacy and safety of the cold loop technique. All myomas were completely removed and intraoperative complication rate was 0.84%.[25] Postoperatively, reports have shown decreased rates of intrauterine adhesions following cold loop resectoscopic myomectomy versus electrosurgical resection, which is ultimately important in patients trying to conceive.[26]

Neodymium-Yttrium-Aluminum-Garnet Laser (Nd:YAG) and GnRH Analogues

Various types of lasers have been used to treat submucosal fibroids, including argon, krypton, neodymium-yttrium-aluminum-garnet (Nd:YAG) and diode laser. Nd:YAG has been the most widespread and was popular in the late 1980s and early 1990s.[27] It was first used by Mergui in France in 1987 to make multiple punctures in myomas, which resulted in tissue death and myoma shrinkage.[28] Since

then, laser has been used to augment the effects of leuprolide. In a study using leuprolide as pretreatment, 75 patients underwent Nd:YAG laser coagulation for thorough devascularization of their myomas. At postoperative transvaginal ultrasound, the myomas reduced in size an average of 50–70% beyond the effect attributable to leuprolide.[29,30] Although the use of preoperative GnRH agonists, such as leuprolide, led to decreased fibroid and uterine size, lower fluid absorption, and restoration of a normal hemoglobin concentration[31,32], it was not shown to improve operating time or surgical outcomes. A meta-analysis shows that there is insufficient evidence to support the routine use of reoperative GnRH agonists. It is beneficial—though as a temporizing agent for the preoperative treatment of anemia secondary to chronic blood loss and it may potentially improve the likelihood of a single-stage hysteroscopic myomectomy of large fibroids. Drawbacks include high cost, menopausal side effects, delay in surgical resection, obliteration of tissue plane, increased perioperative blood loss and operating time, and increased risk of recurrence due to obscured smaller fibroids that re-grow after GnRH wears off.[32,33]

A case series using laser showed that leaving the enucleated submucous myoma in the uterus is a feasible and safe therapeutic option. In this study, ambulatory hysteroscopic myomectomies were performed with diode laser, without anesthesia. Results indicated that when fibroid extraction was not possible, leaving the mass free in the uterus was possible. Patient follow-up showed that most women were asymptomatic and had a high degree of satisfaction with the procedure. There were no reports of painful mass expulsion. Despite promising results, the sample size was small and will require further studies to confirm reproducibility of this technique.[34] Tissue biopsy is typically performed to rule out malignancy. Lasers have shown no advantages over electrosurgery, and are more expensive, slower and require special training and eye protection, so their use has diminished significantly over time.[35]

Vaporization of Submucosal Fibroids

Vaporization technique with a corrugated electrode was used successfully in prostatic hypertrophy with reductions in bleeding, intravasation, duration of surgery and length of time of indwelling catherization. In a 1995 study of 12 women with 3 to 5 cm submucosal myomas, vaporization using grooved ball electrode and grooved cylinder electrode was studied. The most effective current was 220 W to vaporize. The myomas were not vaporized in their entirety, so that portions could be sent for microscopic examination. Results of the study showed less intraoperative bleeding, intravasation of distension fluids, and shorter procedure duration due to the absence of tissue "chips" that interfere with visualization in resectoscopic procedures.[36]

Additionally, vaporization is less expensive than laser ablation and easier to teach than wire loop resection.[37] Care should be taken to frequently suction the resulting air bubbles to decrease the risk of air embolism.

Methods to Decrease Blood Loss during Hysteroscopic Myomectomy

Intralesional Diluted Vasopressin

Vasopressin has been shown to significantly reduce intraoperative blood loss in open myomectomies.[38] In a randomized, double-blind study conducted from 2011 to 2014, 40 premenopausal women with symptomatic submucosal myomas were randomized to transcervical intralesional vasopressin injection or placebo (normal saline) during hysteroscopic myomectomy.

The primary outcome was median duration for myomectomy. Although observed median time was 9 minutes shorter in the vasopressin group, results showed no statistically significant difference between vasopressin and placebo groups. However, there were significant secondary outcomes, including reduced volume of inflow fluid, intravasation, intraoperative blood loss, and improved visualization in the vasopressin group. Due to potential adverse cardiovascular effects, vasopressin should not be used in patients with vascular disease, epilepsy, migraine, asthma, or heart failure.[39] It is important to use diluted solution of vasopressin, avoid intravascular injection, inject the solution slowly, and monitor vital parameters closely. Our preferred dilution is 10 units of vasopressin in 200 mL of normal saline, resulting in a 0.05 U/mL dilution, to minimize the risk of serious cardiovascular complications.

Misoprostol: Rectally or Vaginally

Prostaglandins, such as misoprostol, have uterotonic effects, and have been used to minimize intraoperative blood loss during myomectomy. After oral or sublingual administration, misoprostol reaches its peak in 30 minutes, followed by a rapid decrease in blood concentration.

Following vaginal administration, misoprostol reaches its peak in 1 hour, followed by a progressive decrease in blood concentration. However, it remains at higher blood concentration for at least 6 hours longer than sublingual or oral administration. Rectal administration results in longer half-life compared to oral.[40] In a systematic review, five randomized control studies were analyzed. Preoperative administration of misoprostol showed significant reduction in intraoperative blood loss during abdominal and laparoscopic myomectomies. Misoprostol is safe, well-tolerated and less expensive than vasopressin and GnRH analogs. Diarrhea is the major adverse reaction, but is self-limited.[41]

Tranexamic Acid

Tranexamic acid (TXA) is a synthetic analog of lysine, an antifibrinolytic that inhibits plasminogen and plasmin.[42] It has been associated with reduced perioperative blood loss and transfusion units in cardiac surgery, orthopedic surgery and organ transplant. A meta-analysis from randomized control trials showed intravenous administration of TXA reduced total blood loss, hemoglobin decline, duration of surgery and transfusion requirements following open myomectomy. Additionally, there was no increased risk of deep vein thrombosis or pulmonary embolism.[43] This can be extrapolated to hysteroscopic surgery, particularly when there is high risk of bleeding, such as in large or multiple fibroids, as well as in patients with baseline anemia secondary to chronic blood loss.

CONCLUSION

Hysteroscopic myomectomy has advanced significantly over the last three decades. It is minimally invasive, low-cost, low-risk, fertility-preserving, and has been associated with high patient satisfaction. Currently, techniques such as morcellation and electrosurgical resection are appropriate approaches for submucosal fibroid removal. Morcellation has been associated with decreased operative time and ease of use, however, there is limited data on type 2 fibroid removal. Patients with deep type 2 fibroids would benefit from electrosurgical or cold loop resection, or a combination of both, in the hands of an expert surgeon. Research has been unclear on which technique is superior. Ultimately, the choice should be made on a case-by-case basis, depending on the fibroid classification, number, location, patient goals and the surgeon's level of experience and expertise.

References

1. Lethaby A, Vollenhoven B. Fibroids (uterine myomatosis, leiomyomas). BMJ Clin Evid. 2015;2015

2. Thompson JD, Rock JA, eds. Te Linde's operative gynecology, 7th ed. London, Hagerstrom: JB Lippincott Company, 1992.

3. KK Roy, S Singla, J Baruah, J B Sharma, S Kumar, N Singh, "Reproductive outcome following hysteroscopic myomectomy in patients with infertility and recurrent abortions," Archives of Gynecology and Obstetrics, vol. 282, no. 5, pp. 553–560, 2010.

4. Wamsteker K, Emanuel MH, De kruif JH. Transcervical hysteroscopic resection of submucous fibroids for abnormal uterine bleeding: Results regarding the degree of intramural extension. Obstet Gynecol. 1993;82(5):736–40.

5. Di spiezio sardo A, Mazzon I, Bramante S, et al. Hysteroscopic myomectomy: a comprehensive review of surgical techniques. Hum Reprod Update. 2008;14(2):101–19.

6. Lasmar RB, Barrozo PR, Dias R, Oliveira MA. Submucous myomas: a new presurgical classification to evaluate the viability of hysteroscopic surgical treatment—preliminary report. J Minim Invasive Gynecol. 2005;12(4):308–11.

7. Lasmar RB, Xinmei Z, Indman PD, Celeste RK, Di spiezio sardo A. Feasibility of a new system of classification of submucous myomas: a multicenter study. Fertil Steril. 2011;95(6): 2073–7.

8. Munro MG, Critchley HO, Broder MS, Fraser IS. FIGO classification system (PALMCOEIN) for causes of abnormal uterine bleeding in nongravid women of reproductive age. Int J Gynaecol Obstet. 2011;113(1):3–13.

9. Deutsch A, Sasaki KJ, Cholkeri Singh A. Resectoscopic Surgery for Polyps and Myomas: A Review of the Literature. J Minim Invasive Gynecol. 2017;24(7):1104–10.

10. American Congress of Obstetrics and Gynecologists. Hysteroscopy. Technology assessment in obstetrics and gynecology no. 7. Obstet Gynecol. 2011;117:1486–91.

11. Camanni M, Bonino L, Delpiano EM, Ferrero B, Migliaretti G, Deltetto F. Hysteroscopic management of large symptomatic submucous uterine myomas. J Minim Invasive Gynecol. 2010;17(1):59–65.

12. Zayed M, Fouda UM, Zayed SM, Elsetohy KA, Hashem AT. Hysteroscopic Myomectomy of Large Submucous Myomas in a one-step Procedure Using Multiple Slicing Sessions

Technique. J Minim Invasive Gynecol. 2015; 22(7):1196–202.

13. Neuwirth RS, Amin HK. Excision of submucus fibroids with hysteroscopic control. Am J Obstet Gynecol. 1976;126:95–99.

14. Hallez JP. Single-stage total hysteroscopic myomectomies: indications, techniques, and results. Fertil Steril. 1995;63(4):703–8.

15. Munro MG. Mechanisms of thermal injury to the lower genital tract with radiofrequency resectoscopic surgery. J Minim Invasive Gynecol. 2006;13:36–42.

16. Lieng M, Istre O, Qvigstad E. Treatment of endometrial polyps: a systematic review. Acta Obstet Gynecol Scand. 2010;89(8):992-1002.

17. Cholkeri-singh A, Sasaki KJ. Hysteroscopy safety. Curr Opin Obstet Gynecol. 2016; 28(4):250–4.

18. Emanuel MH, Wamsteker K. The Intra uterine Morcellator: a new hysteroscopic operating technique to remove intrauterine polyps and myomas. J Minim Invasive Gynecol. 2005; 12(1):62–6.

19. Noventa M, Ancona E, Quaranta M, et al. Intrauterine Morcellator Devices: The Icon of Hysteroscopic Future or Merely a Marketing Image? A Systematic Review Regarding Safety, Efficacy, Advantages, and Contraindications. Reprod Sci. 2015;22(10):1289–96.

20. Vitale SG, Sapia F, Rapisarda AMC, et al. Hysteroscopic Morcellation of Submucous Myomas: A Systematic Review. Biomed Res Int. 2017;2017:6848250.

21. Shazly SA, Laughlin-Tommaso SK, Breitkopf DM, et al. Hysteroscopic Morcellation Versus Resection for the Treatment of Uterine Cavitary Lesions: A Systematic Review and Meta-analysis. J Minim Invasive Gynecol. 2016;23(6):867–77.

22. Abbink K, Sendy S, Gaafar TH et al, Gynecol Surg (2015) 12: 267. https://doi.org/10.1007/s10397-015-0905-5

23. Mazzon I. Nuova tecnica per la miomectomia isteroscopica: Enucleazione con ansa fredda. In: Cittadini E, Perino A, Angiolillio M, Minelli L (eds). Testo-Atlante di Chirurgia Endoscopica Ginecologica. Palermo, Italy: COFESE Ed., 1995; XXXIIIb.

24. Di spiezio sardo A, Calagna G, Di carlo C, Guida M, Perino A, Nappi C. Cold loops applied to bipolar resectoscope: A safe "one-step" myomectomy for treatment of submucosal myomas with intramural development. J Obstet Gynaecol Res. 2015;41(12):1935–41.

25. Mazzon I, Favilli A, Grasso M, Horvath S, Di renzo GC, Gerli S. Is Cold Loop Hysteroscopic Myomectomy a Safe and Effective Technique for the Treatment of Submucous Myomas With Intramural Development? A Series of 1434 Surgical Procedures. J Minim Invasive Gynecol. 2015;22(5):792–8.

26. Mazzon I, Favilli A, Cocco P, et al. Does cold loop hysteroscopic myomectomy reduce intrauterine adhesions? A retrospective study. Fertil Steril. 2014;101(1):294–298.e3.

27. Ubaldi F, Tournaye H, Camus M, van der Pas H, Gepts E, Devroey P. Fertility after hysteroscopic myomectomy. Hum Reprod Update 1995;1:81–90.

28. Mergui JL. New Approach to Treatment of Uterine Myomas Video presented at: European Association of Endoscopic Surgery meeting, Lausanne, Switzerland, 1990.

29. Goldfarb HA. Nd:YAG laser laparoscopic coagulation of symptomatic myomas. J Reprod Med. 1992;37:636–38.

30. Goldfarb HA. Myolysis revisited. JSLS. 2008;12(4):426–30.

31. Donnez J, Gillerot S, Bourgonjon D, Clerckx F, Nisolle M. Nd:YAG laser hysteroscopy in large submucous fibroids. Fertil Steril. 1990;54(6):999–1003.

32. Lethaby A, Vollenhoven B, Sowter M. Pre-operative GnRH analogue therapy before hysterectomy or myomectomy for uterine fibroids. Cochrane Database Syst Rev. 2001;(2):CD000547.

33. Sinai talaulikar V, Belli AM, Manyonda I. GnRH agonists: Do they have a place in the modern management of fibroid disease?. J Obstet Gynaecol India. 2012;62(5):506–10.

34. Haimovich S, López-yarto M, Urresta Ávila J, Saavedra tascón A, Hernández JL, Carreras collado R. Office Hysteroscopic Laser Enucleation of Submucous Myomas without Mass Extraction: A Case Series Study. Biomed Res Int. 2015;2015:905204.

35. Emanuel MH. Hysteroscopy and the treatment of uterine fibroids. Best Pract Res Clin Obstet Gynaecol. 2015;29(7):920–9.

36. Brooks PG. Resectoscopic myoma vaporizer. J Reprod Med. 1995;40(11):791–5.

37. Glasser MH. Endometrial ablation and hysteroscopic myomectomy by electrosurgical vaporization. J Am Assoc Gynecol Laparosc. 1997;4(3):369–74.

38. Kongnyuy EJ, Van den broek N, Wiysonge CS. A systematic review of randomized controlled trials to reduce hemorrhage during myomectomy for uterine fibroids. Int J Gynaecol Obstet. 2008;100(1):4–9.

39. Wong AS, Cheung CW, Yeung SW, Fan HL, Leung TY, Sahota DS. Transcervical intralesional vasopressin injection compared with placebo in hysteroscopic myomectomy: a randomized controlled trial. Obstet Gynecol. 2014;124(5):897–903.

40. Tang OS, Gemzell Danielsson K, Ho PC. Misoprostol: pharmacokinetic profiles, effects on the uterus and side-effects. Int J Gynaecol Obstet. 2007;99 Suppl 2:S160–7.

41. Iavazzo C, Mamais I, Gkegkes ID. Use of misoprostol in myomectomy: a systematic review and meta-analysis. Arch Gynecol Obstet. 2015;292(6):1185–91.

42. Goobie SM. Tranexamic acid: still far to go. Br J Anaesth. 2017;118(3):293–95.

43. Wang D, Wang L, Wang Y, Lin X. The efficiency and safety of tranexamic acid for reducing blood loss in open myomectomy: A meta-analysis of randomized controlled trials. Medicine (Baltimore). 2017;96(23):e70–72.

Management of Submucous Fibroids in Office Hysteroscopy

Sergio Haimovich

Myoma—Definition and Classification

Uterine myomas, or fibroids or leiomyomas, are benign neoplasms of the uterus, composed of smooth muscle cells and fibroblasts and rich in extra-cellular matrix.[1]

Myomas are a significant source of morbidity for women of reproductive age. The frequency of uterine myomas in the general population is difficult to estimate because many women with myomas are asymptomatic.

Ultrasound examination of over 1000 randomly selected members of an urban health plan in the USA demonstrated that approximately half of premenopausal women with no previous diagnosis of myomas had evidence of myomas.

Myomas are documented to be the most common indication for hysterectomy in the USA.

The myoma formation starts from the transformation of the single myometrial cell, because of distinct physiological and pathological conditions causing formation of these clonal tumors. It is hypothesized that non-hormonal factors are crucial for initiation of myoma formation while hormonal stimulation is necessary for their further growth.[2] Nevertheless, the exact mechanisms of the myomas' onset, growth, and recurrence remain still unclear.

We know about the crucial role of estrogens and progesterone in the myoma formation. Although reproductive hormones are established to be the main promoters of myoma development many other factors, namely genetic and epigenetic background, micro-RNA, growth factors, cytokines, and chemokines play a role in the myoma formation and growth.

Myoma biology is quite complex, despite looking simple at first glance. Oddly enough, myomas can increase in volume by up to 138% in 6 months but have a low mitotic index.[3] They are clonal smooth muscle cell neoplasms that are growth-responsive to gonadal steroids and have characteristic chromosomal relocations underlying their development. The myometrium contains smooth muscle stem cells known as myometrial stem cells that can transform, under certain conditions, to myoma progenitors cells.[4]

The Extra-cellular matrix (ECM) contributes to growth factor sequestration and solid-state signaling in myomas, rendering the neoplasms stiff.[1]

Myomas seem to consist of at least four components: Smooth muscle cells, vascular smooth muscle cells, and two types of fibroblasts (fibroblasts and fibroid-associated fibroblasts).

According to the direction of growth into the relation with uterine anatomical layers, myomas are divided into subserous, intramural, and submucous myomas.[1] At their onset, all myomas are initially intramural.[1]

During further growth, myometrial muscle forces myomas into the uterine cavity and the endometrial lining of the uterus, or towards the outer margin, as submucous or

subserous myomas[1], thus displacing them. If their growth is directed towards the peritoneal cavity, they can eventually become pedunculated (attached by a stalk to the outer or inner uterine wall).

Classifications

There different classifications, the simplest one is the Wamsteker´s classification (Fig. 8.1) based on the relation of the fibroid and the endometrial cavity.

Lasmar´s **STEP-W** classification by Lasmar (Table 8.1), based on:

Size
Topography
Extension of the base
Penetration into the myometrium
Wall affected

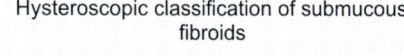

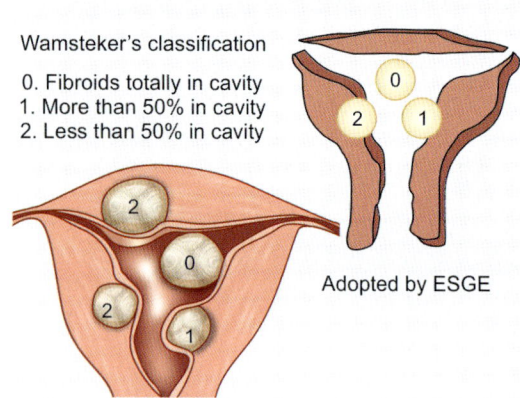

Fig. 8.1: Wamsteker's ESGE classification of submucous fibroids

The purpose of this classification is to give us a score of the difficulty of the hysteroscopy approach.

The Myoma´s Pseudocapsule

During its growth, myoma induces the progressive formation of a sort of pseudo-capsule, due to compression on the surrounding structures and which separates myomas from the healthy uterine tissue.

Table 8.1: Lasmar's STEP-W classification

	Size (cm)	Topography	Extension of the base	Penetration	Lateral Wall	Total
0	>2 to 5	Low	≤1/3	0		
1	>2 to 5	Middle	>1/3 to 2/3	≤50%	**+ 1**	
2	>5	Upper	>2/3	>50%		
Score	+	+	+	+	+	

Score	Group	Complexity and therapeutic options
0 to 4	I	Low complexity hysteroscopic myomectomy
5 to 6	II	High complexity hysteroscopic myomectomy. Consider GnRH use? Consider Two-step hysteroscopic myomectomy
7 to 9	III	Consider alternatives to the hysteroscopic technique

At the ultrastructural level, visualized by transmission electron microscopy, the pseudocapsule cells have the features of smooth muscle cells similar to the myometrium, indicating that the pseudocapsules are part of the myometrium compressed by the myoma.[5] This pseudocapsule causes a dislocation action on the myometrium, which is not destructive since the integrity and contractility of uterine structure is maintained.[6] Pseudocapsule is plentiful of collagen fibers, neurofibers, and blood vessels. Occasionally, bridges of collagen fibers and vessels that anchor myoma to myometrium interrupt the continuous surface of the pseudocapsule. Those phenomena result in the formation of a clear cleavage plane both between myoma and the pseudocapsule, and between the pseudocapsule and the surrounding myometrium as well.

The macroscopic evaluation of the pseudocapsule and of the adjacent myometrium showed

parallel arrays of extremely dense capillaries and of larger vessels forming the capsule, separated from the myometrial vasculature by a narrow avascular cleft.

The general myomectomy dogma is that each surgical fibroid enucleating needs to be gently performed to enhance a correct healing process of the uterine musculature and to facilitate successively the correct uterine musculature anatomical-functional restoring.[7,8]

Intracapsular myomectomy meets the essential postulate of myomectomy: Performing all manipulations as delicately and bloodlessly as it is possible. Thus, if the myoma is dissected entirely through the pseudocapsule opening, using traction on the surrounding myometrium and a gentle selective low energy hemostasis on pseudocapsule vessels, the myometrial bed collapses without excessive hemorrhage once the myoma is removed.[9] The surgical principle for intracapsular myomectomy can be applied to all myomectomies,

This technique allows preservation of the myoma neurovascular bundle, rich of neurofibers containing substances important for adequate myometrial scar healing

The integrity of pseudocapsule and the respect of myometriumare of notable importance for the pregnancy outcomes after myomectomy.

Limiting factors during office hysteroscopy myomectomy

There multiple factors that may limit the success of the myomectomy during an office procedure.

1. *Patient's tolerance:* For some women, the time required to carry out the procedure is the maximum amount of time they tolerate. Some professionals suggest paracervical anesthesia, whereas others indicate sedation. Whenever, the device used during the procedure is of a diameter of 5 mm or less, then procedure can be performed without anesthesia.

   In our outpatient setting, the entire procedure is conducted with noanesthesia. Patients are given only oral analgesic/antispasmodic drug together with a anxiety reducing drug such as diazepam 30 min prior to initiating the procedure.

   The tolerance of the patient is limited also by the time of the procedure. The discomfort is related to the reaction of the uterus to the endocavitarian pressure, the myometrial contractions opposing the pressure translates into a discomfort by low abdominal pain. The intensity of the pain increases in time, this is the reason why office procedures should be short between 15 and 30 minutes depending on the patient tolerance.

2. *Surgeon's skills*: The lack of skills is also a limiting factor. Skills are acquired slowly by completing a learning curve. The first cases should be very low difficulty fibroids,

small and almost completely inside the cavity. With experience comes the confidence and with confidence the surgeon will advance into more difficult fibroids. Skills also will help to over come problems during the procedure such as cervical stenosis.

3. *Myoma´s characteristics:* As seen in STEP-W classification the most limiting factors are size and the depth of penetration into the myometrium wall. Sometimes based on Bettocchi's OPPIuM (Office Preparation of Partially Intramural Myomas), deep myomas will need more than one surgical step. On the first step the mucosa and pseudocapsule is opened allowing the fibroid to migrate into the cavity, this way a Grade 2 myoma can become a Grade 1 or Grade 0 making surgery easier during the second step.

4. *Technique/Devices:* In our practice, we use the myoma mobilization technique with grasping or scissors and mechanical energy. Thus, we perform outpatient myomectomy at the time of examination, since the myoma classification allows for it. According to this technique, we section the endometrium and the fibrous bridges on the entire circumference of the myoma (Figs 8.2 and 8.3).

Then we approach the pseudocapsule, perform mechanical mobilization of the nodule, releasing it from the myometrium (Fig. 8.4). In our opinion, the best myomectomy technique involves working with the myoma pseudocapsule, trying to do the same way that is done in laparotomic or laparoscopic myomectomy.

With this technique the hysteroscopic myomectomy is faster, with less bleeding and pain.

The devices that can be use during an office procedure are:

4.1 Morcellators: There different types of morcellators, mechanical and manual, very small diameter or bigger diameter. The manual morcellators are more for polyps and there is no experience in myomectomy. There is only one small mechanical morcellator adapted to the use during office hysteroscopy and it is the Truclear 5.0 (Fig. 8.5), this morcellator is limited to polyps and some very small completely endo-cavitarian fibroids (G0). Then we have morcellators with a diameter of 6 or more millimeters, those can be applied on bigger fibroids with the limitation of not achieving a complete surgery in case on deep fibroids. The devices are, Truclear 8.0, Myosure Reach and Bigatti Shaver.

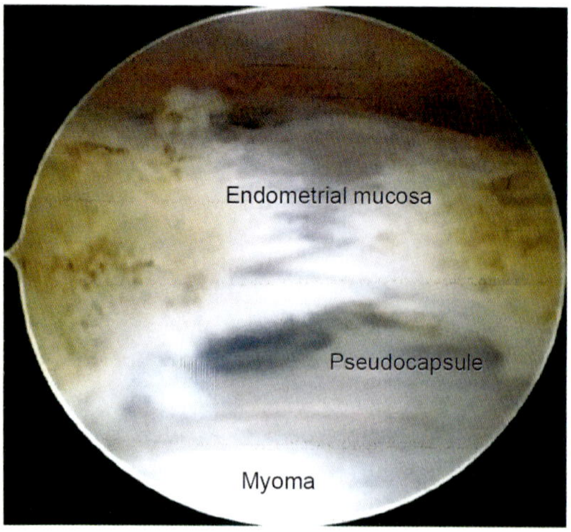

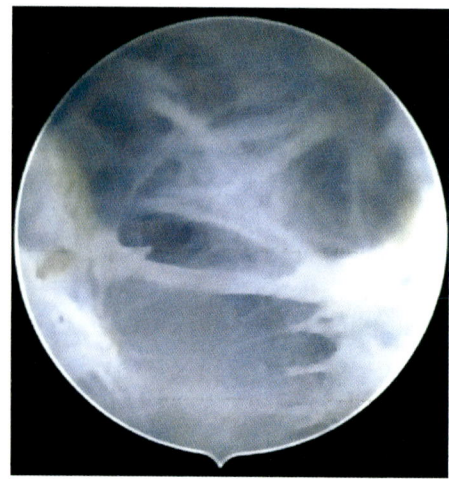

Endometrial mucosa

Pseudocapsule

Myoma

Fig. 8.2: The space between the myoma and the surrounding tissue is the pseudocapsule

Fig. 8.3: The pseudocapsule is full of very laxe connective tissue bridges

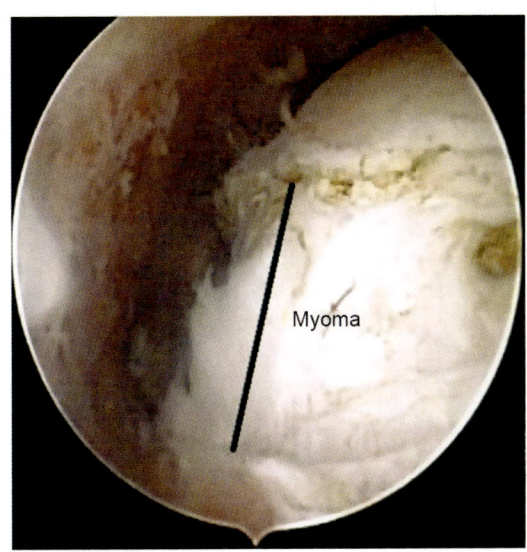

Fig. 8.4: After cutting the pseudocapsule the myoma migrates into the cavity

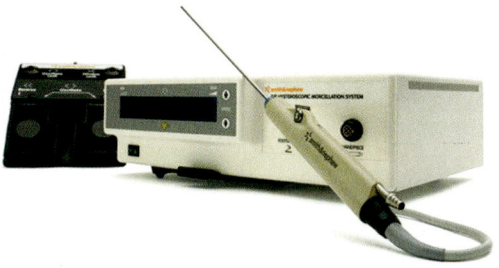

Fig. 8.5: Truclear 5.0 morcellator system

4.2 Mini-resectoscopes: The first one was Gubbini´s 16 Fr mini-resectoscope (Fig. 8.6), recently Storz launched their 15 Fr mini resectoscope (Fig. 8.7). It works similarly to a resectoscope in OR but adapted to office setting. The energy is bipolar so saline can be used. The limitation is the size of the fibroid. If in OR using a resectoscope it can take more than an hour to perform a 3–4 cm myomectomy imagine with a small diameter resectoscope the time it can take. And time is a limiting factor in office settings without anesthesia. The use of bipolar energy, depending on the power intensity, might be painful when reaching the myometrium.

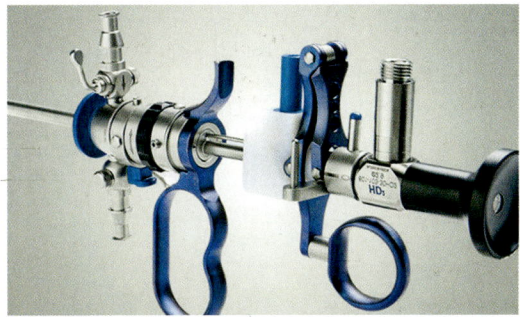

Fig. 8.6: Gubbini's 16 Fr mini-resectoscope

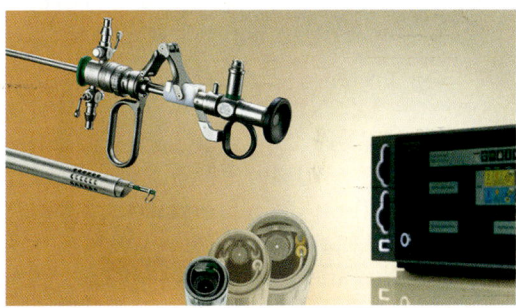

Fig. 8.7: Storz 15 Fr mini-resectoscope

4.3 Mechanical instruments: Cheap and easy to use, but limited to very small fibroids, mostly G0 and G1 (Fig. 8.8).

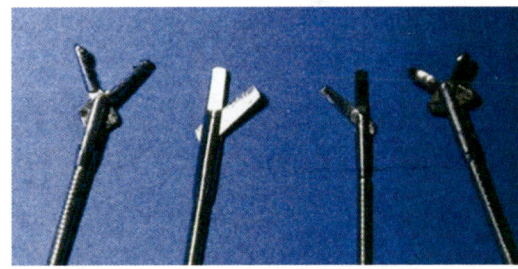

Fig. 8.8: The 5 Fr mechanical instruments

4.4 Bipolar Energy Electrodes (such as Versa point): This is RF energy than can cut in a smooth way, Bettocchi used it for the OPPIuM technique. As with the use of the mini-resectoscope, the dispersion of the energy may affect the myometrium with some pain for the patient (Fig. 8.9).

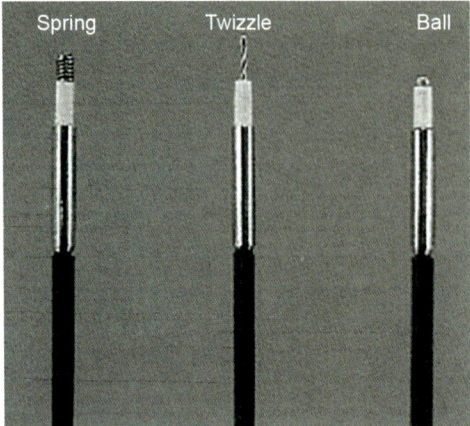

Fig. 8.9 Versa point 5 Fr electrodes

4.5 Diode Laser: This is an energy with 2 characteristics, affinity to water and at the same time affinity to hemoglobin. Thank to these characteristics diode laser can cut and vaporize tissue and simultaneously coagulates any bleeding vessel. The dispersion of the heat is of 0.5 to 1 mm only and does not reach the myometrium. The results is a smooth and clean cut without any pain (Fig. 8.10). The use of laser is for the enucleation of the fibroid cutting a circle around the fibroid (OPPIuM technique) but in cases of deep or big fibroids it can perform a myolysis.

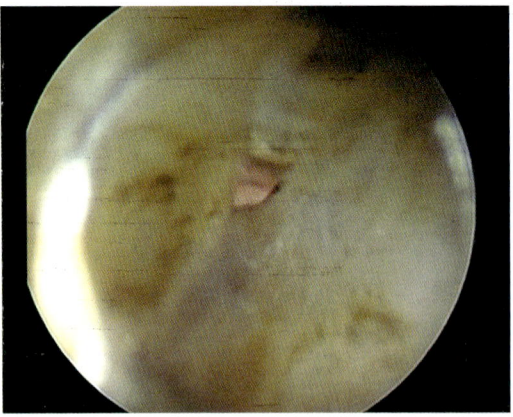

Fig. 8.10: The use of a 1 mm diode laser fiber during a hysteroscopy procedure

Office myomectomy techniques without anesthesia

There are different options for a myomectomy based on the type of the fibroid.

G0: Morcellation of the fibroid with Truclear 5.0 if it is a very small myoma (Fig. 8.11)

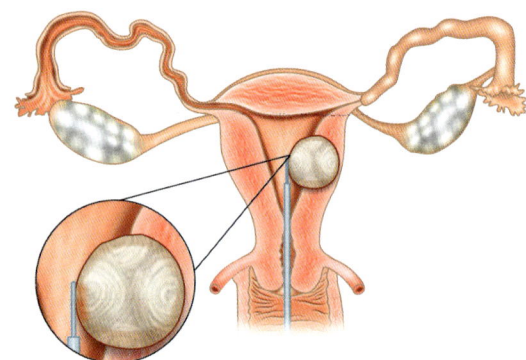

Fig. 8.11: Morcellation of a submucous fibroid

Mini resectoscope is a tool that it can be sure similar to the use of the resectoscope in OR, taking small chips of the fibroid until a complete resection is achieved (Fig. 8.12).

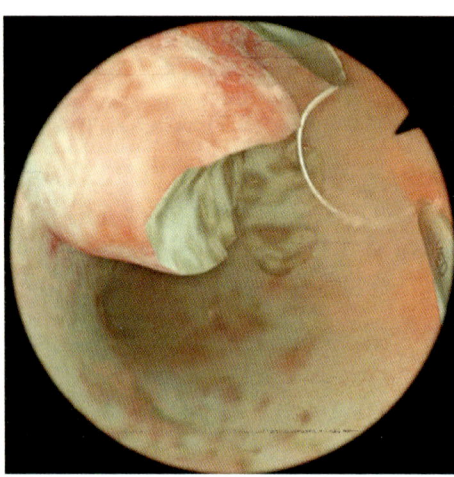

Fig. 8.12: The use of a mini resectoscope for a myomectomy

Cutting the pedicle of the myoma with coagulating energy, in our case with cut it with diode laser and leave the fibroid free inside the cavity. In a matter of minutes the surgery is finished. In a follow up ultrasound 2 months after, 100% of the fibroids disappear. Always take a small sample of the fibroid for histological study. It works for fibroids until 5 cm (Fig. 8.13 a and b).

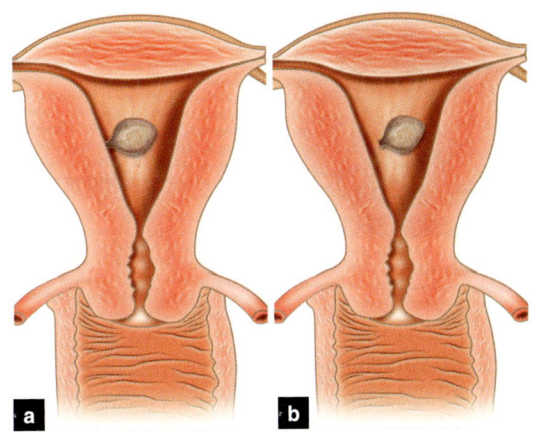

Fig. 8.13a and b: (a) Pedunculated submucous fibroid; (b) Free pedunculated fibroid after cutting the pedicle

G1: This kind of fibroids with more than 50% of endo-cavitarian component. The techniques that can be used in office setting without anesthesia are the same as for G0 fibroids.

The morcellator and the mini-resectoscope are option and the enucleation is another one.

Based on reaching the pseudocapsule the enucleation technique is the most natural way of myomectomy, similar to open or laparoscopic myomectomy.

The fact that this technique respects the pseudocapsule the healing after the myomectomy is faster and without any myometrial scars reducing the probability of adhesions and of affecting fertility.

The opening of the mucosa and the pseudocapsule can be performed by bipolar energy or diode laser energy, then the enucleation is mechanical using grasper or scissors. Sometimes a second step hysteroscopy is needed, specially in big myomas.

The free enucleated fibroid can remain inside the endometrial cavity as described for G0 myoma, with the same follow up. The enucleation is limited to fibroids till 3 cm

G2: These fibroids are actually intramural with a small submucous component of less than 50%, and represent the real challenge of hysteroscopy myomectomy and specially in office setting.

The mini-resectoscope is limited in these kind of fibroids both by the intramural depth but specially by the size.

The morcellator has limitations when it comes to the intramural component. The recommended technique requires 2 steps, first one to eliminate the endo-cavitarian component, giving time to the intramural component to migrate into the cavity and the a second step for finishing the complete removal of the tissue.

The enucleation technique is also limited by fibroids size. Achieving a total liberation of the fibroid can be done in small fibroids and sometime will require a second step.

The turning point is office myomectomy without anesthesia is the myolysis technique. Myolysis is the destruction of the myoma's tissue by energy, it can be perform with RF—radio-frequency (electricity) or by diode laser. There are different studies including randomized controlled trials with the use of RF for myomas even during hysteroscopy, but no device has been developed for the use in office setting.

Diode laser myolysis success is based on the characteristics of the laser, both vaporization and coagulation. By placing the laser fiber inside the fibroid and releasing the energy, within minutes the fibroid is reduced or disappears. Our group has tries it in almost 60 myomas running from 24 mm to 58 mm The mass reduction after one session was between 60 and 100% of the fibroid and the mean procedure time was of 8 minutes. It requires a special fiber developed for this purpose that achieves a 360° dispersion of the heat (Fig. 8.14). Based on the results we believe that it is a very promising technique.

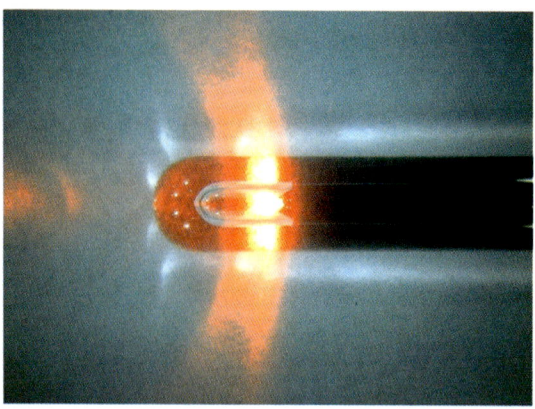

Fig. 8.14: Radial 360° laser fiber

References

1. Bulun SE. Uterine fibroids. N Engl J Med. 2013;369(14):1344-55.

2. Commandeur AE, Styer AK, Teixeira JM. Epidemiological and genetic clues for molecular mechanisms involved in uterine leiomyoma development and growth. Hum Reprod Update.2015;21(5):593-615.

3. Malvasi A, Cavallotti C, Morroni M, Lorenzi T, Dell'Edera D,Nicolardi G, et al. Uterine fibroid pseudocapsule studied by transmission electron microscopy. Eur J Obstet Gynecol Reprod Biol.2012;162(2): 187–91.

4. Peddada SD, Laughlin SK, Miner K, Guyon JP, Haneke K,Vahdat HL, et al. Growth of uterine leiomyomata among premenopausal black and white women. Proc Natl Acad Sci U S A.2008;105(50): 19887–92.

5. Resta L. Uterine myomas and histopathology. In: Tinelli A, MalvasiA, editors. Uterine myoma, myomectomy and minimally invasive treatments. Berlin: Springer; 2015. p. 27-38.

6. Tinelli A, Hurst BS, Hudelist G, Tsin DA, Stark M, MettlerL, et al. Laparoscopic myomectomy focusing on the myoma-pseudocapsule: technical and outcome reports. Hum Reprod.2012;27(2): 427–35.

7. Tinelli A, Malvasi A, Rahimi S, Negro R, Cavallotti C, Vergara D,et al. Myoma pseudocapsule: a distinct endocrino-anatomical entity in gynecological surgery. Gynecol Endocrinol. 2009;25(10):661-7.

8. Tinelli A, Malvasi A. Uterine fibroid pseudocapsule. In: Tinelli A,Malvasi A, editors. Uterine myoma, myomectomy and minimally invasive treatments. Berlin: Springer; 2015. p. 73-93.

9. Tinelli A, Sparic R, Kadija S, Babovic I, Tinelli R, Mynbaev OA,et al. Myomas: anatomy and related issues. Minerva Ginecol.2016;68(3):261–73.

Breakthrough in Office Hysteroscopic Surgery

Giampietro Gubbini, Mario Franchini

Hysteroscopy is the gold standard for diagnosis and treatment of intrauterine pathology. Numerous innovations have resulted in techniques suitable for an office setting. This paper highlights the newer hysteroscopic technologies available and the current use in the clinical setting.

Hysteroscopy has become an important tool to evaluate intrauterine pathology. Office hysteroscopy allows an efficient and accurate diagnosis of intrauterine pathology, including submucosal fibroids, endometrial polyps, cesarean scar defect, potential hyperplasia and cancer.[1, 2]

During the last decades, the introduction of small continuous-flow diameter scopes equipped with 5 Fr working channels has encouraged physicians to increase the number of operative procedures performed in an office setting. Vaginoscopic approach has greatly increased the feasibility and acceptability of office diagnostic and operative hysteroscopy minimizing patient's pain and discomfort.[3–5]

Therefore, knowledge of technologies, increased operator experience and selection of appropriate patients have played a key role in developing hysteroscopic surgery in an office setting.[6, 7]

Today, in most cases, the pathology can be diagnosed and concurrently treated. This 'see-and-treat' philosophy is the essence of one-stop clinics with resultant savings in time, cost and increased patient satisfaction.[8]

Since many hysteroscopic procedures (removal of polyp and submucosal myomas, lysis of adhesions, retrieval of intrauterine device, female sterilization) can be performed in an office setting, a range of scopes (diagnostic and operative) is required in the surgical armamentarium of an ambulatory set-up. This can vary from traditionally available diagnostic (3 mm rigid and flexible) and rigid operative (5–4 mm) hysteroscopes to more complex state-of-the-art modern equipment, including mechanical instrument, bipolar or monopolar electrode.[9,10]

The most recent development in operative hysteroscopy is the advent of a smaller diameter resectoscope and tissue removal system (HTRs) comparing to traditional 22 Fr, 26 Fr resectoscope or 19 Fr, 26 Fr HTRs.[11,12] Polyps and myomas can be treated with these miniaturized instrumentations in an office setting with vaginoscopic approach without any cervical dilatation that is required with scope diameter greater than 5 mm. Therefore, by avoiding cervical dilation, it is possible to reduce the risk of perforation that usually occurs during entry (uterine sounding, initial cervical dilation).

TruClear System

In recent years, an innovative hysteroscopic tissue removal system (HTRs) based on mechanical removal of intrauterine lesions has been developed.[13] Systematic review, meta-analysis and clinical studies have showed that women treated with HTRs for endometrial polyps and myomas have a shorter procedure time than those treated with loop or bipolar electrode resection in an operating room or in an office setting.[14–16]

The small diameter HTRs, TruClear™ 5C system (TruClear 5C, Medtronic, Dublin, EIRE) was first introduced in 2011. The system consists of a 5-mm, rigid oval profile hysteroscope with a fiber zero optic size of 0.8 mm and a vaginal insertion length of 205 mm. The outflow sheath increases the overall diameter to 5.7 mm, but its use is not always necessary. The 2.9 mm small size blade of HTRs (a rigid inner tube, with cutting edges, that rotate within an outer tube, incorporating a 5 mm length side facing cutting window at its distal end) is introduced in the 3.1 mm operative channel hysteroscope (Fig. 9.1). The blade is secured to a reusable handpiece that has two ports: One to a motor control unit, the other connected through a canister to a suction source to aspirate removed tissue. Tissue is captured in the cutting window as the inner tube rotates at 500–1500 revolutions per minute (rpm) and cut into small fragments. The cut tissue is immediately captured in the cutting window and aspirated from the uterine cavity to a canister avoiding any loss or remaining of tissue in the uterine cavity, so that the intrauterine view is maintained and tissue is captured for histological evaluation.

Tips and Tricks

Before beginning the procedure, to reduce the scope diameter to 5 mm, we remove the outer sheath and to avoid cavity collapse, we perform the window-lock procedure to lock

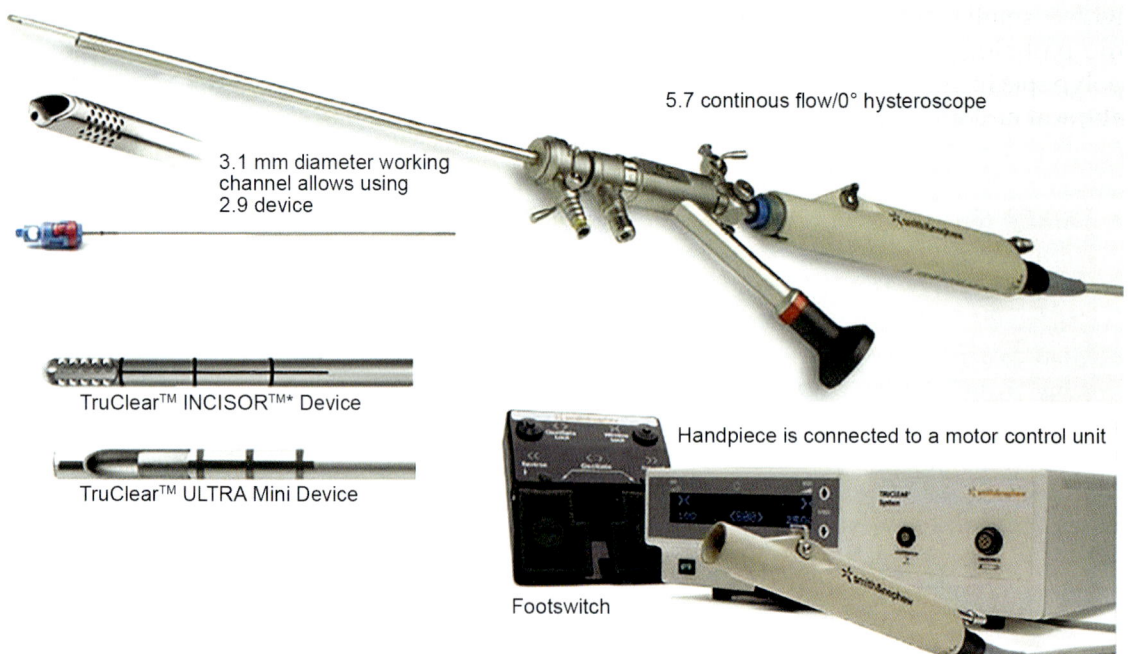

Fig. 9.1: TruClear™ 5C hysteroscopic tissue removal system (HTRs) includes the hysteroscope set (rigid 0° hysteroscope with straight-through, D-shaped working channel with optic offset), the TruClear device, the handpiece connected to a motor control unit and the footswitch

the window. This prevent continuous suction of the distending medium when the inner tube is not activated.

In case of hardness of polyp, we decrease the rotation to 600/900 rpm to achieve a better grip by the rotating blade. Using a suction-irrigating unit we provide a positive pressure of 100/150 mmHg and a continuous flow control of 300–350 mL/min and to apply to the inner tube a suction pressure 0.3/0.4 bar. With this setting any size sessile polyps or those with large flat bases are easily removed with small size HTRs blade even if located in the fundus or in the cornual area of uterine cavity (Fig. 9.2). We start to remove a large polyp, protruding from the cervical ostium, moving under direct visualization from the cervical channel to uterine cavity.[17]

The removal of endometrial polyps using HTRs provides adequate tissue for pathological diagnosis despite the effects of tissue fragmentation. Even if the polyp fragments appeared small in size, we found that HTR with a small diameter blade does not affect the pathological evaluation of endometrial polyp specimens and the detection of complex atypical endometrial hyperplasia.[18]

In 2017, a 2.9 mm blade for myomectomy was introduced and the effectiveness is currently under consideration.

GUBBINI SYSTEM (MINI HYSTERORESECTOSCOPE)

Gubbini system (Gubbini system, Tontarra, Medizintechnik, GmbH, Germany) was introduced in 2010 and the system consists of a 5 mm, rigid oval profile (oblique tip) continuous flow resectoscope with a 2.9 mm 0° optic, a vaginal insertion length of 194 mm.

The system includes two internal sheaths: The first for using 5 Fr bipolar or monopolar electrodes and mechanical forceps in a 5 Fr working channel and the second sheath, with a work slide in titanium, for using different shaped miniaturized loops and rollerballs. The Quick-Lock system of sheath connections enables an easy assembly and a smooth exchange during the procedures shifting from 5 Fr instrumentation to miniaturized loop surgery using the same outer sheath (Gubbini Ellipse System, Tontarra, Medizintechnik, GmbH, Germany) (Fig. 9.3).

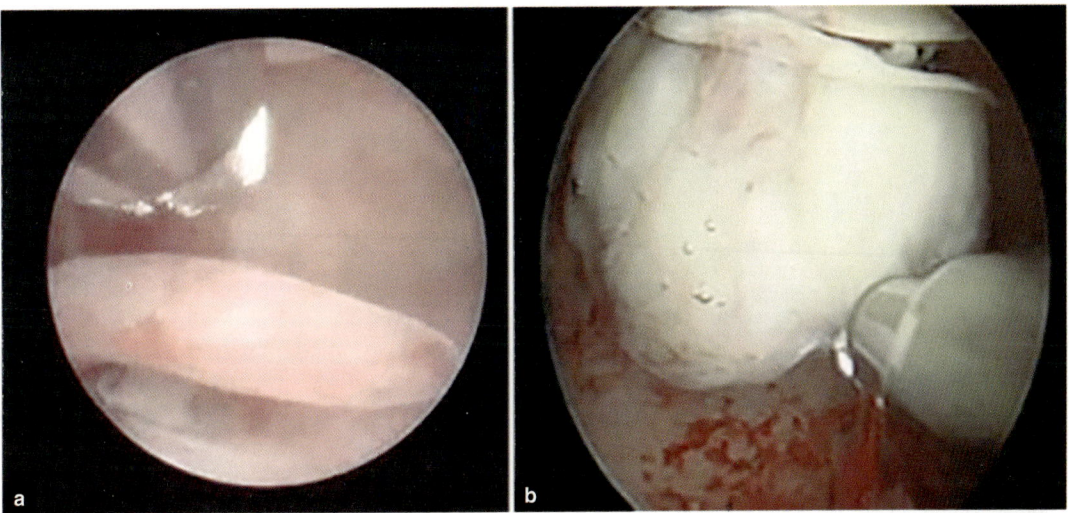

Fig. 9.2a and b: Polypectomy and myomectomy with TruClear system: Tissue is captured in the cutting window, cut into small fragments and aspirated from the uterine cavity to a canister for histological assessment

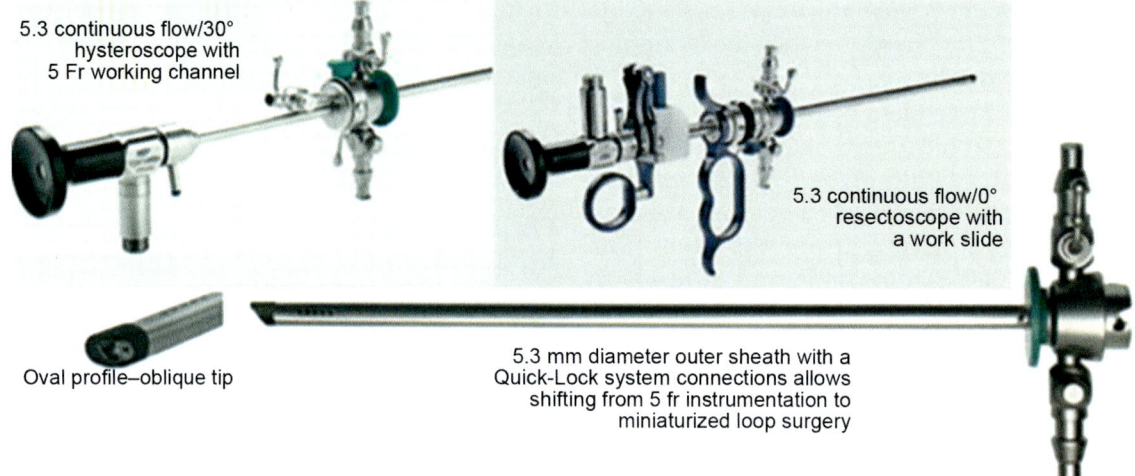

5.3 continuous flow/30°
hysteroscope with
5 Fr working channel

5.3 continuous flow/0°
resectoscope with
a work slide

Oval profile–oblique tip

5.3 mm diameter outer sheath with a
Quick-Lock system connections allows
shifting from 5 fr instrumentation to
miniaturized loop surgery

Fig. 9.3: Gubbini Ellipse system includes two internal sheaths: The first with a 5 Fr working channel and the second sheath, with a work slide in titanium, for using different shaped miniaturized loops. The Quick-Lock system of sheath connections enables an easy assembly during the procedures shifting from 5 Fr instrumentation to miniaturized loop surgery using the same outer sheath

Tips and Tricks

Using mini resectoscope, we perform standard maneuvers resectoscopic surgery with the advantages of miniaturized instrumentation with vaginoscopic approach without any cervical dilatation.[19]

In most cases, endometrial polyps <25 mm and submucous fibroids <15 mm can easily be attempted and treated with classic slicing technique without any anesthesia.

We treat sessile polypoid and myoma G0 lesions starting with their free edge and advancing toward its base of implantation (Fig. 9.4). We proceed directly with resection of the pedicle of pedunculated endometrial polyp when the polyp dimension allows its extraction through the cervical canal.

Our advice is to have sufficient and adequate experience in performing 26–27 Fr resectoscope procedures in the uterine cavity

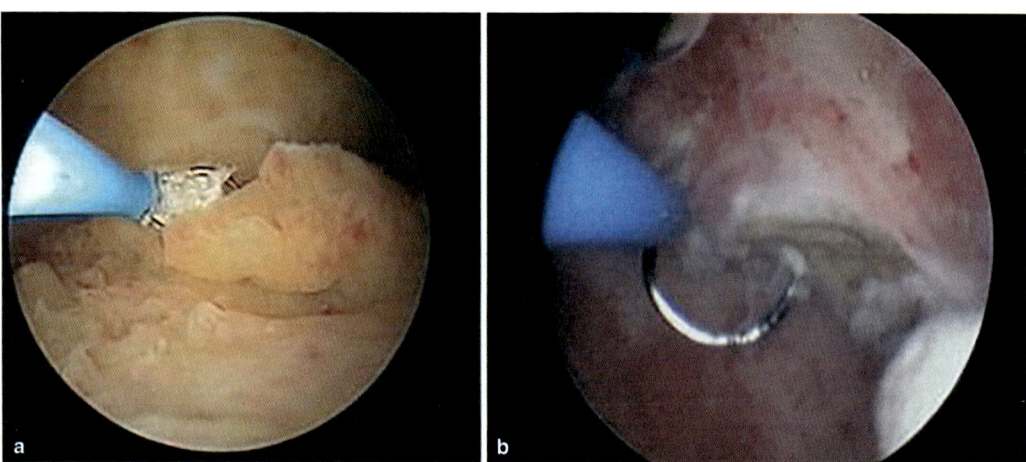

a   b

Fig. 9.4a and b: Polypectomy and myomectomy procedures performed with a "slicing technique" using Gubbini system

and be familiar with electrical energy and fluid management before using mini resectoscope in an office setting.

We use the mini resectoscope under sedation with vaginoscopic approach to treat complete uterine septum and cesarean scar defect (CSD). Avoiding cervical dilatation is a great opportunity for performing the treatment of CSD according to the uterine anatomy without any modification induced by Hegar dilator.[20] Before beginning CSD treatment we fill the bladder with methylene blue solution to enable early identification of bladder injuries.

We use a monopolar or bipolar loop to resect the fibrotic tissue of the proximal part and distal of the niche, and a rollerball electrode to coagulate superficially the entire niche surface. We emphasize to end the procedure with 360° resection (endocervical ablation) of the all residual cervical canal inflamed tissue surrounding the diverticulum in order to replace it with mono-stratified cubic cell-type epithelium (Fig. 9.5).

Conclusion

Since the hysteroscope size has played a pivotal role in the acceptance and the success of an office surgery with vaginoscopic approach, the introduction of the TruClear 5C system and the Gubbini ellipse system enable the implementation of polypectomy and myomectomy in an office setting without substantial patient discomfort.

Moreover, the selection of hysteroscopic equipment for office surgery must be tailored

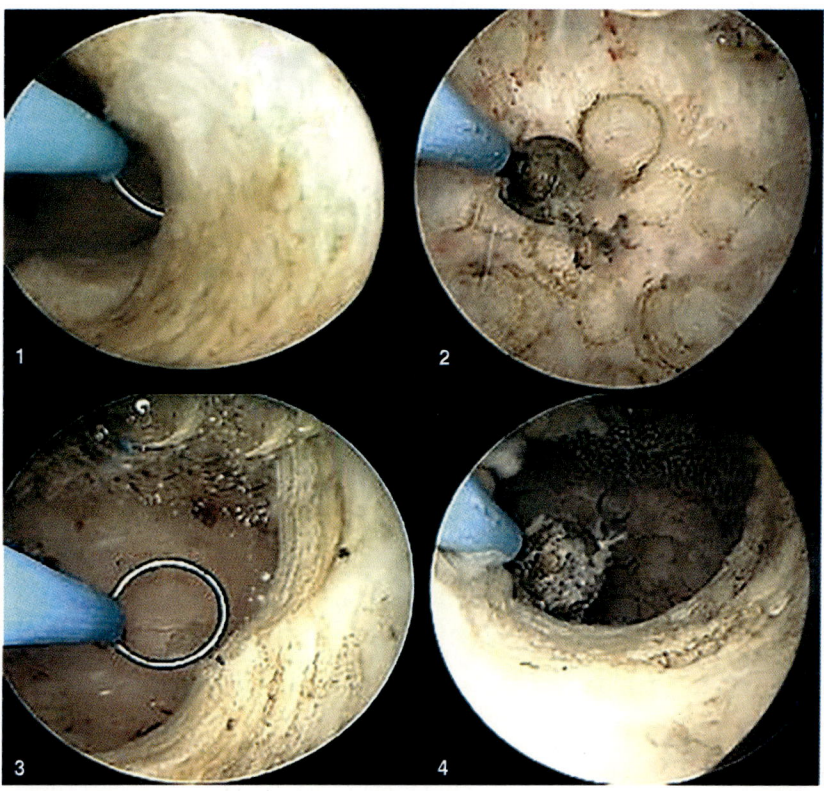

Fig. 9.5: Surgical technique for channel-like resectoscopic treatment with 16 Fr resectoscope. Resection of the fibrotic tissue of the proximal part of the niche (1) and the distal (2). Coagulation of the entire niche surface superficially with a rollerball electrode (3). 360° "endocervical ablation" of the all residual cervical canal inflamed tissue surrounding the diverticulum (4)

to the patient acceptability and skill of the surgeon, this implies that the operator is trained and confident with the hysteroscopic system used to avoid additional cost for failed procedures and patient discomfort.

References

1. Bettocchi S, Nappi L, Ceci O, Selvaggi L. Office hysteroscopy. Obstet Gynecol Clin North Am 2004;31(3)641–54.

2. van Dongen H, de Kroon CD, Jacobi CE, Trimbos JB, Jansen FW. Diagnostic hysteroscopy in abnormal uterine bleeding: a systematic review and meta-analysis. BJOG 2007;114(6):664–75.

3. Bettocchi S, Ceci O, Nappi L, et al. Operative office hysteroscopy without anesthesia: analysis of 4863 cases performed with mechanical instruments. J Am Assoc Gynecol Laparosc. 2004;11:59–61.

4. Guida M, Di Spiezio Sardo A, Acunzo G, Sparice S, Bramante S, Piccoli R, et al. Vaginoscopic versus traditional office hysteroscopy: a randomized controlled study. Hum Reprod 2006;21:3253–7.

5. Campo R, Molinas CR, Rombauts L, Mestdagh G, Lauwers M, Braekmans P, et al. Prospective multicentre randomized controlled trial to evaluate factors influencing the success rate of office diagnostic hysteroscopy. Hum Reprod 2005;20:258–63.

6. Cicinelli E. Hysteroscopy without anesthesia: review of recent literature. J Minim Invasive Gynecol 2010;17:703–8.

7. Cooper NA, Smith P, Khan KS, Clark TJ. Vaginoscopic approach to outpatient hystero-scopy: a systematic review of the effect on pain. BJOG 2010;117:532–39.

8. Kremer C, Duffy S, Moroney M. Patient satisfac-tion with outpatient hysteroscopy versus day case hysteroscopy: randomized controlled trial. BMJ 2000; 320: 279–82.

9. Di Spiezio Sardo A, Bettocchi S, Spinelli M, et al. Review of new office-based hysteroscopic procedures 2003–2009. J Minim Invasive Gynecol 2010;17:436–48.

10. Litta P, Leggieri C, Conte L, Dalla Toffola A, Multinu F, Angioni S. Monopolar versus bipolar device: safety, feasibility, limits and perioperative complications in performing hysteroscopic myomectomy. Clin Exp Obstet Gynecol. 2014; 41:335–38.

11. Dealberti D, Riboni F, Cosma S, Pisani C, Montella F, Saitta S, Calagna G, and Di Spiezio Sardo A.

Feasibility and Acceptability of Office-Based Polypectomy With a 16F Mini Resectoscope: A Multicenter Clinical Study J Minim Invasive Gynecol 2016; 23:418–24.

12. Smith PP, Middleton LJ, Connor M, Clark TJ. Hysteroscopic morcellation compared with electrical resection of endometrial polyps: a randomized controlled trial. Obstet Gynecol. 2014;123:745–51.

13. Emanuel MH, Wamsteker K. The Intra-uterine Morcellator: a new hysteroscopic operating technique to remove intrauterine polyps and myomas.J Minim Invasive Gynecol. 2005;12:62–66.

14. Shazly SA, Laughlin-Tommaso SK, Breitkopf DM, Hopkins MR et al. Hysteroscopic Morcellation Versus Resection for the Treatment of Uterine Cavitary Lesions: A Systematic Review and Meta-analysis. J Minim Invasive Gynecol 2016; 23(6): 867–77.

15. AlHilli MM, Nixon KE, Hopkins MR, Weaver AL, Laughlin-Tommaso SK, Famuyide AO. Long-term outcomes after intrauterine morcellation vs hysteroscopic resection of endometrial polyps. J Minim Invasive Gynecol 2013;20:215–21.

16. Hamerlynck TW, Schoot BC, van Vliet HA, Weyers S. Removal of endometrial polyps: hysteroscopic morcellation versus bipolar resectoscopy, a randomized trial. J Minim Invasive Gynecol 2015;22:1237–43.

17. Ceci O, Franchini M Cannone R, Giarrè G, Bettocchi S, Divina Fascilla F, Cicinelli E. Office treatment of large endometrial polyps using Truclear 5c: feasibility and acceptability. J Obstet Gynaecol Res. 2018, July awaiting to be published online.

18. Franchini M, Zolfanelli F, Gallorini M, Giarre G, Fimiani R, Florio P. Hysteroscopic polypectomy in an office setting: specimen quality assessment for histopathological evaluation. Eur J Obstet Gynecol Reprodud Biol 2015;189:64–67.

19. Ricciardi R, Lanzone A, Tagliaferri V, Di Florio C, Ricciardi L, Selvaggi L, Guido M. Using a 16-French resectoscope as an alternative device in the treatment of uterine lesions: a randomized controlled trial. Obstet Gynecol 2012;120:160–65.

20. Franchini M, Florio P and Gubbini G. Surgical Management of Cesarean Scar Defect in Restoring Fertility. In Tinelli, et al. (eds). Hysteroscopy, Cham (Zug), Springer International Publishing AG, 2018, 409–19.

Hysteroscopy: A Rewarding Touch

Septate Uterus

XiaoLi Ma, Hua Duan

Female congenital uterine anomalies result from abnormal formation, fusion or absorption of the Müllerian ducts during fetal life. Septum uterus is the most common type of congenital uterine anomalies which accounting for approximately 80%~90% of the total uterine anomalies. The true prevalence of the uterine septum is difficult to ascertain as many uterine septum defects are asymptomatic, but appear to range between 1 to 2 per 1,000 and as high as 15 per 1,000. The type of septum can be divided into sub-septus, the septum tissues partly segment the uterine cavity and terminate above the level of internal cervical os, and complete septus, the septum tissues completely segment the uterine cavity and terminate under the level of internal cervical os. Sometimes, the septum tissue terminates at the external cervical orifice which looks like "double cervix" (Fig. 10.1). Septum tissues have fewer blood vessels and relatively high fiber content, and the endometrium covering the septum shows a relatively poor response to hormones, affecting fertilized egg implantation as well as normal growth and development of the placenta. Although this defect does not predispose to increase rates of preterm labor or cesarean delivery, septate uterus is associated with increased rates of first- and second-trimester spontaneous abortion,

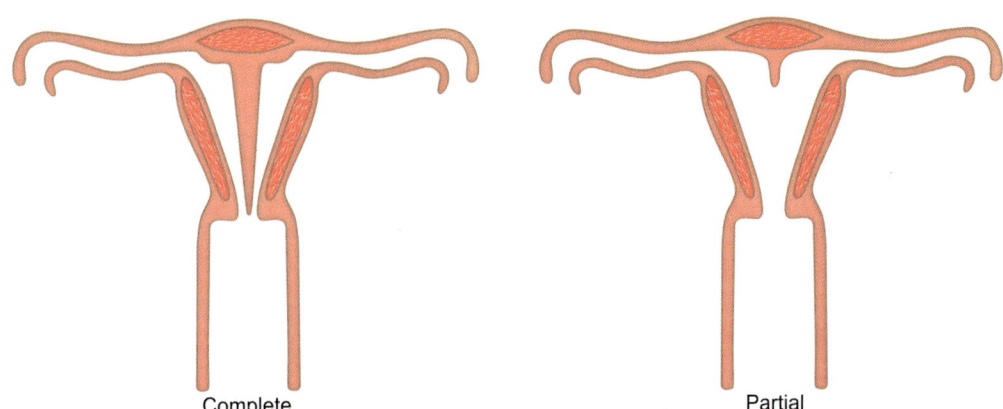

Complete   Partial

Fig. 10.1: Class V Müllerian anomalies include forms of septate uterus. The fibrous or fibromuscular septum may extend partially into the uterine cavity or may extend the entire length

reproductive failure and obstetric complications, seriously damaging women's reproductive function and physical health.

Classification

Accurate classification is important for assessing patient and making reasonable treatment plan. Until now, several classification schemes for female reproductive tract anomalies exist, but the most commonly used systems are AFS (American Fertility Society, 1988) and ESHRE/ESGE (European Society of Human Reproduction and Embryology and the European Society for Gynaecological Endoscopy, 2013) classification.

AFS classification is based on the extent of failure of Müllerian embryonic development and divides uterine malformations into seven main groups, which can provide a classification of the main uterine anomalies appropriate for the vast majority of the patients (Fig. 10.2). However, the limitations of this system include: (i) It is not comprehensive and is inapplicable to combined or complex anomalies. Many congenital uterovaginal anomalies and complex genitourinary anomalies could not be classified in this system; (ii) It does not specify criteria for making the diagnosis of each anomaly or group of anomalies, which hampers precise description of each anomaly and prediction of feasibility and safety of surgical correction; (iii) Class I includes cases with hypoplasia and/or dysgenesis of the vagina, cervix, uterus and/or adnexae, and the grouping of these patients into one category are very general and not functional; (iv) Obstructive anomalies, which are the result of cervical and/or vaginal aplasias and/or dysplasias, in the presence of either a normal or deformed but functional uterus is not represented.

ESHRE/ESGE classification is a new system based on the anatomy of the female genital tract. Anomalies are classified into the following main classes, expressing uterine anatomical deviations deriving from the same embryological origin: *U0, normal uterus; U1, dysmorphic uterus; U2, septate uterus; U3, bicorporeal uterus; U4, hemiuterus; U5, aplastic uterus; U6, for still unclassified cases*. Main class have been divided into subclasses expressing anatomical varieties with clinical significance. Within this system, cervical and vaginal

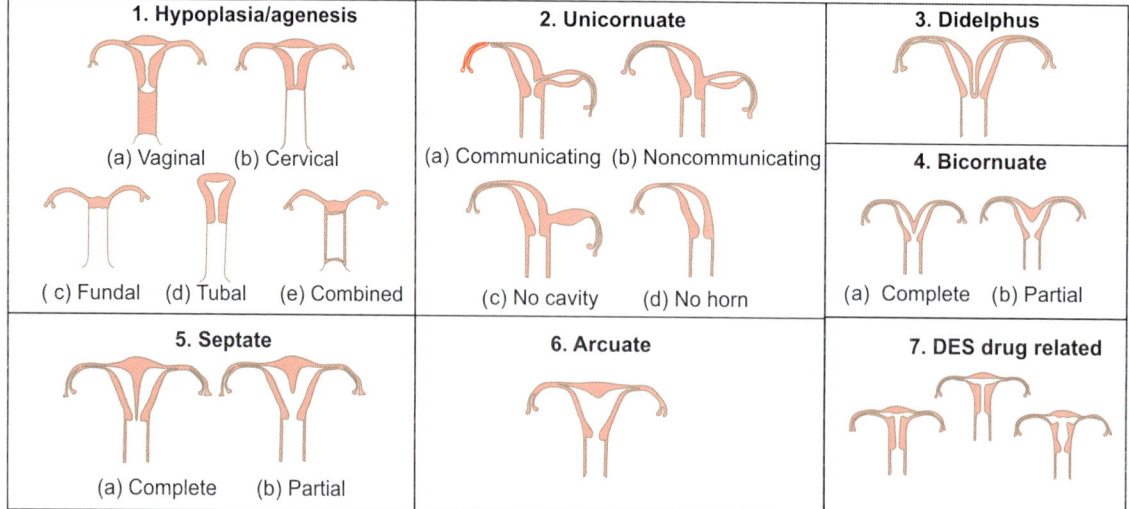

Uterus may be normal or take a variety of abnormal forms.
May have two distinct cervices.

Fig. 10.2: The AFS classification system for female genital congenital anomalies (American Fertility Society, 1988)

anomalies are covered and classified in independent supplementary subclasses, which provide more possibilities for multiple combined or complex anomalies (Fig. 10.3). Furthermore, ESHRE/ESGE classification is based on imageology and described in digital form. Therefore, ESHRE/ESGE classification seems to be more objective, accurate and clear and overcome the limits of the previous systems. However, its clinical value still needs to be proved. Some researchers indicate that this classification may lead to an extraordinary increase in the frequency of diagnosis of septate uterus. Septate uterus diagnosed by this classification system is quantitatively dominated by morphological states corresponding to arcuate uterus or cases where no congenital malformations are identified by the AFS criteria. Surgical treatment in these cases may be unnecessary and may not provide the expected benefits.

Hysteroscopic Metroplasty

Recurrent pregnancy loss and reproductive failure serve as the main indications of metroplasty for whom with requiring fertility. With the development of gynecological endoscopic technology, the treatment techniques are continuously being improved and perfected. Currently, transcervical resection of septa (TCRS) showed advantages as less surgical trauma, shorter hospital stay, and fewer complications, which have become an effective and safe alternative to treat septate uterus.

Surgical Steps

Anesthesia and Patient Positioning

TCRS is typically a day-surgery procedure performed under general anesthesia. The patient is placed in dorsal lithotomy position. Because concurrent laparoscopy is recommended, the abdomen and vagina are surgically

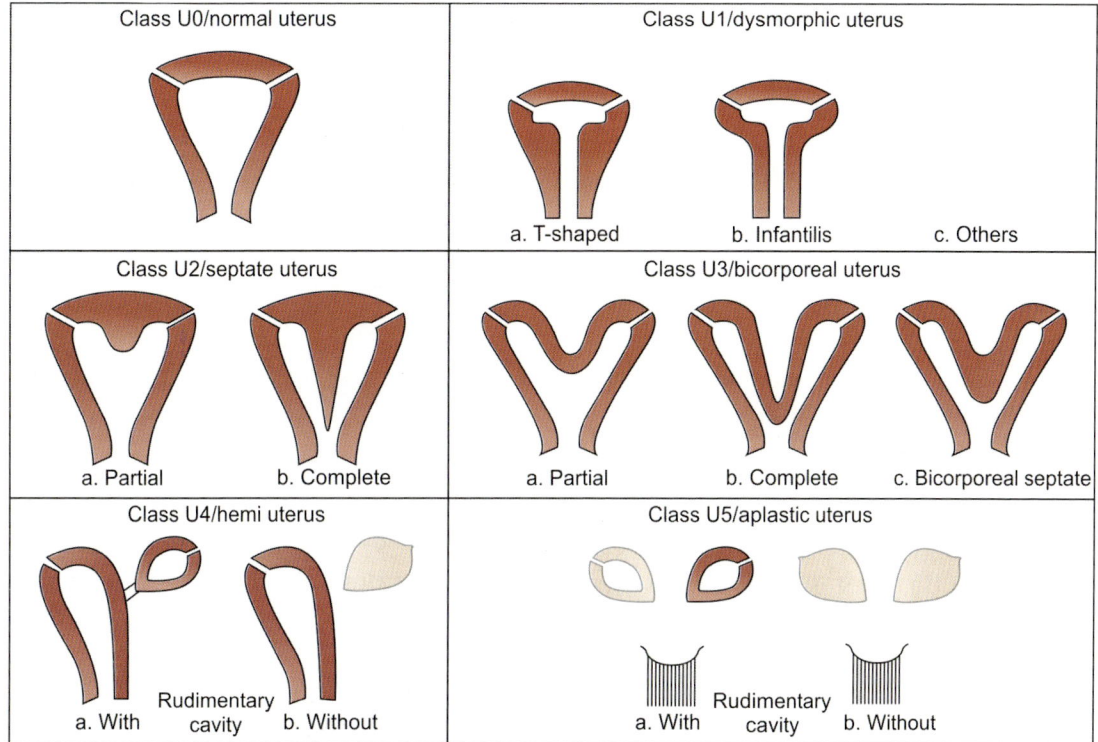

Fig. 10.3: The ESHRE/ESGE classification system for female genital congenital anomalies (Grimbizis, 2013)

prepared. A Foley catheter is inserted into bladder.

Medium Selection

The choice of distending medium is depend on the incising tool used. Sharp incision with scissors, Nd:YAG laser, or bipolar instrument is commonly selected and can be performed in any liquid medium. Monopolar technology will require a hypotonic nonconductive medium.

Combined with Laparoscopy

Because of the potential risk of uterine perforation, concurrent laparoscopy is recommended that can inform a surgeon as to the perforation during TCRS procedure.

Hysteroscope Insertion and Septum Incision

The operative hysteroscope is inserted into the uterine cavity by cervical canal under direct visualization. A panoramic inspection is first performed to identify the septum. When needle electrode issued, a surgeon should attempt to keep the line of incision in the anteroposterior midline of septum. Transection begins caudally, at the septum apex, and continues cephalad toward the fundus. Incision is taken bilaterally and is directed toward the horizontal midline. During incision of the septum, drifting from the vertical midline is common. Incisions typically drift posteriorly in an anteverted uterus and anteriorly in a retroverted one. Thus, a surgeon may pause and reorient periodically.

Septum Resection

In some cases, the septum is broad, wide, and difficult to simply incise. Thus, to achieve the desired uterine cavity, a surgeon must completely excise or resect the septum. In general, scissors maybe used, but in some instances, vaporizing electrodes, loop electrodes, or morcellators are more useful. Instruments are selected according to surgeon skill and preference.

Procedure Completion

After TCRS procedure, the final fluid deficit should be calculated and noted in the operative report.

Tips and Tricks

TCRS is a reconstructive operation of uterine cavity. We should not only remove the septum tissue, but also avoid the destruction of endometrium at the greatest extent. For incomplete septum uterus, incision begins from the apex and continues cephalad toward the fundus. For complete septum uterus, if there is partial communications of the partitioned uterus, the septum should be divided from the os of internal cervix upward to the fundus; if communications dose not exit, a probe can be placed in the contralateral uterine cavity as the indication, and divide the septum to make a connection between the two sides of uterine cavity, and then the incision is carried out as above mentioned. Some noteworthy tips and tricks are summarized as follows.

Symmetrical Incision

Special attention should be paid to the direction and symmetry of septum incision. When needle or annular electrodes are used, a surgeon should attempt to keep the line of incision in the anteroposterior midline. Transection alternates bilaterally along the septal midline toward the bottom of the uterus in a caudad-to-cephalad direction. Try not to bias toward the front or posterior wall of the uterus to avoid damage to the muscle wall of the uterus.

Control the Depth of Incision

It is very important to judge the connection area between septum tissue and myometrium by which a surgeon stop the incision timely to prevent uterine perforation. In general, there is minimal bleeding due to the relative avascularity of the septum's fibroelastic tissue, which retracts upon incision. If the incision is too deep, damage maybe caused to the uterine muscle wall, resulting in heavy bleeding or even uterine perforation, whereas if the incision is uncompleted, residual septum may affect the surgical outcomes. There are some significant signs that indicate the incision is complete, which include the increase of tissue vascularity, serosal transillumination test of hysteroscope combined with laparoscope at uterine fundus, the movement of hysteroscope from one side to the other side without hindrance, reaching a level in line with both tubal ostia, and the thickness of the uterine base is the same as that of the surrounding myometrial wall under ultrasonic monitoring.

Retain Intracervical Septum

For the resection range of the complete septum, the septum should be divided from the internal cervical os upward to the fundus, and the intracervical septum should not be resected to avoid cervical incompetence and the artificially increased probability of miscarriage and premature birth which may caused from it. In addition, whether to resect vaginal septum or not depends on the wishes of the patients. Before the application patients should be fully informed that reserve of vaginal septum may cause vaginal obstruction during delivery.

Concurrent Laparoscopy is Recommended with TCRS Produce

Intraoperative monitoring is essential to prevent the perforation of uterus. Concurrent laparoscopy is recommended with TCRS to help inform a surgeon as to the proximity of the uterine serosa. The advantages are as follows: (i) Surgeon can observe the appearance of the uterus by laparoscopy and easy to make the differential diagnosis of uterine malformation; (ii) Test of serosal transillumination at the uterine fundus can help surgeon determine the depth of incision, indicates the potential uterine perforation. Once perforation occurred, laparoscopy repair immediately to avoid causing severe damage; (iii) To treat the coexisted disease in the abdominal cavity during the same time.

References

1. Barbara L. Hoffman, et al. Williams Gynecology, second edition, 2012, Chapter 18, P 481–505.
2. Cunningham FG, Leveno KJ, Bloom SL, et al. Reproductive tract abnormalities. Williams Obstetrics, 23rd edition. New York, McGraw-Hill, 2010, P 894.
3. Valle RF, Ekpo GE. Hysteroscopic metroplasty for the septate uterus: review and meta-analysis. J Min Invas Gynecol 2013; 20:22–42.
4. Heinonen PK. Complete septate uterus with longitudinal vaginal septum. Fertil Steril 2006; 85(3): 700.
5. Woelfer B, Salim R, Banerjee S, et al. Reproductive outcomes in women with congenital uterine anomalies detected by three-dimensional ultrasound screening. Obstet Gynecol 2001;98(6): 1099.
6. Proctor JA, Haney AF. Recurrent first-trimester pregnancy loss is associated with uterine septum but not with bicornuate uterus. Fertil Steril 2003;80(5):1212.
7. The American Fertility Society classification of adnexal adhesions, distal tubal occlusion, tubal occlusion secondary to tubal ligation, tubal pregnancies, Müllerian anomalies and intra-uterine adhesions. Fertil Steril 1988;49(6):944–55.
8. Grimbizis GF, Gordts S, Di Spiezio, Sardo A, et al. The ESHRE/ESGE consensus on the classification of female genital tract congenital anomalies. Hum Reprod 2013;28 (8):2032–44.

Lateral Metroplasty in T-Shaped Uterus

Pankaj Mate, Mamta Dighe

INTRODUCTION

The size of a normal uterus varies from woman to woman, and many fertile women have a small uterus (a normal anatomic variant) when they are not pregnant. The uterus enlarges normally during pregnancy, allowing them to give birth to a healthy baby.

Any malformation of the uterus in which there is an abnormally reduced volume of uterine cavity due to inward projecting side walls of the uterus, or due to uterine hypoplasia is known as T-shaped uterus. The new classification system of uterine anomalies is developed by the European Society of Human Reproduction and Embryology (ESHRE) and the European Society for Gynaecological Endoscopy (ESGE) (Table 11.1). In this new classification system, Class I

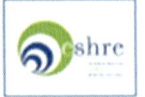

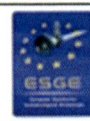

	Uterine anomaly		Cervical / Vaginal anomaly	
Main class		**Sub-class**	**Co-existent class**	
U0	Normal uterus		C0	Normal cervix
U1	Dysmorphic uterus	a. T-shaped	C1	Septate cervix
		b. Infantilis		
		c. Others	C2	Double "normal" cervix
U2	Septate uterus	a. Partial	C3	Unilateral cervical aplasia
		b. Complete		
			C4	Cervical Aplasia
U3	Bicorporeal uterus	a. Partial		
		b. Complete		
		c. Bicorporeal septate	V0	Normal vagina
U4	Hemi-uterus	a. With rudimentary cavity (communicating or not horn)	V1	Longitudinal non-obstructing vaginal septum
		b. Without rudimentary cavity (horn without cavity / no horn)	V2	Longitudinal obstructing vaginal septum
U5	Aplastic	a. With rudimentary cavity (bi- or unilateral horn)	V3	Transverse vaginal septum and/or imperforate hymen
		b. Without rudimentary cavity (bi- or unilateral uterine remnants / Aplasia)	V4	Vaginal aplasia
U6	Unclassified Malformations			
U			C	V

Table 11.1: **ESHRE/ESGE classification Female genital tract anomalies**

incorporates all cases having a uterus with normal outline but with an abnormal lateral wall shape of the uterine cavity (i.e. T-shaped uterus and tubular-shaped/infantilis uteri) (Fig. 11.1). These anomalies in the previous American Fertility Society classification were conversely included in class VII and were mainly related to diethylstilbestrol-related (DES) exposure (American Fertility Society, 1988).

Earlier, this was thought to be a purely acquired abnormality, resulting from in utero-exposure of the female fetus to diethyl stilbesterol (DES). Although it is a rarer than other Mullerian anomalies like septate uterus, bicornuate uterus, etc., acquired forms due to other causes like pelvic tuberculosis and Asherman's syndrome due to prior surgeries also have been described. Intrauterine adhesions at lower end of the uterine cavity can also cause uterine narrowing, forming a T-shaped uterine cavity.[1] There are reported cases of hypoplastic uterus, a cylindrical uterine cavity and bulging of the uterine side walls, combined with a history of primary infertility and recurrent abortions.

Several studies have showed very poor reproductive performance when this uterine malformation is not treated.[2] Reproductive performance after hysteroscopic metroplasty in women with a T-shaped uterus is not well documented: there are only few reports (Nagel and Malo, 1993; Katz et al., 1996; Garbin et al., 1998), compared with numerous reports of surgery for a septate uterus (Homer et al., 2000).

Clinical Presentation

Infertility and obstetric complications are believed to be more common in women with uterine dysmorphism than in those with a normal uterine cavity. T-shaped uterine cavity is associated with infertility, failed implantation, increased risk of ectopic pregnancy, miscarriage and preterm delivery.

Diagnosis

Women are often diagnosed with this condition by exploratory diagnostic procedures, such as magnetic resonance imaging (MRI), 2 dimensional ultrasound, 3 dimensional ultrasound and particularly hysterosalpingography (HSG) (Fig. 11.2a–c).[3-5] In such studies, a widening of the interstitial and isthmus of uterine tube is observed, as well as constrictions or narrowing of the uterus as a whole, especially the lower and lateral portions, hence the "t" denomination compared to a normal funnel-shaped contour. The uterus might be simultaneously reduced in volume, and other abnormalities might be concomitantly present.[6]

On two dimensional ultrasound uterine endometrium shows an abrupt narrowing in the lower two-thirds or lower half of the cavity. 3 dimensional transvaginal sonography (3D-TVS) equipped by an endovaginal volume probe with a frequency of 5-9 MHz provided images of the uterus in three planes, displayed simultaneously, and produced has a high rate of accuracy for both diagnosis and classification of congenital anomalies (Fig. 11.3). 3D-TVS examinations to be carried out during the luteal phase of the cycle (day 21 to 25): This is considered the optimal time to examine patients for the presence of uterine anomalies, because the endometrium appears

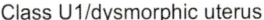

Class U1/dysmorphic uterus

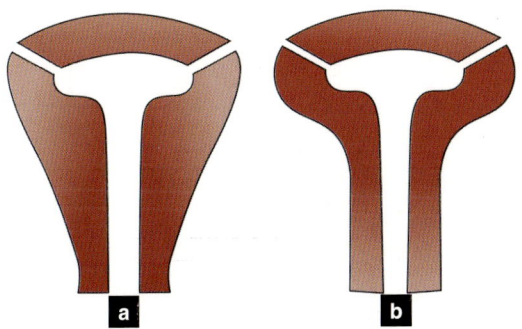

Fig. 11.1: Dysmorphic uteri according to ESHRE and the ESGE classification of female genital tract congenital anomalies (Grimbizis et al., 2013). (a) T-shaped uterus; (b) Uterus infantalis

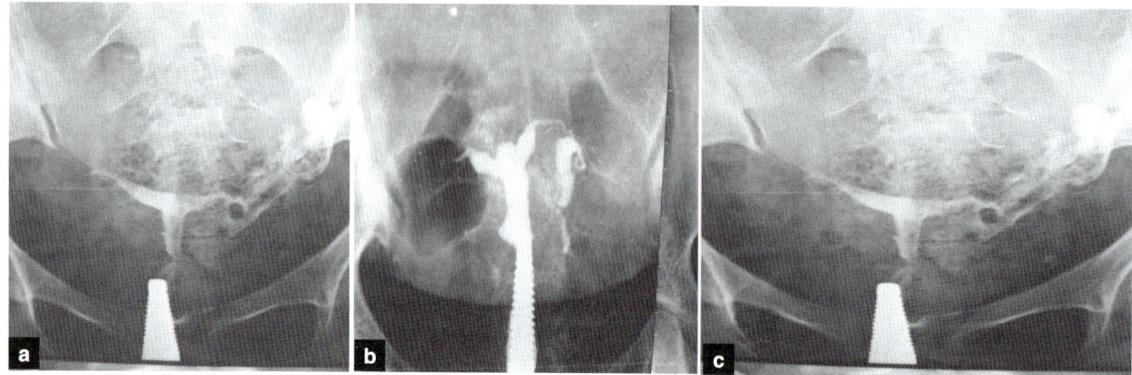

Fig. 11.2a to c: T-shaped uterine cavity on hysterosalpingography

thick and echogenic and the uterine cavity can be clearly differentiated from the surrounding myometrium. During the ultrasonography, it is essential to measure the bulging of the uterine side walls, their thickness and the depth of the healthy myometrium up to the serosa.

Analysis of uterine architecture should be carried out in a standardized plane using the interstitial portions of the fallopian tubes as reference points. The distance between tubal ostia (IO), the transversal diameter at the isthmus (I), I/IO ratio as well as the thickness of the uterine side walls and the depth of the healthy myometrium up to the serosa should be measured (Fig. 11.4a and b).

- Distance between ostia
- Length of the uterine cavity
- Possible section in the width
- Safety margin

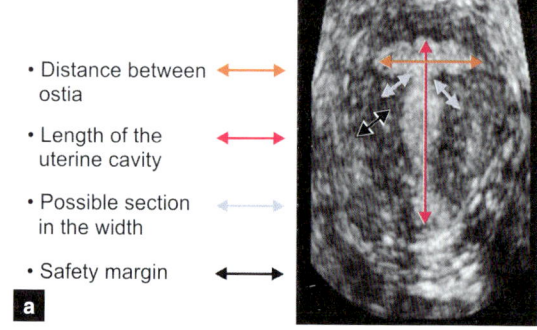

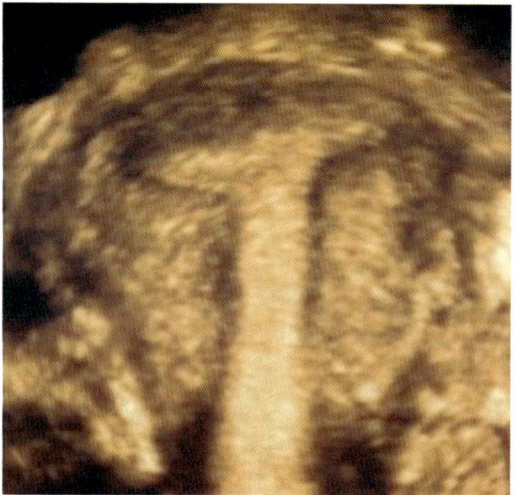

Fig. 11.3: T-shaped uterus on 3D ultrasound

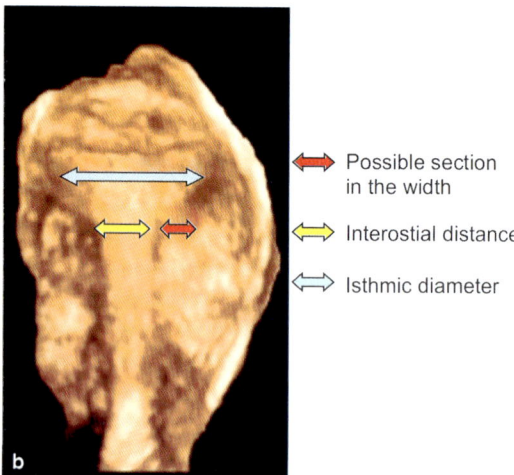

Possible section in the width

Interostial distance

Isthmic diameter

Fig. 11.4a and b: Three-dimensional transvaginal ultrasound imaging referring to the landmarks: the distance between tubal ostia (IO, inter-ostial distance); the transversal diameter at the isthmus (I, isthmic diameter), as well as the depth of the healthy myometrium up to the serosa (of which sections are allowed)

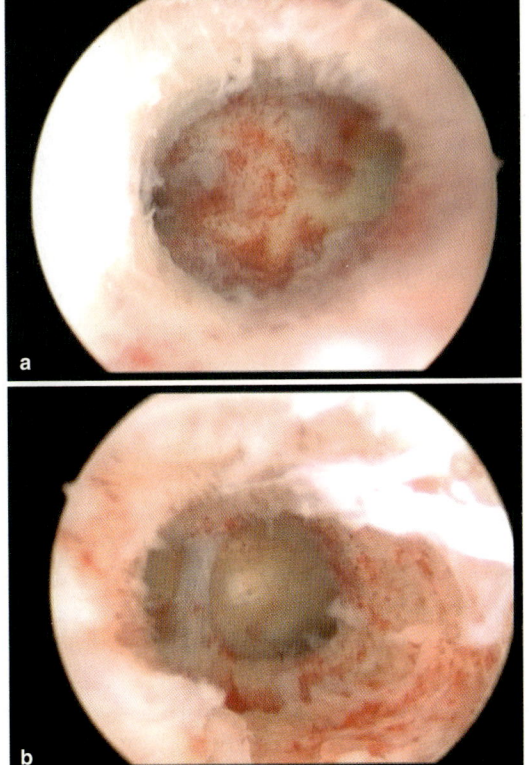

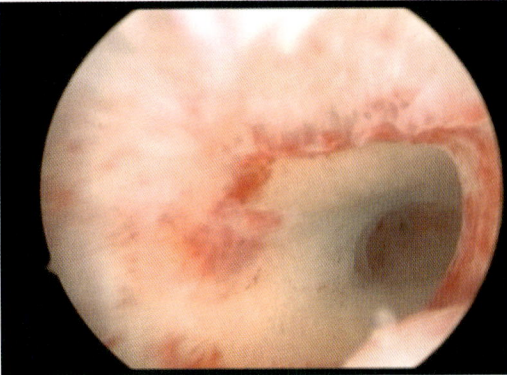

Fig. 11.7: Tubal openings which appear deeply sited on hysteroscopy

Fig. 11.5a and b: Tubular shape of uterine cavity on office hysteroscopy visualized from the level of internal os with difficulty in visualizing tubal ostia

Office hysteroscopy reveals a cylindrical uterine cavity (Fig. 11.5a and b) with a bulging of the uterine side walls and no possibility to visualise the tubal ostia (Fig. 11.6). Hysteroscope can be advanced to observe the positions of

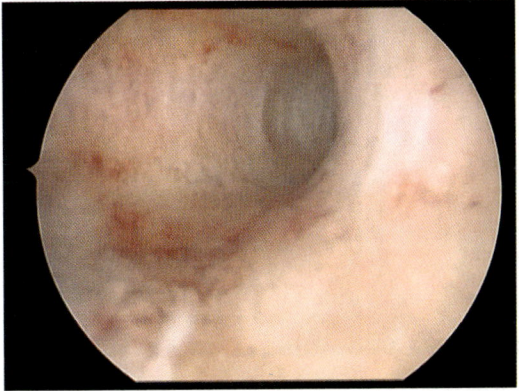

Fig. 11.6: Lateral wall of a dysmorphic uterus

tubal openings which appear deeply sited (Fig. 11.7), to correlate with the preoperative HSG and 3D ultrasoundings, and to assess the depth of uterine wall excision.

At hysteroscopy, the uterus was considered to be dysmorphic if it presented with an enlarged distance between the tubal ostia; with a correlation of two-thirds uterine corpus and one-third cervix (T-shaped uterus) and; inverse correlation of one-third uterine body and two-thirds cervix [tubular shaped (infantilis uterus) (Grimbizisetal, 2013)].

Pre-surgical Assessment of Uterine Cavity

An evaluation of the volume and morphology of the uterine cavity should be carried out by using both office hysteroscopy and three-dimensional transvaginal ultrasound (3D-TVS) assessment. On hysteroscopy, the uterus was considered to be dysmorphic if it presented with an enlarged distance between the tubal ostia; with a correlation of two-thirds uterine corpus and one-third cervix (T-shaped uterus) and; inverse correlation of one-third uterine body and two-thirds cervix (tubular shaped [infantilis uterus]) (Grimbizis et al, 2013). Interostial distance (i.e. distance between the two tubal ostia) as well as the transverse diameter at the level of isthmus, should be assessed using the opening of the jaws of the 5 French (5 Fr) grasping forceps (6 mm) as reference measure.

Management

Several independent studies have shown poor reproductive performance when this kind of uterine malformation is untreated (Berger and Goldstein, 1980; Herbst et al, 1981), as altered volume and shape of the uterine cavity are likely to contribute to defective endometrial receptivity (Revel, 2012).

Different methods and instruments have been used for hysteroscopic metroplasty, including scissors and a resectoscope with a monopolar hook (Garbin et al, 1998; Fernandez et al, 2000; Homer et al, 2000; Barranger et al, 2002). Hysteroscopic surgery should be offered to patients with T-shaped uterine cavity and a history of infertility or adverse pregnancy outcomes. It can also be used to treat patients who failed IVF-ET treatment. Surgery can be performed soon after menstruation to avoid a thickened endometrium which might impact on the hysteroscopic surgery.

The development of operative hysteroscopy has allowed the treatment of these malformations, using monopolar (Fig. 11.8) or bipolar instruments, thus avoiding laparotomy and resulting in lower morbidity.[7]

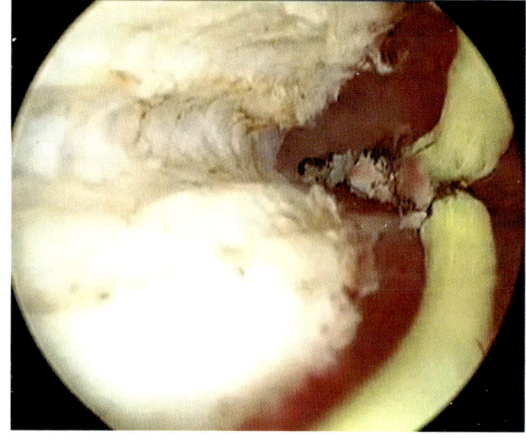

Fig. 11.8: Collin's knife used for lateral metroplasty

The resectoscope electrode needle/hook should be positioned vertically to the lateral uterine wall below the fallopian tube opening. The uterine wall is incised under direct vision from the fundus to the uterine isthmus perpendicularly to the lateral wall of the uterus and decreasing the depth of the incision as the section advanced (Fig. 11.9); according to the preoperative and intraoperative assessment of the depth of uterine wall thickness, the first electrode which cut along the side wall of the uterus would create a

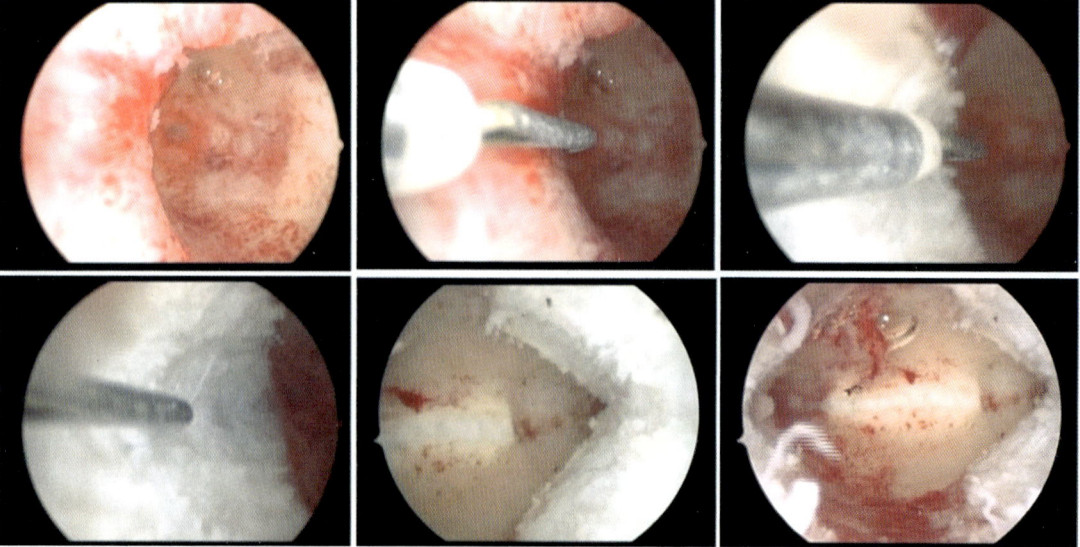

Fig. 11.9: T-shaped uterus with lateral convergent uterine walls with deeply situated ostia: Lateral metroplasty with bipolar hook

groove from the fundus to the uterine isthmus; this should be performed again till the desired effect is achieved. It is important to control the depth of cutting, with deep cut initially, to shallow cut at the end. The cut depth should be controlled within 5–7 mm, to avoid surgical complications like uterine perforation or very thin myometrium. In the same way, the contralateral lateral wall of the uterus is cut; to assess the completeness of the procedure, the hysteroscope can be moved to the middle of the uterine cavity, in order to obtain a symmetrical inverted triangle view of the uterine cavity with bilateral easily observable tubal openings.

It must be emphasized that after two menstrual cycles, a repeat hysteroscopic examination is necessary to assess the effectiveness (Fig. 11.10) of the surgery and to assess whether there are recurrent adhesions, and if necessary, hysteroscopic adhesiolysis can be performed.

Bipolar Instrument

The bipolar electrode or resectoscope is a more recent system developed for use with saline solution. Its efficacy is equivalent to that of monopolar instrument and morbidity is lower. There are no limits to the duration of the procedure, but a strict monitoring of input and output is important as fluid overload can still occur with risk of pulmonary edema or death by excess load. Bipolar instruments have the advantage of being safer, because they can be used with saline, thereby decreasing metabolic complications. In contrast to the monopolar system which penetrates into the tissues and can be partly obscured at certain points, the bipolar system is constantly visible.

Hysteroscopic Scissors

Mechanical scissors are also an attractive option to the resectoscope. Unlike unipolar/bipolar electrode, the incision with scissor

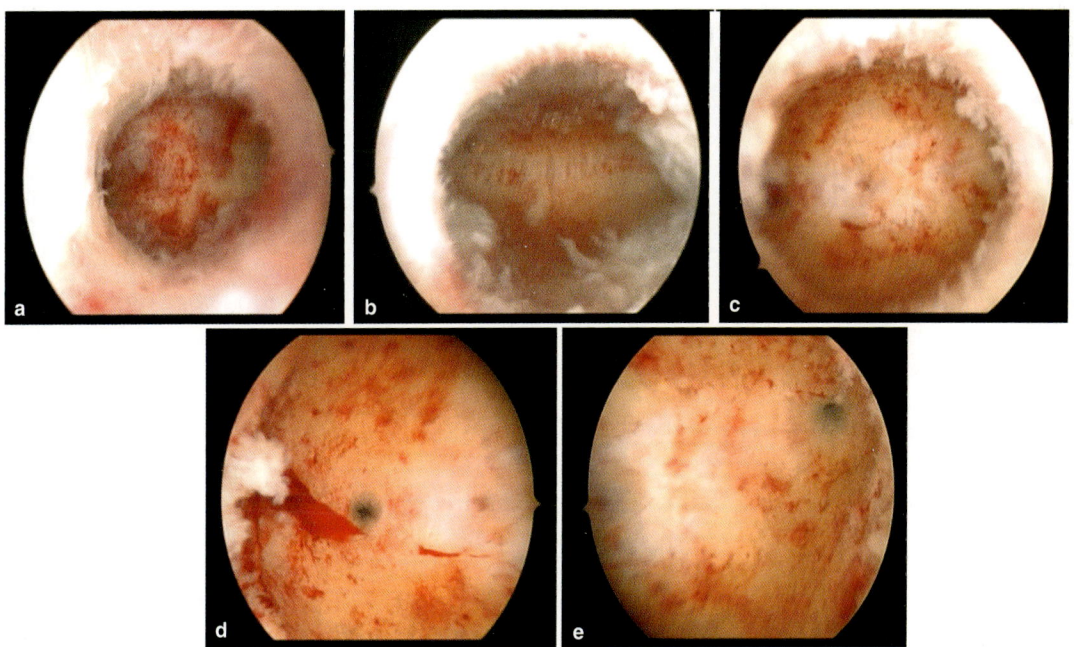

Fig. 11.10a to e: (a) T-shaped uterine cavity; (b) Immediate Post-op after lateral metroplasty; (c) Cavity enhancement achieved noticed on second-look hysteroscopy; (d and e) Both ostia visualized with no protruding/convergent lateral wall on second-look hysteroscopy

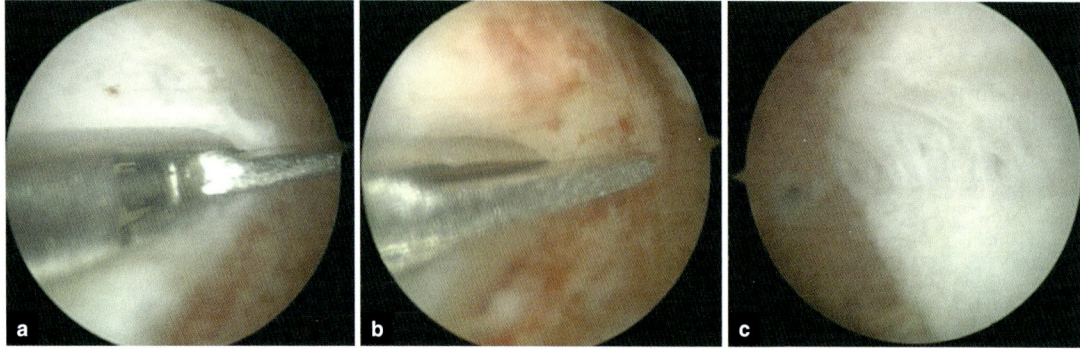

Fig. 11.11a to c: Hysteroscopic lateral metroplasty with mechanical scissors

starts just at the level of internal os and ends below the tubal ostium on both sides. The static blade of the single action scissors is thrust about 2 mm deep within the uterine myometrium (Fig. 11.11a), and the moving blade cuts the tissue (Fig. 11.11b and c). The advantage of using cold scissors, over a resectoscope is that there is no thermal damage to the surrounding endometrium.

Postoperative Care

To prevent secondary intrauterine adhesions after surgery, an intrauterine balloon (pediatric Foley catheter) or IUCD can be inserted and combined estrogen and progesterone cyclical treatment should be given to promote endometrial growth.

Post-surgical evaluation should be conducted by office hysteroscopy and 3D-TVS. The main parameter is the increase in the volume of uterine cavity as measured by 3D-TVS. Office hysteroscopy should be carried out in the early proliferative phase of the following menstrual cycle. The main interest of second-look hysteroscopy is to diagnose and to treat residual synechia to improve the reproductive outcome.

Complications

Immediate complications include severe hemorrhage, however, the risks after the procedure include placenta accreta and Asherman's syndrome.[8, 9]

DISCUSSION

In case of uterine dysmorphism, infertility and obstetric complications are believed to be more common compared with those with a normal uterine cavity. Dysmorphic uterus [both T-shaped and tubular-shaped (infantilis uteri)] is a major concern in reproduction. The hysteroscopic metroplasty seems to be an operation that improves the pregnancy rates for women with a hypoplastic uterus and a history of primary infertility.

Postoperative diagnostic hysteroscopy shows that hysteroscopic metroplasty produced good anatomical results in most cases. This procedure allows the formation of a normal uterine triangular and symmetric cavity. It is considered a low-risk procedure, and can also improve term delivery rate by up to 10-fold, as long as the endometrium is considered to be in good condition.[10–12]

Improved uterine contour may result in an improved pregnancy outcome and term deliveries in women with prior spontaneous pregnancy losses or primary infertility. Vaginal delivery is possible after metroplasty, but in the light of the literature, there should be no hesitation about choosing cesarean as the mode of delivery. Metroplasty probably induces uterine fragility. Obstetric management must be careful, although no uterine rupture is reported in the literature.[13–15] The cases of uterine rupture after hysteroscopic metroplasty concerned septate uterus.[16,17]

References

1. Fernandez H, et al. Surgical approach to and reproductive outcome after surgical correction of a T-shaped uterus. Hum Reprod. 2011;26(7):1730–4.

2. Berger and Goldstein, 1980; Herbst, et al., 1981.

3. Baramki TA (2005). "Hysterosalpingography". Fertil Steril. 83 (6): 1595–606.

4. Viscomi GN, Gonzalez R, Taylor KJ. "Ultrasound detection of uterine abnormalities after diethylstilbestrol (DES) exposure". Radiology 1980;136 (3): 733–35.

5. Van Gils AP, Tham RT, Falke TH, Peters AA. "Abnormalities of the uterus and cervix after diethylstilbestrol exposure: correlation of findings on MR and hysterosalpingography". AJR Am J Roentgenol. 1989;153 (6): 1235–8.

6. Kaufman RH, Binder GL, Gray PM, Adam E. "Upper genital tract changes associated with exposure in utero to diethylstilbestrol". Am J Obstet Gynecol. 1977;128 (1): 51–9. PMID 851159.

7. Fernandez, et al, 2011; Garbinetal, 1998; Herbst, et al., 1981; Katz, et al., 1996; Nagel and Malo, 1993.

8. Meier, Rose; Campo, Rudi (2015). "T-Shaped Uterus". Female Genital Tract Congenital Malformations: 261–270.

9. Fernandez H; Garbin O; Castaigne V; Gervaise A; Levaillant J-M. "Surgical approach to and reproductive outcome after surgical correction of a T-shaped uterus". Human Reproduction. 2011;26 (7): 1730–34.

10. Noyes N, Liu HC, Sultan K, Rosenwaks Z. "Endometrial pattern in diethylstilboestrol-exposed women undergoing *in vitro* fertilization may be the most significant predictor of pregnancy outcome". Hum Reprod. 1996;11 (12): 2719–23.

11. Giacomucci E, Bellavia E, Sandri F, Farina A, Scagliarini G. "Term delivery rate after hysteroscopic metroplasty in patients with recurrent spontaneous abortion and T-shaped, arcuate and septate uterus". Gynecol Obstet Invest. 2011;71 (3): 183–8.

12. Golan A, Langer R, Neuman M, Wexler S, Segev E, David MP. "Obstetric outcome in women with congenital uterine malformations". J Reprod Med. 1992;37 (3): 233–6.

13. Nagel TC, Malo JW. Hysteroscopic metroplasty in the diethylstilbestrol-exposed uterus and similar non fusion anomalies: effects on subsequent reproductive performance. A preliminary report. Fertil Steril 1993;59: 502–6.

14. Katz Z, Ben Arie A, Lurie S, Manor M, Insler V. Beneficial effect of hysteroscopic metroplasty on the reproductive outcome in a 'T-shaped' uterus. Gynecol Obstet Invest 1996;41:41–43.

15. Garbin O, Ohl J, Bettahar Lebugle K, Dellenbach P. Hysteroscopic metroplasty in diethylstilboestrol-exposed and hypoplastic uterus: a report on 24 cases. Hum Reprod 1998;13: 2751–55.

16. Homer HA, Li TC, Cooke ID. The septate uterus: a review of management and reproductive outcome. Fertil Steril 2000;73: 1–14.

17. Gabriele A, Zanetta G, Pasta F, Colombo M. Uterine rupture after hysteroscopic metroplasty and labor induction. A case report. J Reprod Med 1999;44: 642–44.

Proximal Tubal Block—Cannulating Ostium by Hysteroscopy

Sanjeev Khurd, Sadhana Khurd, Aditya Khurd, Vandana Khurd

INTRODUCTION

Tubal factor accounts for 14–30% of infertility cases.[1] Amongst the various tubal pathologies, proximal tubal block, due to tubal obstruction or occlusion accounts for 10 to 25% of the tubal factor. Diagnosis of proximal tubal block has traditionally been made by hysterosalpingography (HSG), since more than 100 years, and subsequently in the later years by laparoscopy, which in present times is combined with hysteroscopy as well. Before *in vitro* fertilization (IVF) arrived on the scene in 1978, with the birth of Louis Brown in England and "Durga" (Kanupriya Agarwal) in India, in the same year, all tubal pathologies were regularly managed surgically. Utero-tubal implantation, with a term pregnancy rate of 11–15% was the standard treatment for cornual tubal blocks,[2] till it was replaced by microsurgical tubo-cornual anastomosis about 4 decades ago. The microsurgical technique improved the live birth rate to 57%, with ectopic pregnancies occurring in about 10% cases.[3] Nevertheless, both these procedures require laparotomy and hence are more morbid, requiring prolonged recovery and hospital stay. The microsurgical tubo-cornual anastomosis can also be done laparoscopically, but requires expertise and skill and only a few expert endoscopic surgeons are able to perform it, thereby limiting its scope.

Tubal cannulation to open proximal tubal blocks, has been a recent addition to our surgical armametrium and has gained a lot of interest and popularity due to it being minimally invasive, less morbid and an effective day care procedure. Although tubal cannulation can be done under fluoroscopic/radiographic, ultrasonographic, falloposcopic and even under tactile guidance, amongst gynecologists and infertility specialists, hysteroscopic cannulation is the preferred modality and is here to stay in the management of proximal tubal block.

ANATOMY OF THE FALLOPIAN TUBE

In order to perform a successful hysteroscopic tubal cannulation for proximal tubal block, we need to understand the anatomy of the intramural portion of the tube. The two fallopian tubes take off from the uterine (endometrial) cavity from the cornua and run a length of about 7 to 14 cm. Each tube is broadly divided into 3 regions viz. intramural (interstitial) portion (1.5–2.5 cm) which traverses through the myometrium, the isthmic part (1–3 cm) and the wider ampullary portion (5–8 cm) with the infundibulum in the terminal region along with the fimbriated ostium. The lumen of the fallopian tube is narrowest (0.2–0.4 mm) in its intramural segment (average diameter 0.8 to 1.2 mm),

1 to 1.5 cm beyond the tubal ostia. It gradually widens: 0.1–1 mm in isthmic region, 1–2 mm at isthmo-ampullary junction, to 1 cm towards infundibulum junction and widest in the region of the infundibulum (> 1 cm).

The tube opens into the uterine cavity at the tubal ostium. Each ostium is situated at the apex of the utero-cornual gutter and can be seen hysteroscopically at the bottom of a saucer-shaped depression as a sharp membranous ring which measures 0.8 to 1.2 mm in diameter. The intramural (interstitial) portion of the fallopian tube is contained within the myometrial wall of the uterine fundus. It is a potential space due to collapse and contraction of muscular oviductal wall. *In vivo*, the intramural lumen is actually 0.8 to 1.2 mm in diameter and can accommodate cannulas 1–1.2 mm in width by stretching marginally due to healthy elasticity, without causing damage to the ciliary epithelium.

The intramural portion of the tube is divided into two segments: A proximal segment approximately 1 cm in length which follows a rectilinear path, and a 1.5 cm distal segment which is nearly always irregular and is continuous with the isthmus portion. In 1962, Sweeny observed that the intramural portion of the tube is sinuous in at least two-thirds of the cases.[9] Thick muscular wall and convoluted intramural course results in the intramural portion of the tube to be a likely site of blockage by debris and mucus plugs. The convoluted intramural course also poses difficulty in cannulation of the fallopian tube.

TUBAL OBSTRUCTION AND TUBAL OCCLUSION AS A CAUSE OF PROXIMAL TUBAL BLOCK

In 1954, Rubin was the first to introduce the concept, later revived by Alan de Cherney of a possible differentiation between tubal obstruction and tubal occlusion.[10] Indeed several authors have reported difficulties in identifying confirmed histopathological lesions as the cause of tubal block in many of these patients who underwent cornual tubal anastomosis for cornual block, but could only find sort of tubal plugs of exudates that simply obstruct the tube. The observations of Sulak et al on 18 patients with proximal tubal block confirmed by numerous diagnostic techniques (HSG, chromosalpingoscopy, laparoscopy, transcervical methylene blue injection, as well as transfundal injection of a dye) are quite interesting.[11] In all cases, these authors surgically resected the occluded tract followed by subsequent microsurgical anastomosis. The surgically sectioned portion of the tube was subjected to histopathological testing. Only in 7 patients, real anatomical-pathological occlusion was found, whereas in the other cases the tubes appeared either totally normal or presented modest fibrotic or inflammatory lesions but were, nevertheless, patent. In particular, in 6 patients the authors detected the presence of some amorphous material comprised for the most part of inflammatory cells. This aggregate was most likely made up of a partially organized exudates which at some points presented actual calcifications.

Therefore, it can be proposed that in some infertile women, there are some sort of 'tubal plugs', which are formed by mucous, debris and organized exudates from tubal secretions and/or material back flowing from the uterine cavity, and may cause obstruction. The real incidence of this pathology is difficult to quantify although approximately 50% of the women diagnosed as having proximal tubal block do infact have an obstruction; the other 50% having true anatomical-pathological occlusions. On the other hand, it is well known that there is a significant percentage of spontaneous pregnancies after some diagnostic procedures which might be capable of removing these intrafallopian 'plugs' by exerting pressure. After hysterosalpingography the rate of pregnancy, for example, is between 13% and 55%. Indeed, some authors have attributed therapeutic capacity to even simple tubal-uterine insufflations, with a pregnancy rate of 20–60%.[12]

Diagnosis of Tubal Block

The fallopian tubes can be well assessed, their normalcy determined and patency confirmed by various modalities, viz. HSG, hysterosal-pingo-contrast sonography (HyCoSy) and laparoscopy combined with hysteroscopy. These also allow us to determine the presence of any tubal pathology and damage resulting in tubal blocks, which may be a causative factor for the couple's infertility.

HSG and laparoscopy are the commonest and most widely performed procedures in our Indian setting. It is important to understand that both HSG and laparoscopy have certain amount of false positive inferences regarding tubal block, hence the diagnosis of tubal block should never be made on the basis of either HSG or laparoscopy-hysteroscopy alone, and one investigation should always be complemented by performing the other, to arrive at a confirmed diagnosis of tubal block.

Ever since it was first performed by Carey in 1914,[4] HSG has been the commonest modality of investigating the fallopian tubes, as it is universally available, non-invasive and least expensive procedure that does not require anesthesia. It is now more than 4 decades that the oil based contrast dye, Lipiodol, introduced by Sicard and Forestier in 1924,[4] has been replaced by aqueous medium, which has greatly reduced the instances of allergic reactions. The timing of HSG and technical quality is important to limit the factors leading to its misinterpretation. HSG, if properly performed and interpreted, can be of great value regarding imparting information about tubal patency, architecture of the tubal lumen—with the rugocity suggesting healthy tubal mucosa, and giving clear delineatation of the level of tubal block. These features allow HSG to score over laparoscopy, which only provides information about the exterior of the fallopian tube. HSG also gives us additional information about the uterine cavity and alerts us on Müllerian anomalies, e.g. uterine septum, unicornuate uterus, etc.

and intra-cavitary distortions due to possible endometrial polyps, fibroids and intra-uterine synechiae. Extravasation and intravasation of the dye may suggest the possibility of genital tuberculosis (GTB).

Making a diagnosis of tubal block merely on the basis of HSG alone however, has limitations due to false positive cases. Insufficient fluid pressure due to leakage of the dye from the cervix may lead to non-filling or incomplete filling of the fallopian tubes, with an erroneous conclusion of tubal block. HSG done soon after menstruation may show intravasation and extravasation of the dye, wrongly suggesting the possibility of GTB. Also, HSG cannot differentiate between a true tubal block caused by a pathology and a physiological block caused by tubal spasm or tubal obstruction due to mucus plugs, debris and organized exudates from tubal secretions and/or material back flowing from the uterine cavity. The pathological tubal block is caused by fibrosis resulting from salpingitis, following pelvic inflammatory disease (PID) or genital tuberculosis (GTB), salpingitis isthmica nodosa (SIN) or endometriosis, which involves the tube and causes tubal occlusion.[5] HSG also does not provide any information about the status of the fimbriae, the tubo-ovarian relationship and presence of peri-tubal adhesions. HyCoSy, like the HSG, has the same limitations in these regards.

A suspected tubal block on HSG must therefore be confirmed by performing subsequent laparoscopy to rule out false positive cases present in 25% to 62% of women undergoing infertility work up. In one large meta-analysis by Swart et al, tubal block was present at laparoscopy in only 38% of cases suggested by HSG.[6] In another study by Bhattacharya et al, false positive HSG was present in 40% of women due to either tubal spasm or mucous plug.[7] A study by Tulandi et al showed that 25% of patients diagnosed with cornual block on HSG actually did not have such block.[8]

Laparoscopy alone for diagnosis of tubal block, like HSG, also has its share of false positive cases. Laparoscopy also has limitations, as it only provides information regarding the exterior of fallopian tubes and does not reveal the precise level of block, as opposed to HSG. Also, laparoscopy cannot differentiate between insufficient filling of fallopian tubes, tubal spasm or blockage due to obstruction.

Laparoscopy combined with hysteroscopy is the gold standard and must compliment HSG to confirm or rule out the suspected tubal block on HSG. Hysteroscopy gives us detailed information of the uterine cavity, cornua and tubal ostia along with the endometrium and cervical canal, in terms of normalcy, as well as presence of pathologies, e.g. endometrial polyps, submucous fibroids, intra-uterine synechiae, etc. Laparoscopy gives us information about the status of the fallopian tubes, fimbriae and tubal patency, presence of peritubal adhesions and distortion of the tubo-ovarian relationship, as well as information about adnexal pathologies.

An important and a significant advantage that laparoscopy combined with hysteroscopy has over HSG, is not only in matters of diagnosis of tubal pathology and block, but strategizing and decision making and offering treatment at the same sitting. The following procedures are therefore performed to benefit the patient.

1. Hysteroscopic tubal cannulation for proximal tubal block.
2. Laparoscopic fimbriolysis for glued fimbriae and adhesiolysis for peritubal adhesions to restore normal tubo-ovarian relationship.
3. Laparoscopic or open neosalpingostomy for terminal tubal block due to hydrosalpinx.
4. Laparoscopic salpingectomy or delinking of hydrosalpinx before IVF treatment.

FALLOPIAN TUBE CANNULATION

The attempt to open the cornual block goes back to the year 1849 by WT Smith.[13] Since then, metal dilators and catheters, balloons, angioplasty guide-wire, ureteric cannulation set, embryo transfer catheters, stiff plastic catheters, infant feeding tubes, epidural catheters, etc. all have been tried by clinicians in an attempt to open the cornual block. Technological advances have led to improvements and in the design of coaxial cannulation set with virtually atraumatic soft guidewires.

Today, all these various cannulation devices have been replaced by coaxial catheters with consistent success. The coaxial catheters have soft atraumatic guidewires, they help in proper alignment according to tubal anatomy, hence the procedure of cannulation becomes smooth and easy.

Selective Salpingography under Fluoroscopy Guidance

In 1985, Platia and Krudy described fluoroscopic cannulation of one of the two proximally blocked fallopian tubes, with the patient becoming pregnant in the third cycle after surgery.[14] Modern day tubal cannulation has evolved since then. Cannulating the tube and performing selective salpingography under tactile or fluoroscopic/radiographic guidance to open up proximal tubal blocks has been the forerunner to tubal cannulation by hysteroscopy. It is done as an outpatient procedure. Catherization of the tubal ostium is done and patency is checked under fluoroscopic imaging after transcervical instillation of contrast medium. Even guidewire cannulation through the catheter can be done if obstruction is observed. In a study by Thurmond et al[15] and Schmitz-Rode et al[16] fluoroscopic guidance is an outpatient, less invasive, cost effective procedure, alternative to tubal microsurgery and IVF, with success rate at recanalization of 71% to 92% and average pregnancy rate of 30%.

Sonographically Guided Transcervical Tubal Catheterization

Sonographically guided transcervical tubal catheterization is a less commonly used technique. Confino and colleagues used catheters with distal balloon to achieve longer lasting mechanical dilatation of the tubal lumen.[17]

HYSTEROSCOPIC FALLOPIAN TUBE CANNULATION

Hysteroscopic fallopian tube cannulation is popular amongst gynecologist and infertility specialists and is done using an operating hysteroscope with a simultaneous laparoscopy guidance. Arrangement of two separate monitors, cameras and light sources for hysteroscopy and laparoscopy each, adds great convenience and comfort.

The hysteroscopes used for tubal cannulation are:

1. *Standard hysteroscope*: It has external diameter of 4 mm with 7.5 mm operating sheath.

    It hence requires cervical dilatation. The angle of vision is 30 degree.

2. *Bettocchi hysteroscope* (*Karl Storz*): It has external diameter of 2.9 mm and 30° angle of vision which helps to operate in the cornu with ease. It has an oval profile which allows for an insertion in a round flexible space. Prior cervical dilatation is usually not required except in cases of cervical stenosis. The authors have been routinely using this hysteroscope.

3. *Modified Bettocchi*: It has external diameter of 1.9 mm.

4. *Versascope system* (*Gynecare division of Johnson and Johnson*): It has external diameter of 1.8 mm and 0 degree angle of vision.

5. The flexible, steerable fiberoptic hysteroscope (Olympus, Fujinon).

Hysteroscopic tubal cannulation should be performed in the immediate postmenstrual period, when the endometrium is thin and vizualisation is better. In the advanced proliferative phase, due to thick mucosa it may be difficult to visualize the ostia. Sometimes dilatation and curettage (D and C) is done prior to cannulation, if the endometrium is polypoidal and visualization is difficult.

Hysteroscopic tubal cannulation is used as a diagnostic as well as therapeutic measure for proximal tubal block. The use of laparoscopy simultaneously helps to negotiate the block and confirm the status of the tubes and fimbriae, as well as helps in direct visualization of tubal patency following tubal cannulation. Laparoscopy also helps in confirming peri-tubal adhesions, distortion of tubo-ovarian anatomy and presence of hydrosalpinx and other factors responsible for infertility, like endometriosis.

It must be emphasized that hysteroscopic tubal cannulation should be performed only for tubes which are apparently normal looking and free from any pathology. They are the ones likely to have tubal obstruction due to debris, mucous and organized exudates forming 'tubal plugs', which can possibly be cleared to open up the blocked proximal tube. Presence of peri-tubal adhesions, distortion of tubo-ovarian anatomy, bipolar tubal disease, hydrosalpinx and presence of moderate/severe endometriosis should prompt the surgeon against proceeding for tubal cannulation to open up tubal block, as they are likely to have tubal occlusion resulting from fibrosis, rather than tubal obstruction caused by 'tubal plugs'. However, one may proceed to laparoscopic management of these pathologies as need be.

Contraindications to Hysteroscopic Cannulation

1. Active pelvic infection
2. Genital tuberculosis
3. Bipolar (proximal and distal) tubal blocks/ multiple tubal blocks
4. Hydrosalpinx/severe tubal damage
5. Previous tubal surgery
6. Associated other infertility factors requiring IVF.

Procedure

Hysteroscopic tubal cannulation is performed under general anesthesia, First, hysteroscopy is performed using Bettocchi hysteroscope (Karl Storz) with external diameter of 2.9 mm and 30 degree angle of vision and a detailed survey of the uterine cavity is done with continuous flow of normal saline or Ringer's lactate to distend the cavity. Particularly the cornu and ostia are evaluated in detail. Sometimes mild adhesions and polyps are present at the cornu, which are then initially tackled. After hysteroscopy is performed and assessment made, laproscope is then introduced to assess the pelvic anatomy, especially the status of both fallopian tubes and fimbriae, along with the general view of abdominal cavity. Before proceeding for hysteroscopic cannulation directly, it is advisable and wise to check patency of both fallopian tubes by injecting methylene blue dye through the hysteroscope sheath, with the tip of hysteroscope placed in close proximity to the tubal ostium (selective transostial chromopertubation) or by using the Rubin's or Leech Wilkinson cannulae. The authors, in their experience, have found that in a subset of about 20% patients, the tube shows up with patency and hysteroscopic tubal cannulation is not required. In those patients, where the tubes do not show any filling at all, even after repeated attempts to demonstrate tubal patency, we proceed to hysteroscopically cannulating the tubes under simultaneous laparoscopy control.

Hysteroscopic cannulation of fallopian tubes through the tubal ostia can be done with use of

1. Catheters
2. Flexible atraumatic guidewires passed through a catheter
   • Terumo guidewire
   • Novy's/Cook's coaxial system
3. Balloon catheters: Catheters with distal balloon to achieve longer lasting mechanical dilatation.

Catheters

Specially designed flexible catheter with an angulated distal segment is passed through the operating channel of the hysteroscope. The flexible catheter straightens while passing through the operating channel and due to its inherent memory, soon returns to its angulated form when advanced into the uterine cavity. The angulation of the catheter helps the surgeon to negotiate its placement in the cornu, since the angulated catheter follows the path of utero-cornual gutter.

Tubal ostium is identified on one side and tip of the hysteroscope is brought in near proximity to the ostium. The tip of the catheter is then further advanced to juxta pose against the tubal ostium under constant hysteroscopic visualization. Methylene blue dye diluted in 20 ml normal saline is then pushed through the catheter to generate higher intratubal pressure to mechanically flush out possible 'tubal plugs'. Simultaneous laparoscopy confirms the filling of the fallopian tube and spillage of the dye through the fimbrial ostium. The catheter is then maneuvered and negotiated to enter the other cornu to open up the tube on the other side.

Simple Cannulation Set using Terumo Guidewire

Cannulation using Terumo hydrophilic coated guidewire (0.64–1 mm) and cannula (7 F) is more economical in comparison to Novy's/Cook's coaxial cannulation set. The ostia are identified and the cannula is introduced through the operating channel of the hysteroscope and aligned with one of the ostia. To prime the catheter, it is flushed with normal saline to ensure smooth movement and low sliding friction of the guidewire within it. The guidewire is then introduced through the cannula and at least 5 cm of the guidewire is kept extended out of the hub of the cannula. The cannula and the hysteroscope should be held still for easy cannulation. Under constant hysteroscopic visualization the guidewire is negotiated into the ostium and interstitial part of the tube, for 1 to 1.5 cm to negotiate the cornual block. The movements should be gentle, untoward force might damage tubal mucosa or cause perforation due to the stiff guidewire. The guidewire should not be pushed further as it may result in perforation due to the sinusoidal track of the intramural portion of the fallopian tube. The Terumo guidewire is relatively stiff and should not be used to cannulate the distal fallopian tube. After introduction of the guidewire into the intramural portion of the fallopian tube, the cannula is railroaded over the guidewire to fix the tip of the cannula into the proximal part of the intramural portion. Guidewire is now removed and the fallopian tube is now flushed with 20 ml of methylene blue diluted with normal saline contained in a syringe attached to the cannula. The easy flow of this solution through the fallopian tube, without backflow into the uterine cavity, confirms the successful recanalization of the fallopian tube. This can be further confirmed by the laparoscopic visualization of methylene blue dye pouring out of the fimbrial end of the fallopian tube. The similar procedure is repeated on the other side and dye injected through the cannula to confirm patency.

Cannulation using a Coaxial Technique

The authors have used many different sets and have found Novy's/Cook's coaxial cannula-tion set to be ideal, although it is delicate and expensive. The coaxial cannulation system keeps the lumen coaxially aligned with the tubal lumen, for advancement of the wire cannula. It has the advantage that the outer catheter (9 Fr) is transparent and has a J-shaped curved terminal portion, i.e. 3 cm of the tip is curved with 30–40 degrees angula-tion, which is ideal for the anatomy of ostium and proximal tube. The inner cannula (3 Fr) is thin, flexible and graduated with centimeter markings. The guidewire (0.6–0.8 mm) is soft and atraumatic and has a platinum tip for better visualization and guides the whole device. The cannulation set is loaded before the introduction of hysteroscope. First the guidewire is loaded into inner cannula, which in turn is loaded into outer catheter. The Bettocchi hysteroscope (Karl Storz) with 30° angle of vision is introduced. The uterine cavity is distended with continuous flow of normal saline or Ringer's lactate. The whole system is now loaded into the operating channel of hysteroscope in such a way that its curve is at right angle to the optics of 30° hysteroscope. The catheter system and the scope should be held still and the outer end of guidewire is held by an assistant to avoid the guidewire from slipping out. The ostia are identified and the outer catheter is aligned with one of the ostia. This alignment is easy due to the J-shaped outer catheter which fits the uterotubal angle at the ostium. The guidewire with inner cannula is gently, pushed to cannulate the ostium for 2 to 3 cm. The guidewire in the Novy's/Cook's cannula-tion set is intended only to facilitate placement of inner cannula. It is not intended for tubal recanalization and should not be advanced beyond tubal isthmus. The movements should be gentle, untoward force might damage tubal mucosa or cause perforation. If there is resistance to passage, the inner cannula is withdrawn and reentry is made at different angle. Methylene dye is injected through the outer catheter to confirm the patency via laparoscopy. The similar procedure is repeated on the other side.

DIFFICULTIES ENCOUNTERED DURING CANNULATION

1. Inability to cannulate the tubes due to resistance: This is particularly true for very soft guidewires. In these cases a relatively more stiff guidewire may overcome the obstruction.

   In case the cannulation is not possible, it is wise to abandon the procedure.
2. Excessive glow as we are working in close proximity of the tissues.
3. Kinking/damage to the catheter.

4. Prolonged procedure leads to mucosal edema and difficulty in visualization of ostia.

Prolonged procedure also has danger of fluid overload.

COMPLICATIONS

Perforation

Perforation of fallopian tubes can occur in up to 6% cases. It occurs in fixed tubes with peritubal adhesions, due to undue force, or due to wrong angulation. It is common with stiff guidewires. In case of perforation the procedure on that side is abandoned and it is left to heal on its own.

Bleeding

If perforation occurs on mesenteric border of tube, there are chances of bleeding and blood collection in broad ligament, which can be confirmed and treated laparoscopically if required.

Infection

Iatrogenic infection is rare if asepsis is maintained. Flare up of pelvic infection can occur if already active pelvic infection is present. Cannulation should not be performed in cases of known pelvic infection.

Ectopic Pregnancy

This is known long-term complication when patient becomes pregnant. All these patients should be warned about the possibility of ectopic pregnancy and they should do the pregnancy scans immediately after missed period. The chances of ectopic with tubal cannulation are significantly less than that with tubal microsurgery. In a study by Das et al, hysteroscopic cannulation and tubal microsurgery in patients with proximal tubal block showed an ectopic pregnancy rate of 10% and 29% respectively.[18]

SUCCESS OF TUBAL CANNULATION

In a review of 1079 patients by Thurmond et al, of selective salpingography under fluoroscopic guidance, the patency rate of 62% and the cumulative pregnancy rate by lifetime probability analysis of 28%, 59%, 73% at the end of 12, 18, 24 months respectively was observed.[19]

In a study by Spiewankiewicz et al,[20] Zhu et al[21] and Burke et al[22] hysteroscopic tubal cannulation with laparoscopic assistance with/without guidewire cannulation, the success rate of recanalization was 76 percent and intrauterine pregnancy rate up to 39 percent.

According to Zhu et al,[21] laparohysteroscopic cannulation for proximal tubal block is an effective method for both diagnosis and treatment of cornual obstruction. In 78% cases a follow up HSG three months later showed patent tubes. Recurrence of tubal block is seen in 50% of patients in six months after cannulation.

CHOOSING TUBAL CANNULATION VERSUS MICROSURGERY VERSUS IVF

In patients with proximal tubal block the options of management are tubal cannulation, tubal microsurgery and IVF. How does one choose the 1st line of treatment? The key is proper evaluation of the cause of proximal tubal block by hysteroscopy combined with simultaneous laparoscopy. When the fallopian tubes are normal looking, free from any pathology at laparoscopy, hysteroscopic cannulation should be the treatment of 1st choice, as the proximal tubal block is more likely to be due to obstruction by 'tubal plugs' formed from mucous, debris and organized exudates, which can be mechanically dislodged and flushed out to open up the blocked tubal lumen. Hysteroscopic cannulation has thus proved to be an effective method both for diagnosis and treatment of proximal tubal block due to obstruction, with good success rates. In case, hysteroscopic cannulation fails to open up the blocked tube, the patient can either go for tubal microsurgery or IVF. Tubal microsurgery or IVF treatments are not influenced adversely by prior tubal cannulation.

However, presence of peri-tubal adhesions, distortion of tubo-ovarian anatomy, bipolar tubal disease, hydrosalpinx and presence of moderate/severe endometriosis should prompt the surgeon against proceeding for tubal cannulation to open up the proximal tubal block, as they are likely to have tubal occlusion resulting from fibrosis, rather than tubal obstruction. These patients should be advised IVF. Dechand et al[23] reported no pregnancy after tubal cannulation, in patients who had severe endo-tubal damage. Combined proximal and distal disease carry a poor prognosis after a surgical repair with microsurgical reconstruction, as shown by a study by Patton et al.[24] There were no live births after a 2-year follow up of these cases. Also, in one study there was no pregnancy reported following fallopian tube recanalization for proximal tubal block and microsurgery for distal tubal block in cases with bipolar disease.[25]

Lee et al during falloposcopy in cases of severe tubal damage reported 67% of the cases had flattened tubal mucosa with adhesions.[26] These cases were suitable for IVF and 27% cases had normal mucosa and they were suitable for microsurgery. Hence, patients with both proximal and distal tubal disease should go for IVF treatment.

It stands to reason that when the patient fails to achieve a pregnancy after a successful tubal cannulation or tubal microsurgery, she should be advised further management with IVF.

CONCLUSION

Hysteroscopic cannulation along with simultaneous laparoscopy should be first choice in the management of proximal tubal block in properly selected cases. It is important to make a distinction between proximal tubal blocks which are caused by obstruction due to 'tubal plugs' formed from mucous, debris and organized exudates and those caused by occlusion due to fibrosis resulting from

salpingitis due to disease processes, viz. PID, GTB, SIN and endometriosis.

Hysteroscopic cannulation has proved to be an effective method for both diagnosis and treatment of proximal tubal block which occurs mainly due to obstruction. It is a simple, minimally invasive, less morbid, cost effective day care procedure and has emerged as an excellent alternative to tubal micro-surgery and IVF. However, in cases of severe tubal mucosal damage, severe tubo-peritoneal adhesions with distortion of tubo-ovarian anatomy, bipolar disease and presence of hydrosalpinx, IVF should be the 1st line of treatment.

References

1. The ESHRE Capri Workshop. Infertility revisited. The state of art today and tomorrow. Hum Reprod 1996; 11: 1779–807.
2. Rock JA, Katayama KP et al. Pregnancy outcome following uterotubal implantation: a comparison of reamer vs sharp corneal wedge resection technique. Fertile Steril.1979; 31: 634–40.
3. Dubuisson JB, Chapron C et al. Proximal tubal occlusion: is there any alternative to microsurgery. Hum Reprod. 1997; 12: 692–8.
4. Imaging techniques for assessment of tubal status-NCBI-NIH by S Panchal, 2014.
5. Honore GM, Holden AEC et al. Pathophysiology and management of proximal tubal blockage. Fertil Steril 1999; 71 (5): 785–95.
6. Swart P, Mol BW, Van Der Veen et al. The accuracy of HSG in diagnosis of tubal pathology: a meta analysis. Fertil Steril. 1995; 64: 486–91.
7. Bhattacharya S, Logan S. Evidence based management of tubal factor infertility. In: The Fallopian Tube. Allahbadia GN, Djahanbakheh O, Saridogan E (Eds) Anshan Publishers, UK 2009. Pp 215–23.
8. Tulandi et al. Reproductive performances after selective tubal catheterization. JMIJ. 2005; 12: 150–2.
9. Sweeney WJ. The interstitial portion of the uterine tube—its gross anatomy, course and length. Obstetrics and Gynecology, January 1962; Volume 19;Issue 1;pp. 3–8.
10. Rubin IC. Forty years progress in treatment of female sterility. Am. J. Obstet & Gynec 68: 324, 1954.

11. Sulak PJ, Letterie GS, Coddington CC, Hayslip CC, Woodward JE and Klein TA. Histology of proximal tubal occlusion, Fertil Steril 1987; 48: 437–440.

12. Tubal flushing for Subfertility. Cochrane doi: 10.1002/14651858. CD 003718.pub4.

13. Smith WT. New method of treating sterility by removal of obstructions of the fallopian tubes. Lancet I. 1849; 529–30.

14. Platia MP, Krudy AG. Transvaginal fluoroscopic recanalization of a proximally occluded oviduct. Fertil Steril. 1985; 44: 704–6.

15. Thurmond AS, Machan LS, Maubon AJ et al. A review of selective salpingography and fallopian tube catheterization. Radiographics. 2000; 20: 1759–68.

16. Schmitz-Rode T, Neulen J. Gunther RW. Fluroscopically guided fallopian tube recanalization with a simplified set of instruments. Rofo. 2004; 176: 1506–9.

17. Confino-E, Tur-Kaspa I, Gleicher N. Sonographic transcervical balloon tuboplasty. Hum Reprod. 192; 7: 1271–3.

18. Das K, Nagel TC, Malo JW. Hysteroscopic cannulation for proximal tubal obstruction: a change for the better? fertile Steril. 1995; 63: 1009–15.

19. Thourmond AS. Selective salpingography and fallopian tube recanalisation. Am J R Roentgenol. 1991; 56: 33–8.

20. Spiewankiewicz B, Stelmachow J. Hysteroscopic tubal catheterization in diagnosis and treatment of proximal oviductal obstruction. Clin Exp Obstet Gynecol 1995; 22: 23–7.

21. Zhu Gj Luo LL, Lin H. Diagnosis and treatment of cornual obstruction by transcervical Fallopian tube cannulation under hysteroscopy (Article in Chinese). Zhonghua Yi Xue Za Zhi. 1994; 74: 203–5.

22. Burke RK. Transcervical tubal catheterization utilizing flexible hysteroscopy is an effective method of treating cornual obstruction: a review of 120 cases. J Am Assoc Gynecol Laparosc. 1994; 1 (4 Pt 2): S 5.

23. Dechand H, Daures JP, Hedon B. prospective evaluation of falloposcopy. Hum Reprod. 1998; 13.

24. Patton PE, Williams TJ, Coulam CB. Results of microsurgical reconstruction in patients with combined proximal and distal tubal occlusion: double obstruction. Fertil Steril, 1987; 48 (4): 670–4.

25. Letterie GS, Luetkehans T. Reproductive outcome after Fallopian Tube canalization and microsurgery for bipolar tubal occlusion. J Gynecol Surg. 1992; 8: 11–13.

26. Lee K K. Diagnostic and therapeutic value of nonhysteroscopic transvaginal falloposcopy with a linear everting catheter. Zhonghua Yi Xue Za Zhi (Taipei). 1998; 61: 721–5.

Selective Pertubation during Office Hysteroscopy

Péter Török

INTRODUCTION

During infertility work-up organic and functional factors can be detected standing in the background of the problem. Tubal factors can be diagnosed in 30–50% of infertile patients.[1] Assessment of the tubal patency is advised to be performed in early phase of work-up, prior to apply any assisted reproductive techniques or tubal reconstructive surgery. Laparoscopic chromopertubation is accepted as gold standard to evaluate tubal patency, but X-ray [hysterosalpingography (HSG)] and ultrasonography (hysterocontrast-sonography (HyCoSy)) could be used for this procedure. Due to the available data lower specificity and sensitivity of HSG and the HyCoSy are well known.[2] As being an operation, laparoscopic surgery needs general anesthesia, hospitalization. Operating room is compulsory also, which increases the costs of the procedure and strain for the patient.[3] As a part of the infertility work-up uterine cavity should be visualized, as well. For detecting intrauterine pathologies hysteroscopy is accepted as gold standard method. Hysterolaparoscopy gives the most comprehensive information, while looking for the cause of infertility.[4]

Having a new method which combines the otherwise used office hysteroscopy[5] with tubal patency test was the conception that had led to develop office hysteroscopy guided selective chromopertubation (OHSC-SPT). This procedure is less invasive, nevertheless effective and reproducible method, which can be performed in an outpatient setting without anesthesia. In case of negative results more invasive and expensive laparoscopy is needed only in positive cases for verification or tubal reconstructive surgeries.

Tubal flushing effect is a published phenomena of hysterosalpingography in connection with tubal patency test.[6] In a subsequent study this effect of the OHSC-SPT was analyzed comparing tubal flushing effect of the hysterosalpingography.

Method

The procedure is performed in an ambulatory setting. Patient is in dorsal lithotomy position. Modified no-touch technique is performed using Cusco instrument and thorough disinfection of the vagina and the portio. Insertion of the hysteroscope happens without grasping, or dilatation of the cervix. A 30°, 2.7 mm rigid optic is used for the examination, with a 5.5 mm sheath (EMD Endoscopy Technologies). Normal saline (0.9% sodium chloride) is used for the distension, at controlled intrauterine pressure of 80–100 mm Hg. First step of the examination is a routine office hysteroscopy, during which any deformity of the uterine cavity and the endometrium can be visualized.

Technique of Pertubation

In the second step a 1.7 mm plastic catheter (Cavafix, B-Braun) is inserted through the working channel of the sheath and the tip is placed to the tubal ostium (Fig. 13.1). During selective pertubation, each fallopian tube is considered as a diagnostic unit. By rotating the hysteroscope, the direction of the catheter can be modified toward the ostium. The cone shape of the tubal ostium will help in leading the tip of the flexible catheter into the ostium. The catheter should not to be inserted into the tube, only the tip should be placed at the entry of it. Through the catheter 2–10 mL of methylene blue dye (Patente Blue, 2 mL in 1000 mL saline) is injected slowly. In case of a patent fallopian tube no blue fluid will appear in the uterine cavity. Dye gets through the catheter and tube to the abdominal cavity. Normal color of the endometrium can be seen, while the transparent catheter turns blue, due to the methylene blue flowing inside it (Fig. 13.2). Occluded fallopian tube changes the uterine cavity into blue, due to

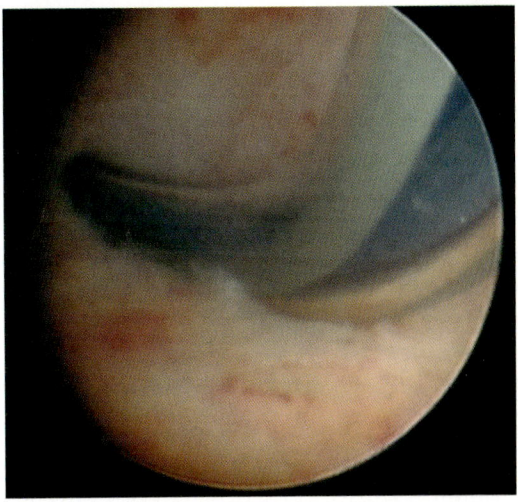

Fig. 13.2: Patent tube, blue dye in the catheter

the back-flow of the methylene blue (Fig. 13.3). In case of corneal occlusion, blue dye will flow back immediately. If the blockage is at the distal part of the tube, the first fraction of the blue dye will disappear and after some time of the injection will the back-flow be detectable. 10 mL of dye is more than the volume of a normal tube. After the evaluation of tubal patency, blue dye clears up within 5–10 seconds and the whole procedure can be repeated on the other side. To be more exact and precise and to exclude hydrosalpinx

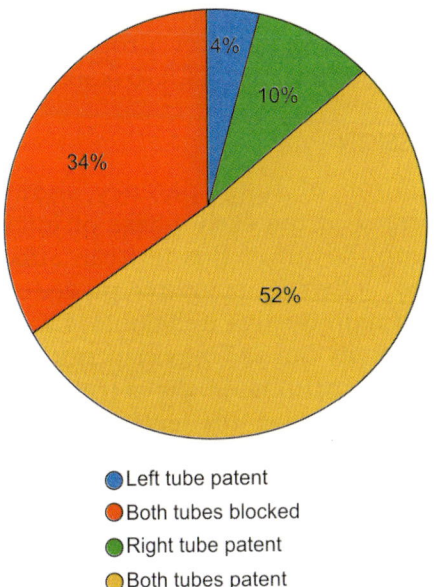

○ Left tube patent
● Both tubes blocked
● Right tube patent
○ Both tubes patent

Fig. 13.1: Tip of the catheter in the tubal osmium

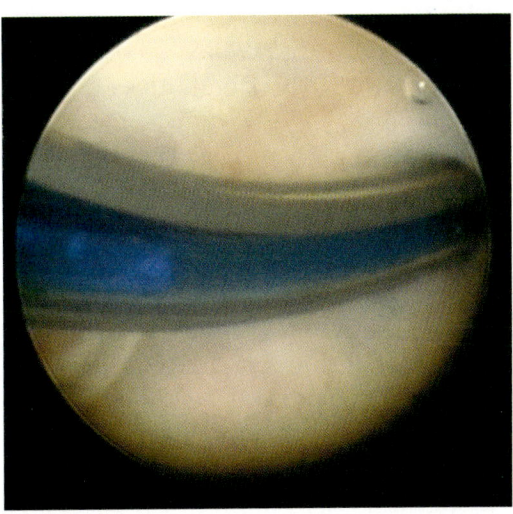

Fig. 13.3: Blocked tube, back-flow of the blue dye

transvaginal ultrasonographic examination should be performed before and after the hysteroscopy. By detecting free fluid around the fimbrial part of the tubes or in the pouch of Douglas, the result of the perturbation can be verified. Total examination time is 4–8 minutes. As usual after office hysteroscopy, there is no need for postoperative observation, and the procedure can be performed with a high patient compliance.[6]

Results

In a series of 120 cases, average age was 33,55 ± 4,02 years, BMI was 23,71 ± 4,27. Among patients indication of the patency test was primer infertility in 68%, secondary infertility was in 32%. Result of the test considered negative in case of at least one patent tube. In case of both blocked fallopian tubes, result of the test was considered as positive. In 79 cases (65,83%) result was negative, in 41 cases (34,17%) both tubes were blocked. In case of negative result average age was 32,63 ± 3,63 years, BMI was 23,77 ± 4,62. Primary infertility could be found in 68%, secondary infertility in 32% of the cases. In case of positive result average age was 35,37 ± 4,18 years, BMI was 23,62 ± 3,78, primary and secondary infertility could be found in 67% and 33% at the background. Among patients with negative results in 5 cases (6.3%) left tube was patent, in 12 cases (15,2%) right-sided tube was patent and in 62 cases (78,5%), both tubes proved to be patent.

Verification has been performed in cases of positive result (41 patients) by laparoscopic perturbation. Applying laparoscopy negative result could be achieved in 5 cases, which is considered as false positivity (12%) (Fig. 13.4). Due to these results specificity of the method is 94% (79/(79+5)), sensitivity is 100% (36/(36+0)), positive predictive value is 0,88 (36/(36+5)), negative predictive value is 1,00 [79/(79+0)].

In another study tubal flushing effect of the outpatient method: Selective chromopertubation

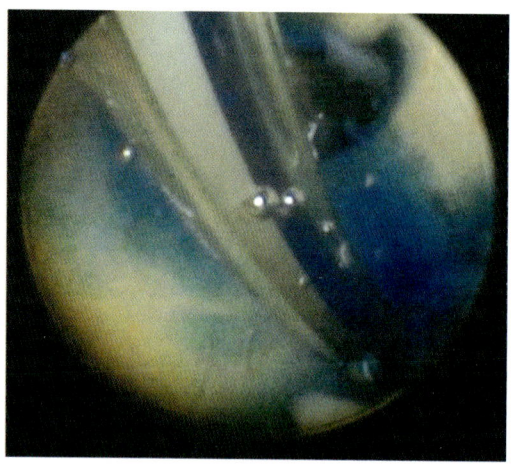

Fig. 13.4: Results of OHSC-SPT

via office hysteroscopy (OHSC-SPT) was evaluated, and compared to that of HSG.

Out of the 60 OHSC-SPT subjects, both tubes were blocked in 24 cases, and at least one of the tubes was patent in 36 cases. Out of these 36 cases, 7 (19.4%) spontaneous pregnancies were conceived; in three (8.3%) cases, pregnancy was conceived after intrauterine insemination (IUI) performed on male indication. The number of pregnancies observed in the HSG group (163 examined subjects) was 37 (32 spontaneous, 5 IUI-assisted) out of 153 followed-up subjects (24.4%). The pregnancy proportion ratio estimate was 1.15 (90% CI: 0.70–1.90; p = 0.671).

DISCUSSION

Evaluation of tubal patency should be performed at the early phase of infertility work-up. Result of this test can affect the therapy, either by operative procedures or assisted reproductive techniques. Evaluating uterine cavity can add important information, that also influences the success of the treatment. By using this developed method of OHSC-SPT, uterine cavity, tubal patency can be evaluated reliable in an outpatient setting, with low costs. Due to the data in literature and above mentioned results, first method of evaluating tubal patency should be an out-patient one. In case of positive result, more invasive method could be performed as a second step, to verify the result or use reconstructive surgery in special cases.

References

1. Watrelot A, Hamilton J, Grudzinskas JG. Advances in the assessment of the uterus and fallopian tube function. Best Pract Res Clin Obstet Gynaecol 2003 Apr;17(2):187–209.

2. Papaioannou S, Bourdrez P, Varma R, Afnan M, WJ Mol B, Coomarasamy A. Tubal evaluation in the investigation of subfertility: A structured comparison of tests. BJOG 2004;111:1313.

3. Marsh F, Kremer C, Duffy S. Delivering an effective outpatient service in gynaecology. A randomised controlled trial analysing the cost of outpatient versus day case hysteroscopy. BJOG 2004;111: 243.

4. Jayakrishnan K, Koshy AK, Raju R. Role of laparohysteroscopy in women with normal pelvic imaging and failed ovulation stimulation with intrauterine insemination. J Hum Reprod Sci 2010 Jan;3(1):20–4.

5. Campo R, Van Belle Y, Rombauts L, Brosens I, Gordts S. Office mini-hysteroscopy. Hum Reprod Update 1999;5:73–81.

6. Mohiyiddeen L, Hardiman A, Fitzgerald C, Hughes E, Mol BW, Johnson N, Watson A. Tubal flushing for subfertility. Cochrane Database Syst Rev. 2015 May 1;(5).

Practical Experience in Office Hysteroscopic Polypectomy

Amy Garcia

Polypectomy performed with small caliber operative hysteroscopes in the office environment provides patients with the benefits of awake procedures and less risk than that associated with use of general anesthesia in an operating room or ambulatory surgical center. Operative hysteroscopy, however, does require surgical skill beyond what is required for basic diagnostic procedures. The operative hysteroscopist must be comfortable with the hysteroscope angled or fore-oblique lens during cervical entry, uterine cavity navigation and utilization of operative instruments used through the operative sheath. And because patients are more likely to be awake, in office polypectomy can seem daunting to the beginning hysteroscopist.

This chapter will first focus on the basic physics of the operative telescope and sheath to understand how controlling the hysteroscope can be mastered. Second, specific techniques of surgical removal of endometrial polyps will be addressed that will facilitate polypectomy, especially for large polyps, numerous polyps and those with sessile and fundal attachments.

THE OPERATIVE HYSTEROSCOPE

Continuous Flow Sheath

The hallmark of the operative hysteroscope is the continuous flow mechanism of the sheath

that allows simultaneous inflow and outflow for procedures (Fig. 14.1). Occurring through separate channels, this dynamic fluid flow creates uterine distention by allowing the inflow to occur at a given pressure while outflow occurs with some resistance until the intrauterine pressure has adequately risen to a point that will distend the uterine cavity and force fluid into the fenestrations of the operative sheath. In this way, clean fluid is brought into the visual field, often over the lens to clear the view of debris and blood while the outflow channel carries away fluid that would otherwise obscure the visual field. One example of a continuous flow mechanism is seen in Fig. 14.2. So, the surgeon has the capacity to actively and assertively clear the visual field, adding safety to the procedure, all while maintaining uterine distention under direct control. It is also this direct fluid control that allows the gynecologist to dictate the amount of fluid entering the uterine cavity and the amount of pressure that is created. The

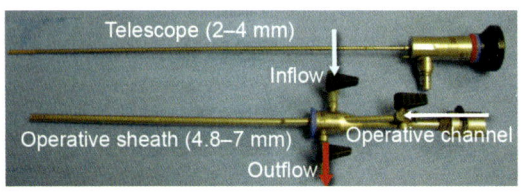

Fig. 14.1: Operative hysteroscope sheath and telescope. *Courtesy:* Amy Garcia.

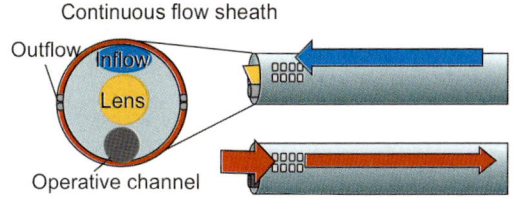

- Inflow clears visual field
- Low-resistance inflow
- High-resistance outflow
- Creates uterine distention
- Facilitates visualization

Fig. 14.2: Continuous flow operative hysteroscope sheath. *Courtesy:* Amy Garcia.

degree of uterine distention and therefore, intrauterine pressure that is necessary for an operative procedure is enough to create an appropriate visual field. Acute awareness of the amount of intrauterine pressure, which will be experienced by the patient as uterine cramping and pain, is essential for a comfortable in-office experience and the surgeon must keep the intrauterine pressure at the minimum needed for a successful procedure.

Fore-oblique Lens

Understanding the fore-oblique lens is essential to improve hysteroscopic skill. The visual field created by the angle of the lens adds to the utility of the hysteroscope as a tool that is used for visualization. The field-of-view is created by the lens angle, which allows the surgeon to see more of the area in front of the lens, including the operative instrument as it exits the operative sheath. The increased field-of-view will also allow the hysteroscopist to navigate within the uterine cavity with minimal movement of the hysteroscope against the cervix (Fig. 14.3a)

A fundamental component of the telescope is the attachment of the light post. The light post is always fixed to the telescope in the physical relationship which is opposite to the angle direction of the fore-oblique lens. Essentially, the field-of-view will always look in the direction which is opposite the position of the light post attachment. For example, in order to look up, the light post is rotated down (Fig. 14.3b). By rotating the position of the light post, one can fully assess the entire uterine cavity, including the cornua with simple rotation of the hysteroscope lens or light post. This maneuver, when mastered, will facilitate complete evaluation and operative navigation of the endometrial cavity with less overall discomfort for the patient. An important note is the fore-oblique lens will always look down at the operative instrument (Fig. 14.3c) Choosing the best angle of approach to pathology will be determined by the fore-oblique angle visual field, the exit angle of the operative instrument and the rotation of the lens or light post.

It is possible to know exactly where the light post is located and the direction of the visual field by locating the notch in the

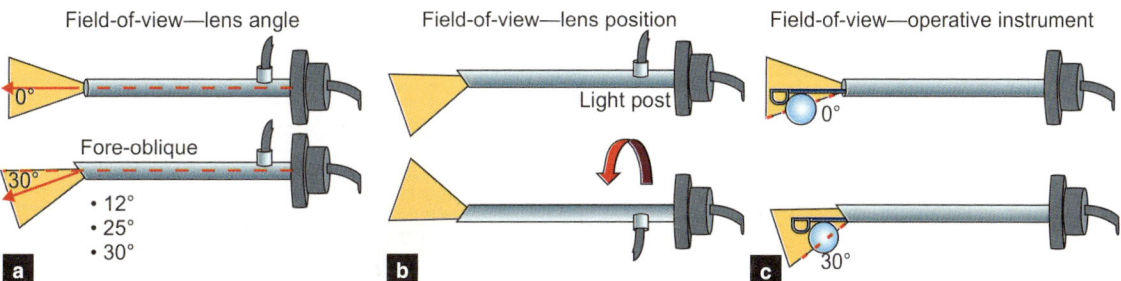

Fig. 14.3a to c: (a) Field-of-view created by the fore-oblique lens; (b) Relationship of the light post and fore-oblique lens direction to navigate the hysteroscope field-of-view; (c) A fore-oblique lens allows increased visualization of pathology and operative instruments more proximal to the hysteroscope. *Courtesy:* Amy Garcia.

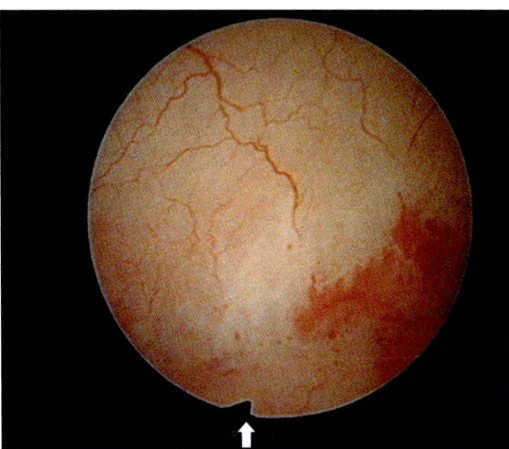

Fig. 14.4: Arrow indicates the notch created in the hysteroscopic image that corresponds to the position of the light post and, therefore, indicates the direction of the visual field. *Courtesy:* Amy Garcia.

hysteroscopic image seen on the monitor. The notch in the image will correspond to the position of the light post and in this example, the post is down and, therefore, the lens looks upward. If ever the operator is disoriented to the direction of the field of view, locating the light post will aid orientation (Fig. 14.4).

The visual field created by the fore-oblique lens will appear off-center to that of the zero degree lens. One must maintain the appropriate entry angle into the cervical canal to prevent unnecessary trauma to delicate tissues, bleeding and patient pain (Fig. 14.5). Adjusting to the off-set visual field is imperative for hysteroscope insertion parallel with the cervical canal.

Camera Orientation

Disorientation within the uterine cavity occurs not only with an incomplete understanding of the fore-oblique lens but also by an unawareness of the camera position on the hysteroscope. Most camera heads will have a locking mechanism to secure the telescope lens to the camera. It is recommended that the camera head not be fixed to the hysteroscope but rather allowed to rotate freely. While one is navigating the fore-oblique lens with rotation of the light post and, therefore, the visual field, the camera must remain in an upright orientation. If the camera head is fixed, it rotates with movement of the light post. If both the camera head and the visual field created by the lens are allowed to change, it can become very difficult to maintain correct position within the uterine cavity (Fig. 14.6).

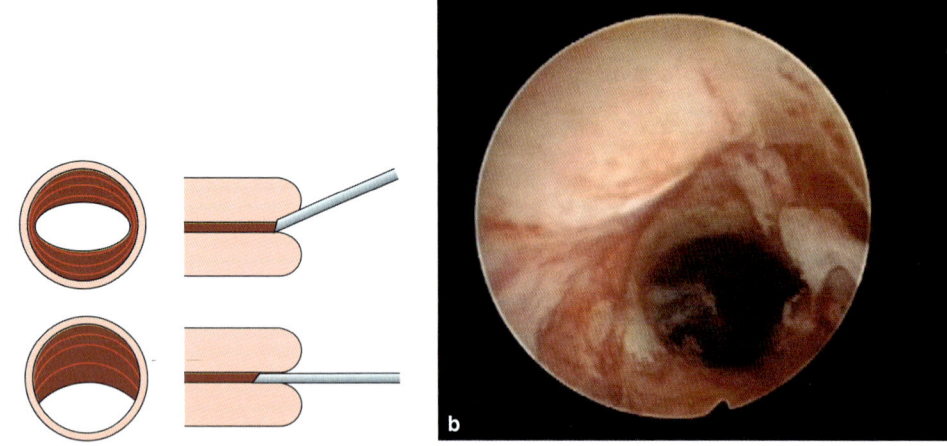

Fig. 14.5a and b: (a) Incorrect and correct placement of the hysteroscope within the cervical canal and associated visual field; (b) Hysteroscopic off-set image that correlates with correct parallel placement of the hysteroscope within the cervical canal with the light post down as evidenced by the notch in the image with the visual field looking up. *Courtesy:* Amy Garcia.

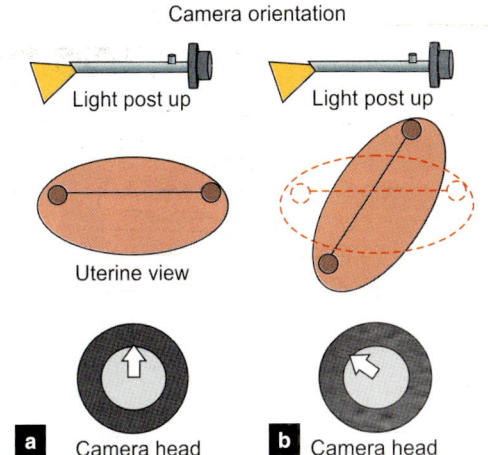

Fig. 14.6a and b: (a) Maintaining the camera head in an upright position by allowing the lens to rotate without rotating the camera head off of its upright axis. (b) If the camera head is fixed to the lens, then the camera head will also rotate when the lens moves and the orientation of the visual field will be incorrect. Actual orientation of the visual field should be the dotted red line. *Courtesy:* Amy Garcia.

POLYPECTOMY

Operative Instrument Orientation

Placing the operative instrument into the visual field, one can determine the best angle of approach to pathology based on size and location of polyp attachment to the uterine wall. In general, the best approach to pathology will be in parallel to the uterine wall with the operative instrument having access to the polyp base at right angles. This approach maximizes the amount of tissue accessible to the instrument and creates the best fulcrum point for movement of the hysteroscope away from the uterine wall. It is extremely important to remember that one must move the instrument and hysteroscope together (Figs 14.7 and 14.8).

When the operative instrument transects the base of the polyp, exposure to the remaining attached tissue is made possible by using the instrument/hysteroscope and stretching out the attachment parallel to and away from the uterine wall. This maneuver will expose the base, allowing transection of the attachment to occur (Fig. 14.9).

Polyp Size

Removal of polyps after separation from the uterus can become challenging if the polyp is significantly larger than the diameter of the internal cervical os, cervical canal or external cervical os. A decision for polypectomy, therefore, must includes a plan for tissue retrieval. Ideally, if the polyp was separated intact, keeping it intact at removal is preferable

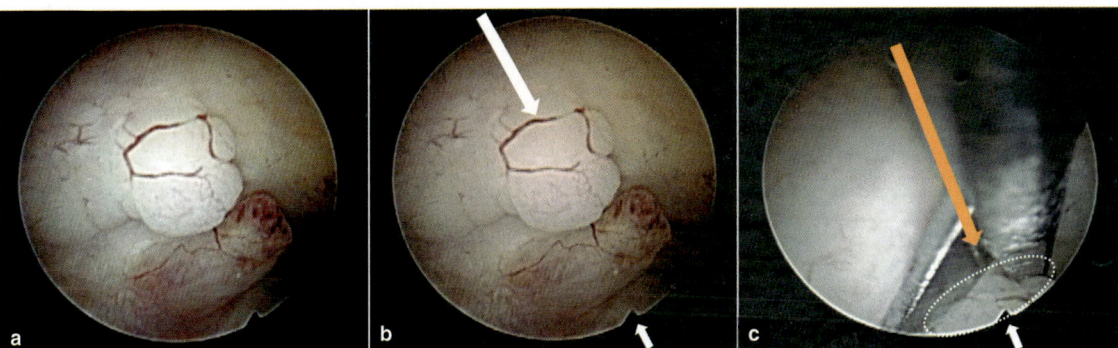

Fig. 14.7a to c: (a) 1.5 cm anterior wall soft density polyp/mass; (b) The anticipated angle of exit of the operative instrument (a large arrow) confirmed by the location of the notch (a small arrow) which indicates not only the angle of the visual field, but the location of the operative instrument as it exits the operative sheath. (c) Orange arrow indicates the entry angle of the operative instrument which is parallel with the hysteroscope and perpendicular to the tissue attachment plane at the base of the polyp (dotted circle). Note, a change in orientation of the operative instrument is created by rotation of the light post. *Courtesy:* Amy Garcia.

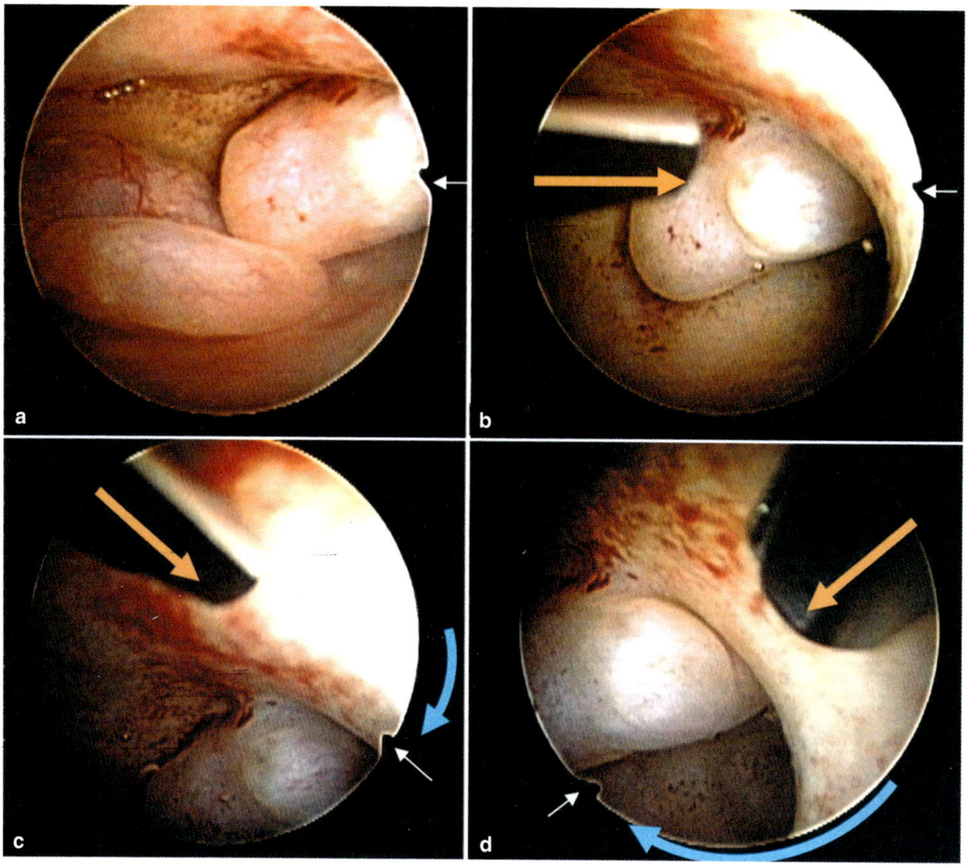

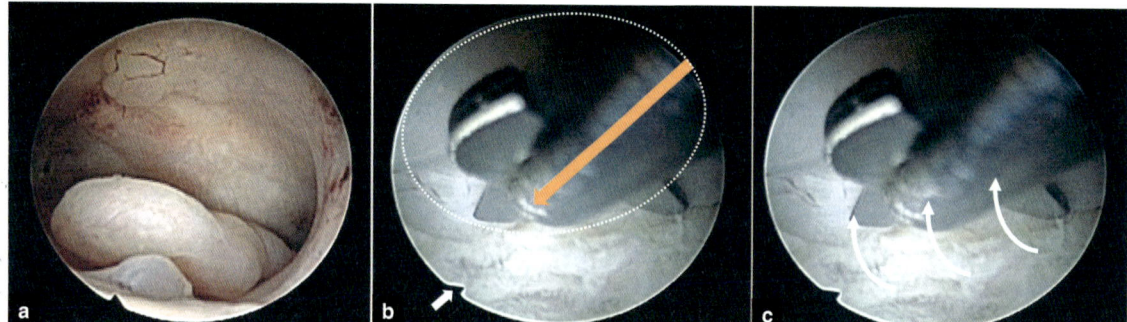

Fig. 14.8a to d: (a) Several benign polyps with the lens looking to the right. White arrow indicates the notch or location of the light post; (b) Orange arrow indicates the entry angle of the operative instrument which is opposite to the notch/light post; (c and d) In order to have a more effective approach to the polyp base, the light post or lens must be rotated (blue arrows) changing the instrument exit angle and position. *Courtesy:* of Amy Garcia.

Fig. 14.9a to c: (a) 2.0 cm × 2.5 cm posterior wall benign polyp; (b) Approaching the posterior polyp, the angle of exit of the operative instrument (orange arrow) confirmed by the location of the notch (small arrow) which indicates not only the angle of the visual field, but the location of the operative instrument as it exits the operative sheath and approaches the polyp base (dotted line); (c) Curved arrows indicate the direction of motion with the instrument/hysteroscope to lift the base away from the attachment to the posterior wall of the uterus, exposing the base for transection. *Courtesy:* Amy Garcia.

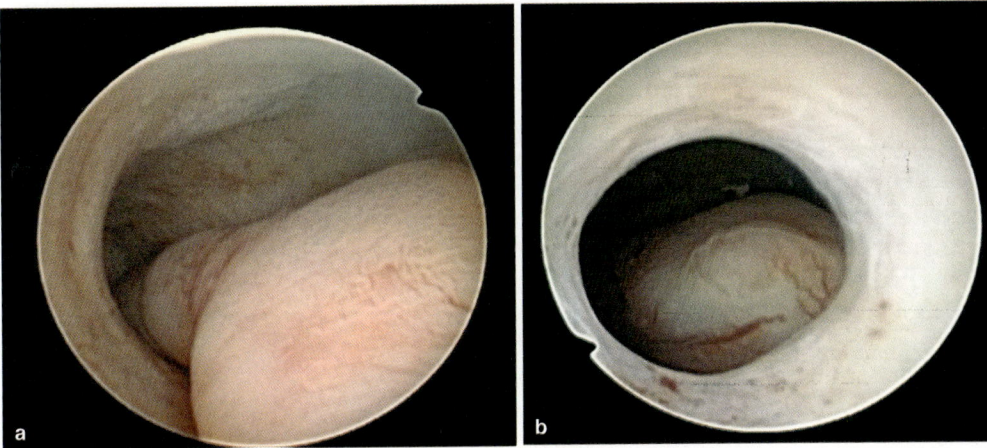

Fig. 14.10a and b: (a) A large benign endometrial polyp fills the length and width of the uterine cavity in a postmenopausal patient; (b) The large polyp is viewed in the same patient from the cervical canal to illustrate the size discrepancy between the cervix and the polyp. *Courtesy:* Amy Garcia.

for pathologic evaluation. However, the particular clinical circumstance may ultimately dictate how complete removal of the polyp is accomplished (Fig. 14.10).

The large polyps must be removed in pieces if necessary. This will require segmental transection of the polyp into separate pieces (Fig. 14.11a). Near total segmental transection prior to complete separation from the uterus allows for the tissue to conform to the cervical dimensions as it is pulled through the cervical canal (Fig. 14.11b). A gentle continuous rotation of the tissue while pulling can

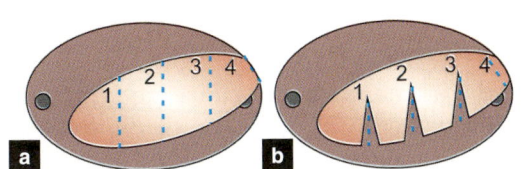

Fig. 14.11a and b: (a) A large endometrial polyp must sometimes be sequentially segmented and individual segments removed. The dotted lines indicate the order in which the segments would be transected. (b) It is sometimes possible to segment the polyp without complete separation of pieces. Incision of the polyp sequentially can disrupt the integrity of the tissue adequately to allow it to conform to the dimensions of the cervix upon removal. *Courtesy:* Amy Garcia.

sometimes be helpful to contract the tissue further for removal (Fig. 14.17).

Estimation of Polyp Size via Hysteroscopy

There are several ways to estimate the dimensions of endometrial polyps, which are potentially quite inaccurate give the magnified visual field. Because of the magnification, and estimate of polyp size will generally be much larger than the actual size. A good way to learn how to estimate size is by using a known measurement, such as the diameter of the hysteroscopic sheath or distance between the tips of operative instruments, to directly and incrementally measure polyp dimensions under visualization during removal (Figs 14.12 to 14.14). Of course, most polyps can be measured once removed from the uterine cavity using a small millimeter ruler.

Polyp Density

Tissue density is important in several ways. Dense tissue will require instruments such as scissors to be sharp (Fig. 14.12a to d). Dull instruments may not be efficient or may be entirely inadequate. Dense tissue will often take more time to transect as it is not as amenable to manipulations with the hysteroscope or instrument as softer tissue. Dense tissue may not

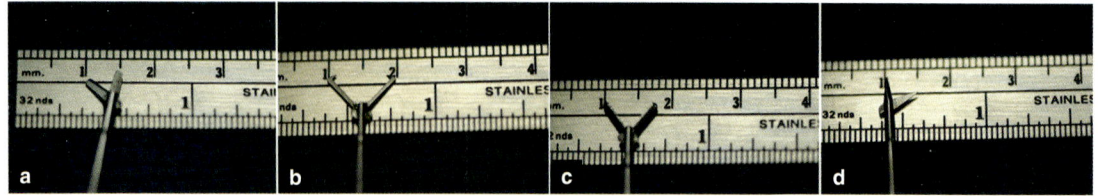

Fig. 14.12a to d: Multiple 5 French operative instruments and open-tip diameter. (a) Flat scissor tip 5 mm; (b) Tenaculum tip 10 mm; (c) Grasper tip 8 mm; (d) Sharp scissor tip 5 mm. *Courtesy:* Amy Garcia.

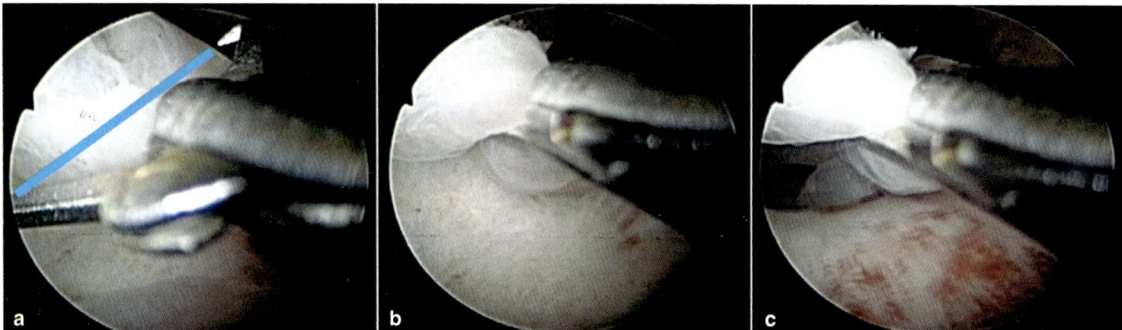

Fig. 14.13a to c: (a) The blue line indicates the inter-tip distance which is a known diameter of 10 mm with this particular instrument. The polyp is 10 mm in diameter across the width. (b) Once the polyp is grasped, tissue diameter is significantly compresses. (c) Polyp removal through the cervix is facilitated by tissue compression. *Courtesy:* Amy Garcia.

conform to the cervical openings as easily as tissue of similar size which is softer and more compliant. The tenaculum is an optimal instrument for grasping more dense tissue because the tips of the instrument open wider and will penetrate into dense tissue for a tenacious hold (Fig. 14.12b). Fragile tissue is generally a sign of abnormality such as hyperplasia or carcinoma and special care with tissue manipulation is warranted to maintain the tissue integrity during removal. Fragile tissue or soft polyps are better removed with a grasper whose serrated jaws can hold tissue more gently than can a tenaculum because the tips of the latter instrument will easily pull through fragile or soft tissue (Fig. 14.12c).

Polyp Attachment

Sessile Polyp

Broad based and sessile polyps are generally attached at the widest dimension of the polyp. A larger area of attachment requires more

transection than for a pedunculated attachment (Fig. 14.14). The sessile attachment requires a technique of lifting the tissue away from the uterine wall after transecting in order to continually expose the base of the polyp. Once separated, the polyps are removed in a similar fashion as other polyps based on the tissue density and the dimensions.

Fundal Polyp

Fundal attachment poses an added difficulty for tissue removal. The axis of the hysteroscope and, therefore, the operating instrument will be at right angles to the plane of tissue resection. Unlike polyps attached to the sidewalls or the anterior or posterior walls, the fundal wall is an impediment to being able to transect tissue with the blade of the scissors and the tip must be used instead. It is recommended to use blunt-tipped scissors for fundal pathology removal to avoid unnecessary tissue trauma that could be created with a

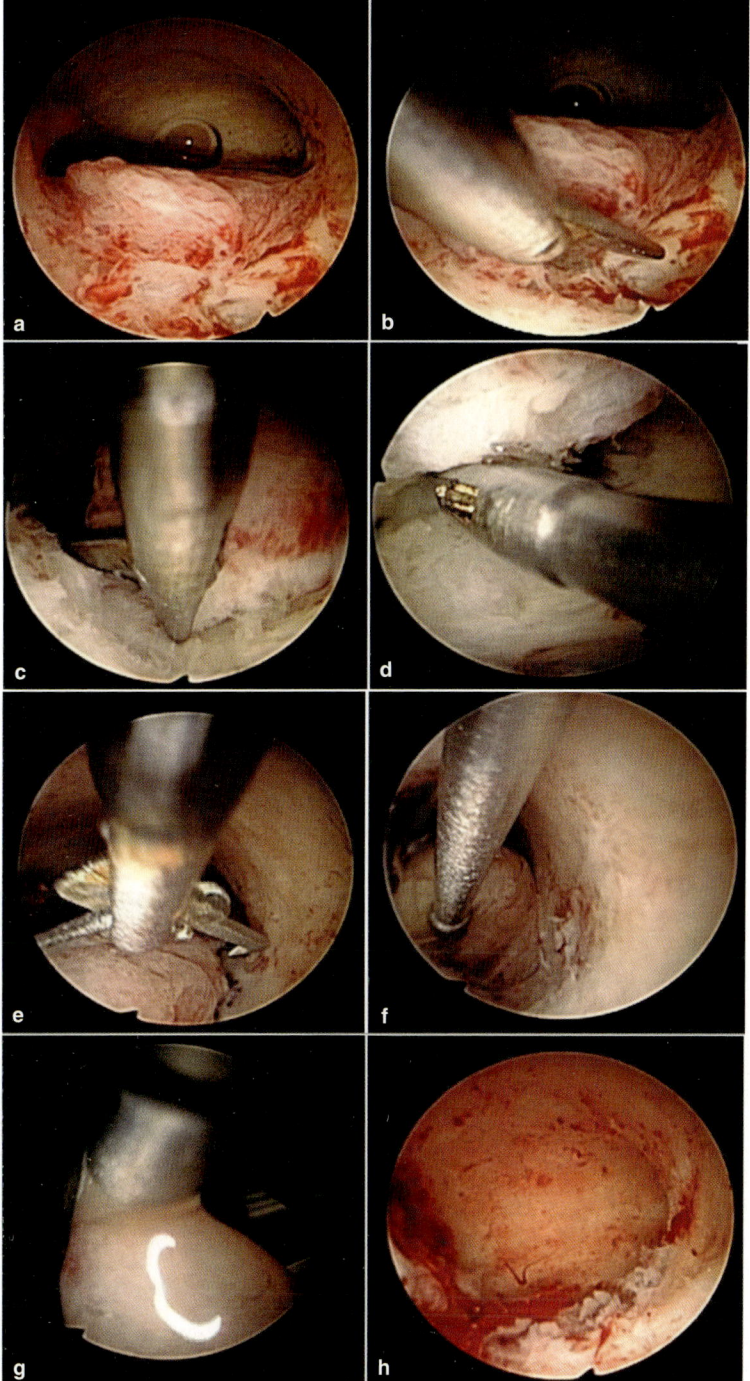

Fig. 14.14a to h: (a) A large sessile polyp attached to the posterior uterine wall; (b) Approaching the polyp base with flat scissors; (c) Using scissors to transect the base; (d) Using the instrument, the polyp is constantly lifted away from the uterus to expose the polyp base; (e) Once separated, the polyp is grasped at the end with the least diameter; (f) The polyp is brought through the cervix under visualization; (g) The polyp has been removed; (h) Inspection of the uterine cavity following polypectomy. *Courtesy:* Amy Garcia.

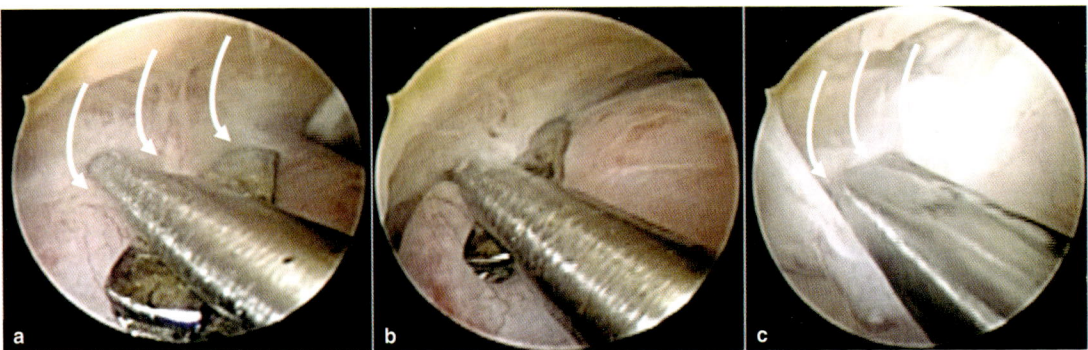

Fig. 14.15a to c: (a) The base of a polyp attached at the fundus is initially exposed by downward pressure against the polyp; (b) Transection of tissue is accomplished with small incisions made at the tip of the scissors; (c) Continual exposure of the polyp base by pushing down on the polyp. *Courtesy:* Amy Garcia.

sharp-tipped instrument. The base of the polyp is exposed by using the hysteroscope/instrument to pull the tissue down and away from the fundus. By using just the tips of the scissors to make small incisions tissue is released off the uterine wall (Fig. 14.15).

Polyp Retrieval

Grasping tissue for retrieval is made easier by the following steps. First, it is important to closely control the fluid inflow and outflow through the hysteroscope. Small tissue pieces can move significantly and if totally separated from the wall of the uterus, will float and swirl in the inflow current. By decreasing the inflow or closing the channel entirely, disruptive currents are inhibited and it is easier to grasp pathology for removal. Simultaneously closing the outflow temporarily during retrieval will maintain uterine distention for visualization. Second, leaving the polyp attached by just a small fragment of tissue will keep the polyp in place for subsequent grasping and removal. The final separation of the polyp from the uterine wall, in this scenario, requires only a slight twist or tug from the retrieving instrument. This often requires less time for removal than waiting for free-floating pieces to settle. Third, once the tissue is grasped by the operative instrument, removal is accomplished by holding the tissue in the instrument and removing the hysteroscope and

instrument from the uterine cavity and cervix as one unit (Fig. 14.16).

Pathology generally cannot be pulled through the hysteroscope operative channel due to its small diameter. One must also keep in mind the size relationship of the pathology to the cervical diameter and tissue density in order for the tissue to pass through easily. Whenever possible, the polyp should be grasped for removal at the most narrow dimension which will allow the edge of the

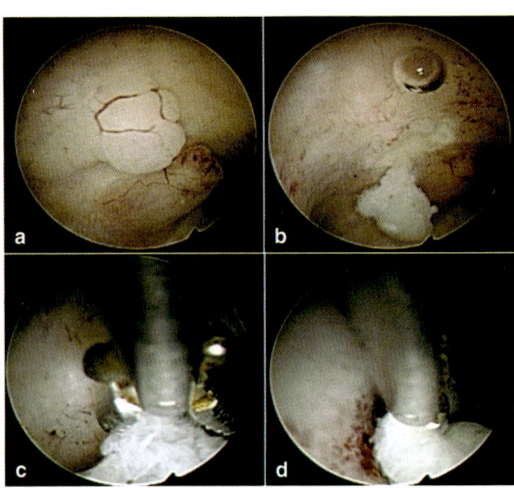

Fig. 14.16a to d: (a) 1.5 cm anterior wall soft density polyp/mass; (b) After transection of the majority of the polyp, it is left attached to the uterine wall by a small fragment; (c) Graspers are used to grasp and remove the very soft tissue; (d) The tissue is removed through the endocervical canal. *Courtesy:* Amy Garcia.

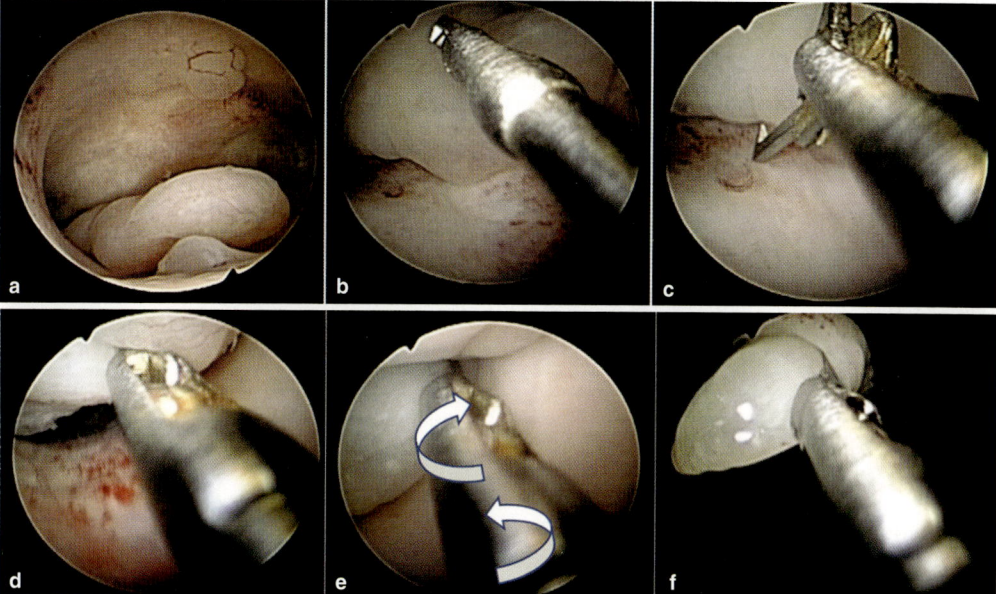

Fig. 14.17a to f: (a) 2.0 cm × 2.5 cm posterior wall benign polyp; (b) Approaching the polyp after separation with the tenaculum; (c) Grasping the polyp in a perpendicular fashion; (d) Bringing the polyp into the cervical canal; (e) Slight rotation of the instrument back and forth to aid in compression of the polyp and removal. *Courtesy:* Amy Garcia.

polyp with the smallest diameter to be pulled into the canal of the cervix first. This allows the polyp to elongate in the cervix and improves the likelihood of successful removal. And finally, if the inflow channel has not previously been closed, it should be closed during the removal of the hysteroscope. Many a tenuous grasp on specimens has been lost due to the rushing flow of fluid.

Multiple Polyps

If there are multiple polyps, then it is recommended to transect as many as possible, leaving a small attachment on each. It is most efficient not to change the type of instrument in the operative channel unless really necessary. Once retrieval is needed the instrument is changed to a grasping instrument. Multiple insertions and removals of the hysteroscope may be needed when there are many polyps. Instruments such as the tenaculum may facilitate grasping more than one polyp at a time for removal depending on the size and density of the polyps (Fig. 14.12b).

Bleeding

Bleeding after polypectomy always occurs, however, significant bleeding is not usual. Intrauterine pressure from uterine distention generally will tamponade minor bleeding. The continuous flow hysteroscope allows the surgeon to balance inflow and outflow to adequately provide tamponade but to also keep the visual field clear of blood. At the end of the procedure, the intrauterine pressure can be decreased by decreasing the inflow of fluid and watching for significant bleeding. Remember, because of the magnification with hysteroscopy, the amount of bleeding present will often be over-estimated. Once the uterine cavity has been evacuated of fluid and allowed to contract, bleeding likely will not be significant. If one is performing polypectomy with electrosurgical instruments, bleeding is generally avoided. Communicate with the patient that she will have minor bleeding for several days and perhaps mild to moderate cramping amenable to over-the-counter analgesics.

Intrauterine Adhesions

Sha Wang, Hua Duan

An intrauterine adhesion (IUA) is caused by the damage on basal layer of endometrium which results in the histopathological findings of hyperplasia of connective tissues and may partially or completely obliterating uterine cavity.[1] These cases may lead to a series of clinical problems including hypomenorrhea or secondary amenorrhea, infertility, recurrent miscarriage, and premature labor.[2–4] Aetiological agent of IUAs may include postpartum or post-abortive curettages and previous uterine surgeries.[5] Reported prevalence of IUAs is as high as 25–30% in the repeated artificial abortion and curettage.[6–7]

CLASSIFICATION

Severity of IUAs should be classified because of the damage on menstruation and fertility directly affects the treatment strategies and outcome prognosis. Although a number of classification systems have been proposed, but global usage and validated are not uniform. As the different classifications used by different countries make the comparison of therapeutic effects between studies and studies are quite different. Recently, experts in branch of obstetrics and gynecology affiliated by Chinese Medical Association proposed and formulated a new classification systems of IUAs (Table 15.1) which on the one hand, the characteristics of IUA in China were taken as the basis. On the other hand, it refers to the standard of AFS and ESGE.

Diagnosis

1. Hysteroscopy

Hysteroscopy allows direct visualization of morphologic characteristics of uterine cavity and also the distribution, extent, range and location of residual endometrium as well as the morphology of fallopian tube and cervical canal. It is the accurate method for diagnosis of IUAs. Meanwhile, it can identify the stage of IUAs and provide the references for prognosis evaluation. Hysteroscopy is considered as the preferred method of diagnosis of the disorders in uterine cavity.[8]

2. Transvaginal sonography (TVS)

Although TVS is a simple, non-invasive and repeatable method in diagnosing the uterine disorders but the sensitivity of TVS is not as good as hysteroscopy for IUAs, when compared with hysteroscopy, especially for the peripheral type of IUAs as the sensitivity was only 52%.[9] In recent years, the advantages of three-dimensional (3D) TVS application have become more and more obvious. 3D TVS can display the whole uterine cavity and endometrial morphology, and even measuring the endometrial thickness and blood flow by which can improve the sensitivity to IUA

Table 15.1: Stage of IUAs in China

Items	Content	Score
Extent of cavity involved	<1/3	1
	1/3–2/3	2
	>2/3	4
Type of adhesions	Filmy	1
	Fibrous	2
	Muscular	4
Oviductal orifice	Unilateral invisible	1
	Bilateral invisible	2
	Bilateral uterine horn disappear	4
Endometrial thickness (late proliferative phase)	≥7 mm	1
	4–6 mm	2
	≤3 mm	4
Menstruation pattern	Menstrual volume≤1/2 normal	1
	Spot	2
	Amenorrhea	4
Reproductive history	Spontaneous abortion once	1
	Recurrent abortion	2
	Infertility	4
Intrauterine operation	Artificial abortion	1
	First trimester curettage	2
	Second-Third trimester curettage	4

Note: According to the score, stage mild: 0~8; moderate: 9~18; severe: 19~28

diagnosis.[10] For all this, the value of 3D TVS in IUAs diagnosis is still uncertain.[11]

3. Hysterosalpinography (HSG)

HSG can simultaneously detect the uterine cavity and fallopian tube at the same time, but the positive predictive value of HSG was only about 50% and the false positive rate as high as 74%[12] when compared with hysteroscopy. More than that, HSG was limited to use in that completely closed uterine cavity or cervical adhesions. It is a reasonable alternatives when hysteroscopy is not available.

4. Sonohysterography (SHG)

SHG has the higher sensitivity and specificity in diagnosing abnormal morphology of uterine cavity than transvaginal sonography.[13, 14] But its sensitivity and specificity on IUAs diagnosis was only 75% when compared with hystero-scopy.[15] As an imaging diagnosis, SHG also cannot make surgeon to look directly into the uterine cavity, it is only be taken as an alternative examination when hysteroscopy is not available.

5. Magnetic Resonance Imaging (MRI)

MRI can evaluate the upper part of uterine cavity with cervical adhesions. The adhesion tissue appears to be low signal intensity on T2-weighted images. However, because of the high price limits its use.

Treatment

1. Purpose of Surgical Operation

Surgical treatment is not recommended for asymptomatic patients or patients with no fertility request. Transcervical resection of adhesion (TCRA) should be considered as the first choice for the patients with infertility, recurrent abortion, hypomenorrhea and fertility requirements. At present, TCRA is regarded as the standard treatment for IUAs patients. During TCRA procedure, the surgeon can clearly identify the characteristics of adhesions, the bilateral uterine horn and oviduct orifice under direct visualization. The aim of TCRA is to restore the morphology and volume of uterine cavity, to relieve associated symptoms, to prevent the re-adhesion formation, and also to promote the endometrial regeneration as well as to restore fertility.[16, 17]

2. Surgical Steps

i. Anesthesia and patient positioning

TCRA usually be performed under general anesthesia. The patient is placed in dorsal lithotomy position. Because concurrent laparoscopy is recommended, the abdomen and vagina are surgically prepared. A Foley catheter is inserted into bladder.

ii. Medium selection

The choice of distending medium is depend on the incising tool used. Sharp incision with scissors, Nd:YAG laser, or bipolar instrument is commonly selected and can be performed in any liquid medium. Monopolar technology will require a hypotonic nonconductive medium.

iii. Combined with laparoscopy

Because of the high potential risk of uterine perforation, concurrent laparoscopy is recommended that can inform a surgeon when perforation happened during TCRA procedure.

iv. Hysteroscopy adhesionlysis

The point of surgery is to protect the remaining endometrium during TCRA procedure as the residual endometrium will play an important role to repair the uterine cavity wound and to improve the surgical efficacy. Currently high-frequency electric is the main energy selection in hysteroscopy operation, which include mono-polar and bipolar. Usually, the adhesive tissues can be separated or incision by needle electrode and be cut or removed by annular electrode. The use of needle electrodes can minimize damage to the residual endometrium and also can make the residual endometrium to form a flap, a surgical skill, which can retain the blood supply and has a mediating effect on wound repair. In some severe cases, specially for the type of mixed adhesions, cold scissors can also be selected to separate adhesive tissues or alternate between electrodes and lasers. It is very important to judge the connection area between adhesion tissues and myometrium by which to prevent the heavy blooding and uterine perforation. There are some significant signs that can indicate the adhesion tissues were removed completely which include the increase of tissue vascularity, serosal transillumination test by laparoscope on the surface of uterine body and fundus.

3. Perioperative Management

So far there is no effective method on restoration of reproductive function for severe IUAs patients. The re-adhesion ratio following TCRA was 62.5%[18] with the pregnancy rate only about 22.5–33.3%.[19–20] Therefore, comprehensive ancillary measures are recommended after TCRA procedure as the part of the treatment.

i. Re-adhesion management

Many approaches have been proposed to prevent adhesion reformation after adhesion-lysis, which includes placement of intrauterine device (IUD) or intrauterine stents or balloon as well as the use of anti-adhesion gel such as hyaluronic acid gel in the post-operative period.[21, 22] These methods may have a local therapeutic effect, but there are also have corresponding disadvantages. IUD as a foreign body provokes excessive inflammation and increases the risks of abnormal uterine bleeding, infection, IUD embedment and uterine perforation. Nowadays a new kind of balloon device, which matches the morphology of the uterus cavity, and can block the attachment of the uterine cavity, has been applied to our clinic practice. This device can significantly reduce the rate of re-adhesion and has been recommended by "Chinese expert consensus on the diagnosis and management of intrauterine adhesions", which recommended placement time of the device is 5–7 days and the preferred volume of balloon is no more than 5 ml.

ii. Promoting endometrial regeneration

To promote the damaged endometrium regeneration is the key point after TCRA procedure. Currently, estrogen therapy is widely used in clinical practice to promote the proliferation of residual endometrial cells. However, there are no unified criteria for estrogen dosage choice in the treatment of IUAs. CMA recommended estradiol valerate 2–4 mg/d or its equivalent. Moreover, other measures had been attempted to promote endometrium regeneration, such as stem cell therapy and amnion graft. The transplantation of autologous bone marrow stem cells[23-24] and menstrual blood stem cells[25] were found to have positive effect on pregnancy rate.[26] Meanwhile, the usage of fresh[27] and freeze-dried amnion graft[28] were also proved to be effective to improve the menstruation and pregnancy rate. However, the number of the researches and samples involved in the studies are limited. Current evidence is not sufficient to demonstrate the value of stem cell and amnion graft in promoting endometrial regeneration after TCRA.

4. Follow-up and Reproductive Prognosis

i. Second-Look Hysteroscopy

Second-look hysteroscopy is the precondition to evaluate the curative effect of surgery. According to the published papers, the time of second-look hysteroscopy is ranged from 1 week[29] to 3 months after TCRA[30,31]

procedure. Currently, most widely accepted reassessment time is 2–3 months post-operatively which recommended by CMA and AAGL.

ii. Fertility Related Matters

For those severe IUAs patients, especially when residual endometrial area is less than 1/3 of the uterine cavity area, assisted reproductive-technology (ART) should be considered and recommended. The endometrial thickness of patients receiving IVF treatment should be achieved 7 mm in the late proliferative phase.[32] However, for severe IUAs patients, the endometrial thickness can hardly reached 7 mm even in the normal uterine anatomic morphology. In the view of reported the thinnest thickness of endometrium that can be impregnated was 3.7 mm as so far,[33] ART on the basis of endometrial thickness should be individualized.

iii. Fertility Outcomes

It has been reported that the overall conception rate after TCRA is 40.4–64.7%, live birth rate is 38.9–86.1%. The conception rate was higher in mild IUAs (58–64.7%) compared with moderate and severe IUAs (30–33.3%, 14–33%, respectively), although the endometrial status was improved significantly after TCRA in severe IUAs patients, but pregnancy-related complications are still a concern which may cause by repeated implantation failure or abnormal placental blood supply.[19,20,34] Therefore, special emphasis should be placed on prenatal management, to observe dynamically growth and development of embryo, and to deal with the complications in time.

References

1. Di Spiezio, Sardo A, Calagna G, Scognamiglio M, et al. Prevention of intrauterine post-surgical adhesions in hysteroscopy. A systematic review. Eur J Obstet Gynecol Reprod Biol. 2016; 203:182–192.

2. Gilman AR, Dewar KM, Rhone SA, et al. Intrauterine adhesions following miscarriage:

look and learn. J Obstet Gynaecol. 2016; 38(5):453–457.

3. Hanstede MM, van der Meij E, Goedemans L, et al. Results of centralized Asherman surgery, 2003-2013. Fertil Steril. 2015; 104(6): 1561–1568.

4. Chen L, Zhang H, Wang Q, et al. Reproductive outcomes in patients with intrauterine adhesions following hysteroscopic adhesiolysis: experience from the largest women' s hospital in China. J Minim Invasive Gynecol. 2017; 24(2): 299–304.

5. Rein DT, Schmidt T, Hess AP, et al. Hysteroscopic management of residual trophoblastic tissue is superior to ultrasound-guided curettage. J Minim Invasive Gynecol. 2017; 18(6): 774–778.

6. Hooker AB, Lemmers M, Thurkow AL, et al. Systematic review and meta-analysis of intra-uterine adhesions after miscarriage: prevalence, risk factors and long-term reproductive outcome. Hum Reprod Update.2014;20(2): 262–278.

7. Rein D T, Schmidt T, Hess A P, et al. Hysteroscopic management of residual trophoblastic tissue is superior to ultrasound-guided curettage. J Minim Invasive Gynecol. 2011; 18(6):774–778.

8. Expert consensus on the diagnosis and management of intrauterine adhesions in China. Zhonghua Fu Chan Ke Za Zhi.2015; 50(12):881–887.

9. Salle B, Gaucherand P, de Saint Hilaire P, et al. Transvaginal sono hysterographic evaluation of intrauterine adhesions. J Clin Ultrasound.1999; 27(3):131–134.

10. Mohamed Amer MI, Omar OH, E Sherbiny Hamed M, et al. Subendometrial blood flow changes by 3-dimensional power Doppler ultrasound after hysteroscopic lysis of severe intrauterine adhesions: preliminary study. J Minim Invasive Gynecol. 2017; 22(3):495–500.

11. Saravelos SH-Li TC. Virtual hysteroscopy with HD live. Ultrasound Obstet Gynecol. 2017; 49(2):284–286.

12. Acholonu UC, Silberzweig J, Stein DE, et al. Hysterosalpingography versus sonohystero-graphy for intrauterine abnormalities. JSLS. 2011; 15(4):471–474.

13. Bingol B, Gunenc Z, Gedikbasi A, et al. Comparison of diagnostic accuracy of saline infusion sonohysterography, transvaginal sonography and hysteroscopy. J Obstet Gynecol. 2011; 31(1):54–58.

14. Ahmadi F, Javam M. Role of 3D sonohystero-graphy in the investigation of uterine synechiae/Asherman's syndrome: pictorial assay. J Med Imaging Radiat Oncol. 2014; 58(2):199–202.

15. Soares SR, Barbosa dos Reis MM, Camargos AF. Diagnostic accuracy of sonohysterography, transvaginal sonography, and hysterosalpingo-graphy in patients with uterine cavity diseases. Fertil Steril. 2000; 73(2):406–11.

16. AAGL practice report: practice guidelines for management of intrauterine synechiae. J Minim Invasive Gynecol. 2010; 17(1):1–7.

17. Thomson AJ, Abbott JA, Deans R, et al. The management of intrauterine synechiae. 2009; 21(4):335–41.

18. Yu D, Wong Y M, Cheong Y, et al. Asherman syndrome-one century later. Fertil Steril. 2008; 89(4):759–779.

19. Yu D, Li T C, Xia E, et al. Factors affecting reproductive outcome of hysteroscopic adhesiolysis for Asherman's syndrome. Fertil Steril. 2008; 89(3):715–722.

20. Roy K K, Baruah J, Sharma J B, et al. Reproductive outcome following hysteroscopic adhesiolysis in patients with infertility due to Asherman's syndrome. Arch Gynecol Obstet. 2010; 281(2):355–361.

21. Lin XN, Zhou F, Wei ML, et al. Randomized, controlled trial comparing the efficacy of intra-uterine balloon and intrauterine contraceptive device in the prevention of adhesion reformation after hysteroscopic adhesiolysis. Fertil Steril. 2015; 104(1)235–240.

22. Cai H, Qiao L, Song K, et al. Oxidized, regenerated cellulose adhesion barrier plus intrauterine device prevents recurrence after adhesiolysis for moderate to severe intrauterine adhesions. J Minim Invasive Gynecol. 2017;24(1):80–88.

23. Johary J, Xue M, Zhu X, et al. Efficacy of estrogen therapy in patients with intrauterine adhesions: systematic review. J Minim Invasive Gynecol. 2014; 21(1)44–54.

24. Nagori CB, Panchal SY, Patel H. Endometrial regeneration using autologous adult stem cells followed by conception by in vitro fertilization in a patient of severe Asherman's syndrome. J Hum Reprod Sci. 2011; 4(1):43–48.

25. Singh N, Mohanty S, Seth T, et al. Autologous stem cell transplantation in refractory Asherman's syndrome: a novel cell-based therapy. J Hum Reprod Sci.2014;7(2):93–98.

26. Tan J, Li P, Wang Q, et al. Autologous menstrual blood-derived stromal cells transplantation for severe Asherman's syndrome. Hum Reprod. 2016;31(12):2723–2729.

27. Gargett CE, Schwab KE, Deane JA. Endometrial stem/progenitor cells, the first 10 years. Hum Reprod Update.2016; 22(2):137–163.

28. Wang X, Duan H. Clinical evaluation of amniontic products after transcervical resection of intensive degree of intrauterine adhesions. Zhonghua Fu Chan Ke Za Zhi, 2016; 51(1):27–30.

29. Pabuccu R, Onalan G, Kaya C, et al. Efficiency and pregnancy outcome of serial intrauterine device-guided hysteroscopic adhesiolysis of intrauterine synechiae. Fertil Steril. 2008; 90:1973–1977.

30. Robinson JK, Colimon LM, Isaacson KB. Postoperative adhesiolysis therapy for intra-uterine adhesions (Asherman's syndrome). Fertil Steril, 2008; 90(2):409–414.

31. Yang JH, Chen MJ, Chen CD, et al. Optimal waiting period for subsequent fertility treatment after various hysteroscopic surgeries. Fertil Steril. 2013; 99(7):2092–2096.

32. Kasius A, Smit JG, Torrance HL, et al. Endometrial thickness and pregnancy rates after IVF: a systematic review and meta-analysis. Hum Reprod Update. 2014; 20(4):530–541.

33. Check JH, Cohen R. Live fetus following embryo transfer in a woman with diminished egg reserve whose maximal endometrial thickness was less than 4 mm. Clin Exp Obstet Gynecol. 2011; 38(4):330–332.

34. Thomson AJ, Abbott JA, Kingston A, et al. Fluoro-scopically guided synechiolysis for patients with Asherman's syndrome: menstrual and fertility outcomes. Fertil Steril, 2007; 87(2):405–410.

Hysteroscope:
The Wonder Scopy

Hysteroscopy and Infertility

José Metello, José Jiménez, Sushma Deshmukh

Hysteroscopy in infertility
Is rewarding surgery
Specially in unexplained infertility
Disturbing polyps, myomas, IA it checks
Clear proximal tubal blocks
Disclosing uterine angles and curvatures
Helpful even in embryo transfer
Diagnosis of endometritis, adenomyosis
So helping gestosis

INTRODUCTION

Hysteroscopy is an amazing technology which has given opportunity to view the uterine cavity. Due to direct assessment of cavity, its application has become routine in infertility. With the advent of reliable accessory instruments, hysteroscopic surgeries play important role in restoring fertility. It plays major role in fertility enhancing surgeries with laparoscopy. Nowadays hysteroscopy is used as 'See and Treat' technology.

Evaluation of Uterine Cavity

Endometrium evaluation is part of the standard work up in infertility. Usually the first exam is done by transvaginal ultrasound (TVUS) which allows the evaluation of the myometrium, endometrium and cavity in a non-invasive way. 3-D USG, hysterographies, sonohysterography (SHG) or hysterosalpingo-

graphy (HSG) (Figs 16.1 to 16.5) are other techniques sensitive to detect the so called physical anomalies of the uterine cavity, like uterine malformations, cavity indentations suggesting polyps or fibroids or cavity irregularities like adhesions. The addition of color-flow or power Doppler respectively may improve the diagnostic capability of TVUS. Color flow Doppler may demonstrate the single feeding vessel which is typical of endometrial polyps and in fibroids we can appreciate peripheral vascularity. So it becomes easy to differentiate between polyp and submucous myoma (Fig. 16.6).

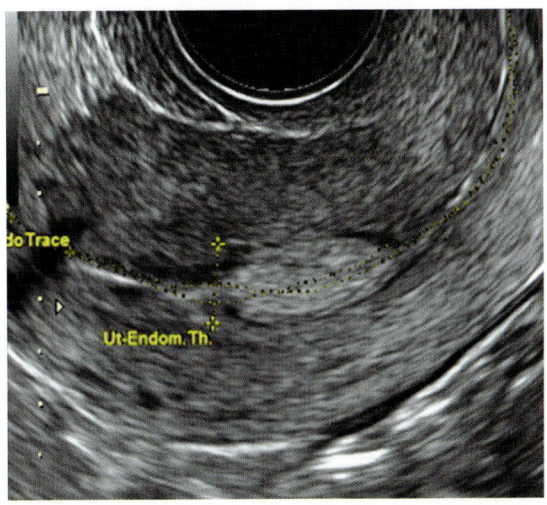

Fig. 16.1: TVUS—endometrial polyp

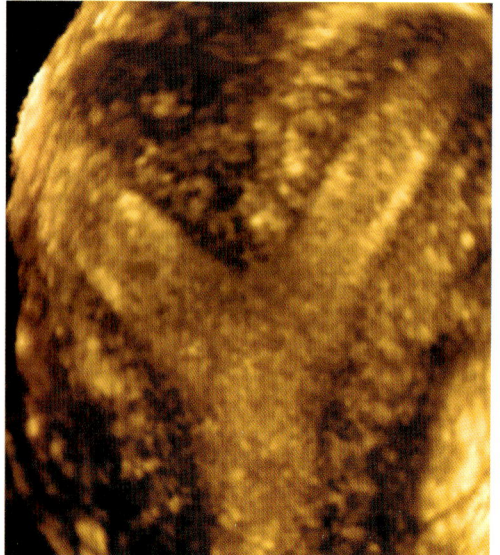

Fig. 16.2: 3-D USG—septum

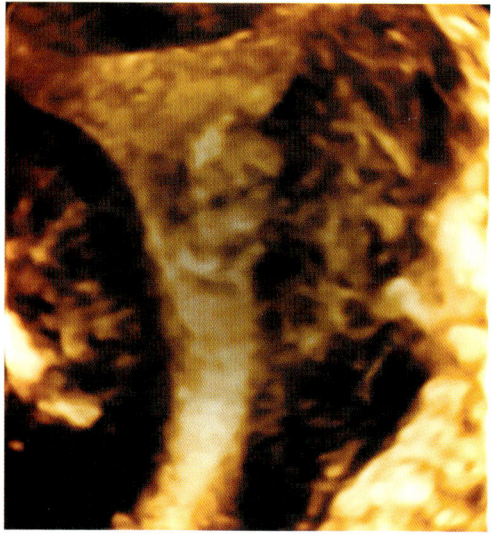

Fig. 16.3: 3-D USG—submucous myoma. *Courtesy:* Dr Sonal Panchal.

These are dynamic exams and they might be helpful to define the exact impact of lesion in relation with the endometrium.

Let us discuss all the conditions one by one.

1. Polyps

Polyps are benign localized, overgrowths of endometrial glands and stroma covered by endometrial epithelium

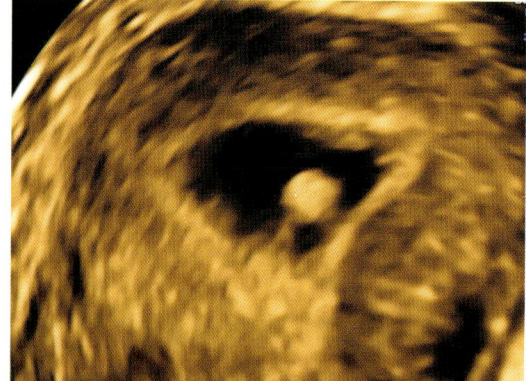

Fig. 16.4: SSG—polyp in the endometrium. *Courtesy:* Dr Sonal Panchal.

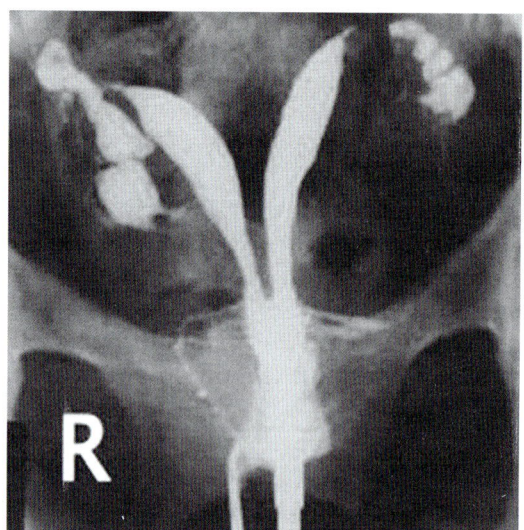

Fig. 16.5: HSG—septate uterus. *Courtesy:* Dr Sandeep Mahajan.

Polyp is one of the most common endometrial abnormalities. 9–25% in the general population.

Infertility and Polyp

The polyps are often asymptomatic but they can sometimes cause menstrual irregularities such as intermenstrual bleeding. They are commonly identified during the investigation for abnormal uterine bleeding and infertility.

Instead, there are a lot of postulations about a single or multiple mechanism by why the polyps affect the endometrial receptivity, is

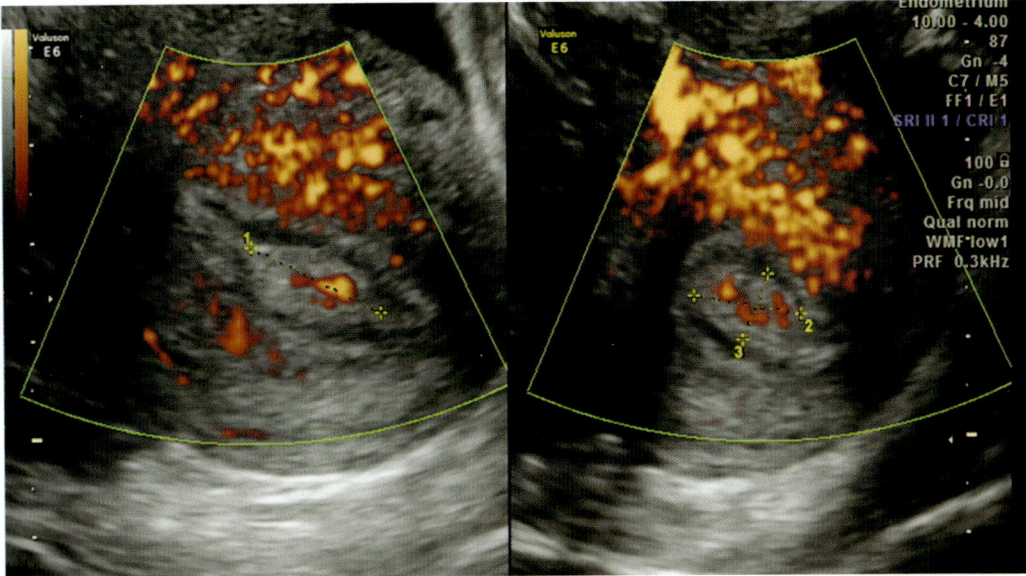

Fig. 16.6: Color Doppler TVUS polyp—single feeding vessel. *Courtesy:* Dr Sandeep Mahajan.

clear that the polyps produce alterations at various levels, anatomic, genetic expression, immunologic modulation, etc. and its removal is necessary to reverse this changes

Movarek et al reported a prevalence of 15.3% in infertile patients. Several studies have shown higher frequency of endometrial polyps in the patients with endometriosis compared to those without the disease. Several authors agree that polyps may interfere with fertility, both by natural conception and IUI (Perez Medina et al, Human reprod, 2005). There are only few reports assessing the effect of endometrial polyps on in vitro fertilization/ ICSI. In a study by Isikoglu et al, endometrial polyps less than 1.5 cm. did not affect implantation and PR in IVF (2006 RB.M).

Management

Majority of publications points to the hysteroscopic removal of polyps in all the patients, especially in the infertile group and previous treatment for infertility.

- *Expectant management:* The class II evidence states that polyps may spontaneously regress in approximately 25% of cases, specially polyps <10 mm

- *Surgical by hysteroscopy:* Hysteroscopic procedures are best performed when the endometrium is thin because there is a decreased operative time, decreased fluid absorption, and easiness of surgery. So hysteroscopy immediately after a menstrual flow is the ideal time for surgery.

Surgery can be done—by forceps, scissors, bipolar system, resectoscope/morcellator.

There is no universal rule to select the best surgical approach to remove endometrial polyp larger than internal uterine orifice.

Outpatient Hysteroscopic Treatment

Small polyps (<0.5 cm) should be removed using 5 Fr mechanical instruments (sharp scissors and/or grasping forceps), principally for reasons of cost (Fig. 16.7). The most widely diffused technique involves the use of grasping forceps. The polyp is approached by positioning the forceps, with opened jaws, at its implantation base. By gently closing the jaws, the forceps finally pushed toward the uterine fundus. The procedure is repeated several times until the polyp's base is completely detached from its parietal implantation.

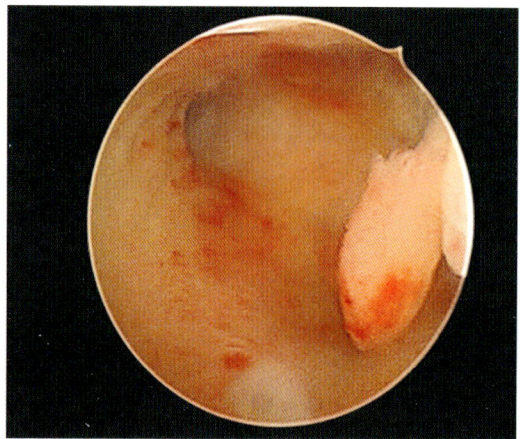

Fig. 16.7: Hysteroscopy: Lateral wall polyp

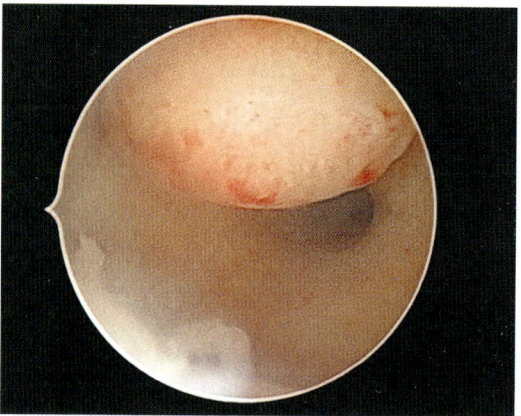

Fig. 16.8: Anterior sessile polyp

Larger polyps (>0.5 cm) can be removed en bloc (or by resecting the lesion's base of implantation with a forceps or a bipolar electrode) only if the internal uterine orifice (IUO) is wide enough to permit extraction. Alternatively, the polyp must be sectioned by the electrode into adequately small fragments that are subsequently extracted from the uterine cavity with a grasping forceps (alligator or tenaculum forceps). Among other factors, one must take into account its morphology and location within the uterine cavity, which can vary considerably.

Results: Spiewankiewicz et al obtained 70% PR in 1 year after hysteroscopic removal of end. Polyp among 25 infertile patients.

In a large study by Perez-Medina et al in 2800 infertile pts. trying to conceive for 2 yrs. and planned for IUI, polyps were detected in 452 (16.1%) patients. After hysteroscopic removal of polyps cumulative PR was 63% as compared with 28% in the control gr.

Problems

- Inaccessible polyps, specially midcavity lat. Wall, fundal, sessile (Fig. 16.8) premenstrual phase
- In the case of sessile polypoid lesions, the resectoscopic technique involves a method of continuous resection (slicing) of the polyp, starting from its free end and advancing toward its base of implantation).
- Usually, resectoscopic treatment of endometrial polyps should be reserved to patients who are reluctant to tolerate an ambulatory operative procedure, or where the size and/or number of polyps are more.

Suggestion: Pretreatment of endometrium before surgery with GnRh.

2. Proximal Tubal Occlusion (PTO)

15% a married couples experience infertility. Of these 30% have infertility due to tubal causes. And 15–20% of patients with tubal infertility have proximal (utero-tubal) obstruction.

Evidence of tubal obstruction found in 15–20% of all hysterosalpingograms and 16–40% of these are false positive.

Based on histology three forms of occlusion have been labeled:

    I. "Nodular" in cases of salpingitis isthmica nodosa (SIN) or endometriosis

    II. "Non-nodular" or fibrotic, and

    III. "Pseudo", related to hypoplastic tubes.

Rahimunnisa, et al. Int. J Ob-Gy 2009, Hou Hy, et al Minim Invasive Gynecol 2014 show mean successful cannulation rate of 70% with at PR33% (13–55%).

Diagnosis

The diagnosis of tubal patency is usually done with HSG or laparoscopy. Unfortunately HSG has a high percentage of false negative and positive results. A meta-analysis by Swart comparing HSG and laparoscopy estimated a sensitivity of 65% and a specificity of 83%. Several reasons help to explain this: Tubular muscular spasm, tubal kinking, air bubbles, mucus plug, or just inadequate interpretation of the exam.

To confirm a treat a PTO there are several options that include falloposcopy and histeroscopy/laparoscopy.

Treatment

There are various methods:

1. Tubal cannulation involves the insertion of a fine catheter under direct guidance or fluoroscopy. Thurmond reviewed the results of selective salpingography in 1466 patients and concluded that successful recanalization could be achieved in around 71–92% with around 30% pregnancy rates.

2. A possible alternative would be the US guided hysteroscopic cannulation, but it seems that its accuracy is inferior to the other options.

3. Concerning hysteroscopy/laparoscopy, a review of the literature showed a mean successful cannulation rate of 70% with a pregnancy rate of around 33% (13–55%). Although fluoroscopy is cheaper it needs radiation exposure and on the other hand a hysteroscopy/laparoscopy approach has several advantages, as it allow for a direct visualization of the pelvis and uterus and it is possible to correct adhesions or other pathology.

   - Various cannulation sets are there Terumo guide wire, Cook cannulation set. Very nicely done in office setting with 2.9 mm Bettocchi office hysteroscope but ideal is hystero-laparoscopy under general anesthesia. So that we can evaluate uterus, tubes, ovaries and adnexa.

- 2.9 mm 30° fore oblique hysteroscope placed in the uterine cavity.
- Right ostium is located and guide wire introduced and advanced under vision towards the ostium and negotiated into the lumen in a gentle way.
- The same procedure repeated on the left side (Fig. 16.9).
- Confirm with laparoscopy by instillation of methylene blue.

Problems

Unable to cannulate due to failure to visualize and negotiate internal tubal ostia. This is due to thick endometrium.

Gautam A et al suggested use of dcapeptyl (3.75 mg) subcuctaneously 20 days before the procedure. It ensures thin endometrium and easier nontraumatic access to the ostia.

3. Intrauterine Adhesions

Incidence varies geographically. True incidence unknown. 0.3 in general population, 21% after postpartum curettage is required.

In developing countries the incidence is increasing due to:

1. Higher number of therapeutic and illegal abortions

2. Use of sharp curettage for performing the same

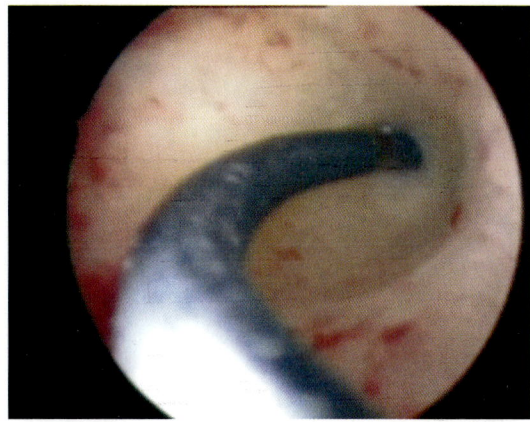

Fig. 16.9: Cannulating the left ostium with Terumo Guidewire

3. Higher incidence of genital TB and puerperial infection.
4. Lower awareness of this clinical condition.
   - Trauma to non-gravid endometrium
   - D&C, abdominal myomectomy, cervical biopsy/polypectomy, IUD, hysteroscopic surgery, septal resection, resection of fibroids.

Diagnosis

- USG (Fig. 16.10)
- HSG-sensitivity-75–81%, and specificity 80% (Fig. 16.11)
- Hysteroscopy

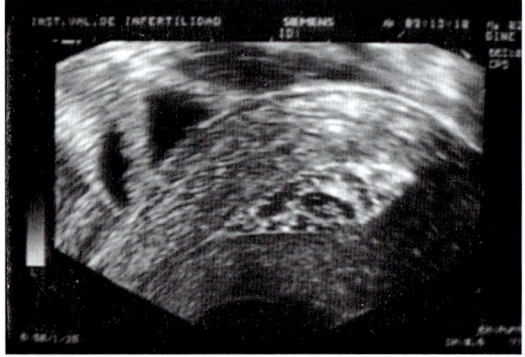

Fig. 16.10: TVUS—intrauterine adhesion

Hysteroscopy

Hysteroscopy has been established as the criterion standard for diagnosis of IUA. It provides access to the endometrial cavity and more accurately confirms the presence, extent, and morphological characteristics of adhesions and the quality of the surrounding endometrium. It provides a real-time view of the cavity, enabling accurate description of location and degree of adhesions, classification, and concurrent treatment of IUAs (Figs 16.12 and 16.13).

Classification

- American Fertility Society, 1988 /Nasr, et al 2008
- Mild–moderate–severe score
- No clear consensus of the proposed classification.

Treatment: Hysteroscopy

Goals

- Restoration of the triangular cavity
- Visualization and confirmation of permeability of the ostium.
- Avoid destruction to normal endometrium

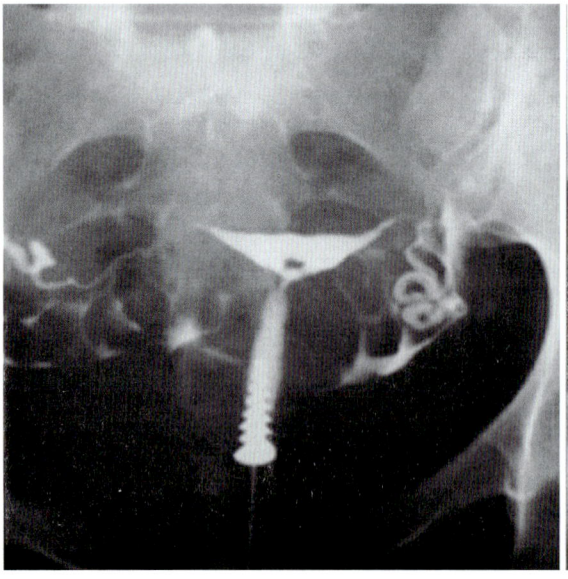
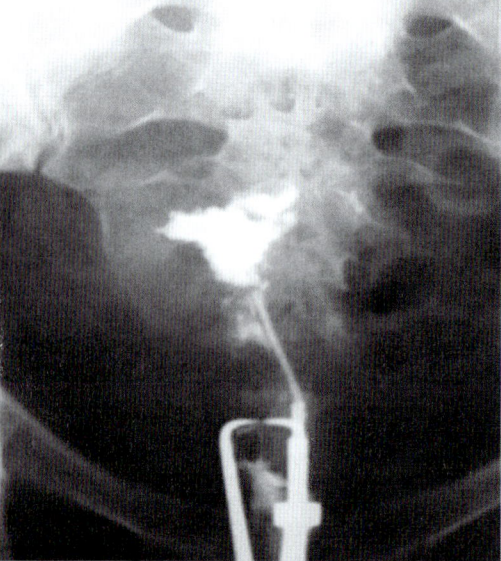

Fig. 16.11: HSG—intrauterine adhesion. *Courtesy:* Dr Sandeep Mahajan.

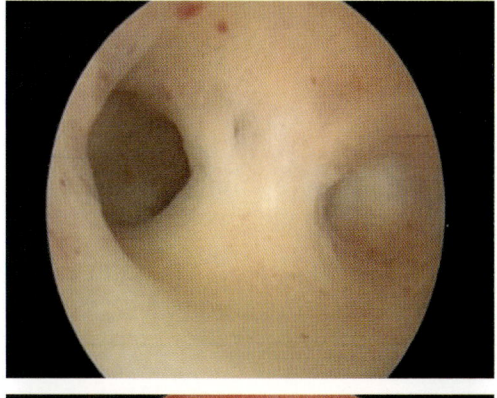

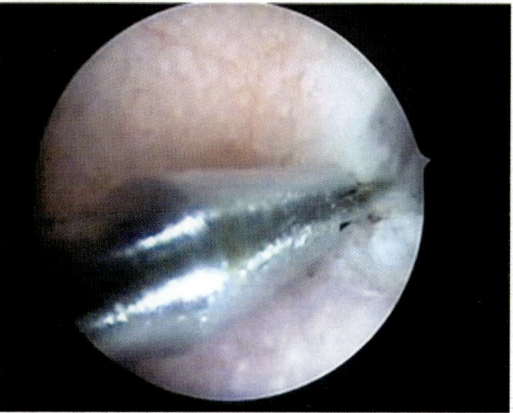

Fig. 16.14: Breaking the adhesions with scissors

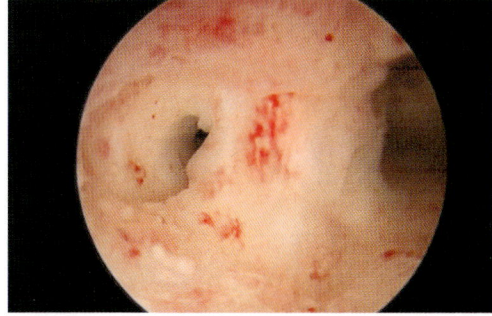

Figs 16.12 and 16.13: Hysteroscopy—intrauterine adhesion

- Minimal manipulation
- Avoid uterine perforation

Hysteroscopic treatment enables lysis of IUAs under direct vision and with magnification. Just the uterine distention required for hysteroscopy may lyse mild adhesions, and blunt dissection may be performed using only the tip of the hysteroscope. Thus, in favorable cases the restoration of cavity can be obtained through "no touch" hysteroscopy in outpatient setting without general anesthesia. Figure 16.14. scissors are most commonly preferred.

Monopolar and bipolar electrosurgical instruments and the Nd: YAG (neodymium-doped yttrium aluminum garnet) laser have been described as techniques used to lyse adhesions under direct vision, with the advantages of precise cutting and good hemostasis. Disadvantages include potential visceral damage if uterine perforation occurs, further endometrial damage predisposing to recurrence of IUAs, cost, and the degree of cervical dilation required to accommodate the operative instruments.

Prevention of IA

1. ***Physical barriers:*** The use of a Foley catheter for 3 to 10 days after surgical lysis of IUAs is similarly reported to act as a physical intrauterine barrier

   A new intrauterine stent was also described as a mechanical method to prevent adhesions recurrence . It is a silicon made, triangular shape device which fits the normal triangular shape of the uterine cavity (Cook medical Inc, Bloomington, USA). In several cases treated for IUA in which the treatment protocol had included intrauterine balloon stent immediately after the procedure, good results in terms of fertility outcome were achieved.

2. ***Anti-adhesion barriers:*** Hyaluronic acid is one of the most widespread component in human tissue and it is involved in many biological function such as mechanical support, cell migration and proliferation

3. ***Stem cells:*** Endometrial tissue had an intrinsic capacity of regeneration

4. ***Platelet rich plasma:*** PRP (rich of growth factor).

4. Tuberculosis

Prevalence of this infection has been seen in 5–10% of infertility cases. But the range varies

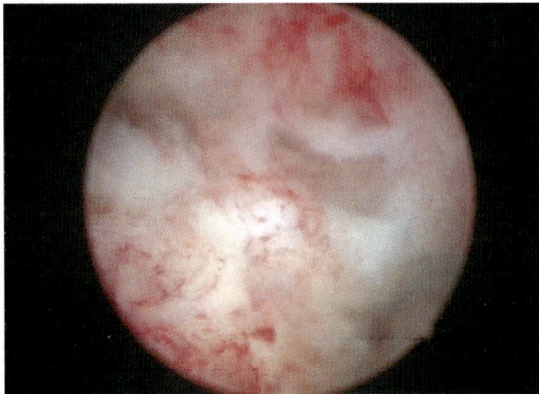

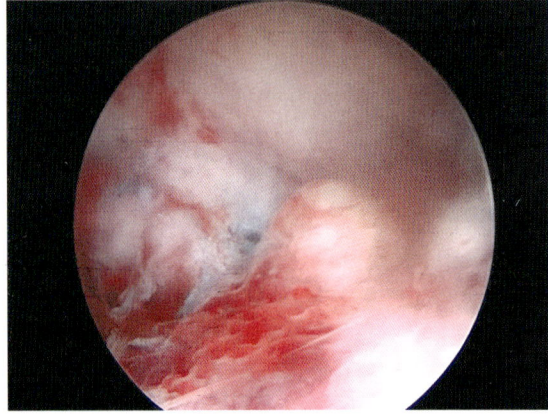

Figs 16.15 and 16.16: Hysteroscopy showing bizarre pale endometrium with nodule

from less than 1% in the USA to 10% and may be more than that in developing countries.

Genital organs most frequently affected by tuberculosis in order of frequency are fallopian tubes (95–100%), endometrium (50–60%), and ovaries (20–30%), cervix (5–15%) and rarely vulva and vagina (1–2%).

Classical hysteroscopic findings of endometrial TB is a rough dirty looking bizarre pale endometrium with gland openings not seen and with overlying whitish deposits (Kumar A, Kumar A) (Figs 16.15 and 16.16).

5. Fibroids and Infertility

A review by Pritts et al (2009) concluded that fibroids causing intracavitary distortion result in decreased rates of clinical pregnancy, implantation and live birth as well as ↑ rate of spontaneous miscarriage.

1. Most prevalent benign solid lesion tumor ranging from 20 to 80% in reproductive age women.
2. Fibroids can be found in up to 10% of infertile women.
3. Minimal invasive surgery is now the gold standard for women who wish to preserve their fertility and hysteroscopic myomectomy is the best treatment option for women with submucosal leiomyomas.

There are various classifications:

The European Society of Hysteroscopy advocates.

- G0—located completely in the uterine cavity.
- G1—more than 50% contained within the uterine cavity
- G2—less than 50% contained within the uterine cavity.

Another STEPW (size, topography, extension, penetration and wall).

Depending upon the patents divided in
- Low complexity (0–4 score)
- High complexity (5–6 score)
- Required alternatives (more than 5–6) to hysteroscopic myomectomy

Diagnosis

USG (TVS), SSG, Doppler (discussed in detail elsewhere)

Problems

Bleeding, fluid overload, perforation

Hysteroscopic Techniques

- Office hysteroscopic myomectomy for (1.5 –2 cm)
- Office preparation of partially intramural myomas (OPPIuM)
- Electrosurgical (thermal loops and vaporizing electrodes) (Figs 16.17 and 16.18)
- Mechanical instrument (cold loops)
- Lasers
- Intrauterine morcellators two main brands 1—Myosure, 2—TRU CLEAR, and third one is Bigatti Shaver.

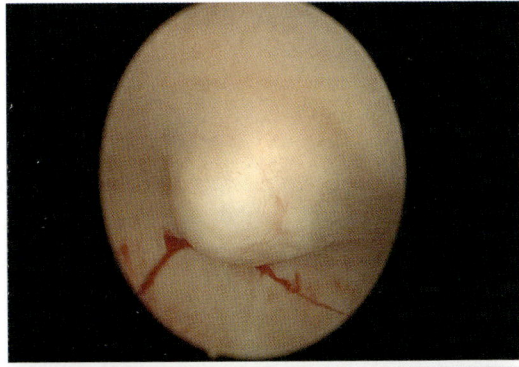

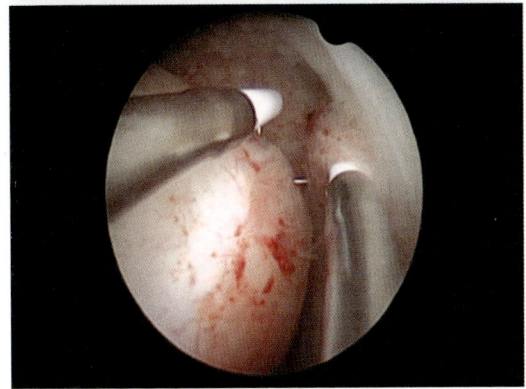

Figs 16.17 and 16.18: Hysteroscopic view and electrosurgical resection

Both of there use mechanical energy instead of high frequency electrical energy.

In nutshell:

- Submucosal fibroids are known to have a negative impact on spontaneous pregnancy rate and ongoing pregnancy/live birth.
- Hysteroscopic management up to 2 cm submucosal fibroid significantly enhances PR and 3 cm and more enhances birth rate
- Post operative fertility outcome is adversely affected by:
  - Multiple infertility factors
  - Fibroid characteristics (no., size, intramural portion and presence of concomitant intramural fibroids)

6. Uterine Septum

- Incidence 2–15 per 1000 women
- Adverse reproductive outcomes infertility, pregnancy loss, poor obstetrical outcome like malpresentation, preterm delivery.

- However many women with uterine septa do not experience any reproductive difficulties.
- Many studies suggest that uterine septum does not play a role in the process of conception as such.
- One of the larger studies (Gergolat M et al 2012) compared 153 women with all types of uterine anomalies. The 33 women diagnosed with septate uterus there was a high incidence of infertility (21.9% *vs* 7.7%). However, this difference did not reach statistical significance.

Classification

- Incomplete (Class U2a)
- Complete (Class U2b) (Fig. 16.19)

(By ESHRE and ESGE) the septate uterus classified as class U2) and Defined as the uterus with normal outline and an internal indentation at the fundal midline exceeding 50% of uterine wall thickness.

U2a—partial septate uterus dividing the uterine cavity above the internal OS.

U2b—complete septate uterus dividing the uterine cavity up to the level of internal OS

Treatment

Currently, there are 2 main hysteroscopic treatment options available for a septate uterus: resectoscopic surgery (with collin's knife) and operative minihysteroscopy with miniaturized instruments.

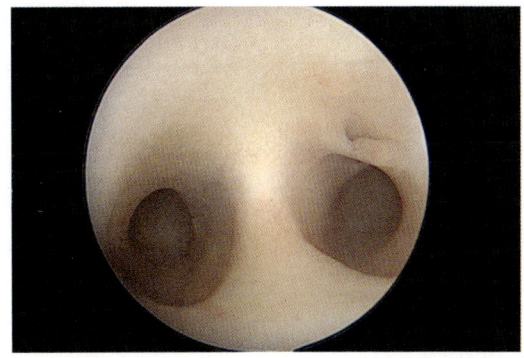

Fig. 16.19: Hysteroscopy showing complete septum

There are few papers that compared the use of scissor, with receptoscope with unipolar power, and with Versapoint® 5 mm electrode bipolar, for the treatment of uterine septum, but in all the reproductive outcomes such as pregnancies, abortions, term deliveries, and preterm deliveries were not significantly different between the techniques

Valle et al[7] descriptive meta-analysis show a 63.5% pregnancy rate and a 50.2% live-birth rate after hysteroscopic metroplasty of septate uterus.

7. Chronic Endometritis

- Asymptomatic condition. Present in 0.2–46% amongst infertile women. Trials from Kasius et al. with 606 patients identified CE in only 2.8% in a population of asymptomatic infertile pts (Fig. 16.20).
- The study by same group concluded that women with CE show altered endometrial contractility in both preovulatory and midluteal phases which may explain symptoms such as pain, abnormal uterine bleeding and infertility.
- In patients of recurrent implantation, plantation failure, CE was identified in 30.3% with low implantation rate 11.5%

Treatment

Treatment can be done with antibiotics. Several options have been described. If no culture is done a treatment similar to pelvic inflammatory disease with Ceftriaxone 250 mg IM in a single dose plus Doxycycline 100 mg orally twice a day for 14 days with Metronidazole 500 mg orally twice a day for 14 days, has been suggested , with good cure rates-normal examination after appropriate antibiotic treatment.

8. Adenomyosis

Adenomyosis referes to the presence of ectopic glandular tissue, located deep in the myometrum. The prevalence ranges from 1–70% and increases with age.

The most common symptoms are abnormal uterine bleeding and dysmenorrhea in up to 65%[5] of patients.

Infertility

A 2014 review by Verciline[6] concluded that adenomyosis was associated with a 68% reduction in the likelihood of pregnancy in women seeking conception after surgery for rectovaginal and colorectal endometriosis. The same author reviewed the outcome of adenomyosis associated with IVF/ICS to conclude that women with adenomyosis had a 28% reduction in the likelihood of clinical pregnancy at IVF/ICSI compared with women without adenomyosis and a higher rate of spontaneous abortion.

Histeroscopy allows for the direct visualization of the uterine cavity, however its ability to diagnose adenomyosis is limited. Several hysteroscopic patterns have been described:

- Irregular endometrium or endometrial defects with superficial openings suggesting a disruption of endomyometrial surface
- Abnormal hypervascularization under low pressure
- Cystic hemorrhagic lesions, with a brownish fluid draining into the ednometrium

Dakkly et al. analysed the diagnostic accuracy of histeroscopy and TVS for the

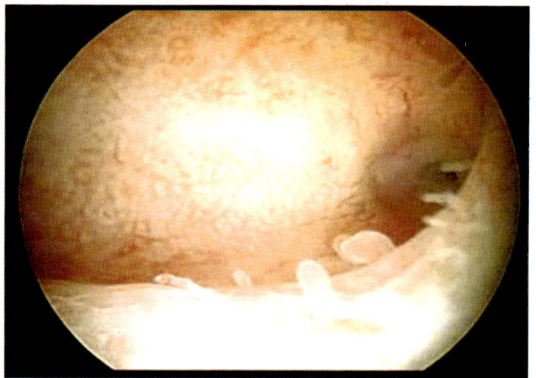

Fig. 16.20: Endometrial cavity-micropolyps and straweberry pattern (*Courtesy*: Dr Luis Alonso Pacheco).

diagnosis of adenomyosis on a cohort of 292 patients. He concluded that hysteroscopic appearance of the endometrial cavity had low sensitivity (40.74%) and specificity (44.62%). Endometrial biopsy had a sensitivity of 54%, but was more specific (78.46%). Contrasting with this was the accuracy of TVS with a high sensitivity

Treatment

While hysteroscopic ablation or uterine artery embolization might be useful in women not looking for childbearing, other options have to be considered in infertile couples.

If submucous cystic adenomyotic are seen bulging into the uterine cavity, it is possible to dissect the myometrial wall of the cyst using a 5 frech scissor[17] or to do an ablative technique that destroys the inner cystic wall. Gordts agrees with the idea that the ablative approach is preferable to cysts localized deeper in the intramural portion.

However as opposed to what happens after a myomectomy where after resection a normal uterine cavity is expected, the resection or ablation of adenomyotic cysts usually results in a visible defect of the myometrium.

9. Niche in the Cesarean Scar (Isthmocele)

Sometimes the healing process of the cesarean section scar is incomplete, with a disruption of the myometrium. The real incidence is unknown however it might range between 24 and 56%.

During the last 30 years the rate of cesarean deliveries has increased. Globally this has not resulted in decreased neonatal morbidity or mortality. However, important maternal complications have been reported like infertility, pelvic adhesions, and pelvic pain and a higher rate of perinatal complications in a subsequent pregnancy such as uterine rupture prematurity, low Apgar scores, Neonatal Intensive Care Unit (NICU) admissions and higher perinatal death.

Symptoms

Frequently it is asyntomatic, but sometimes is responsible for menorrhagia, abdominal pain, dyspareunia and dysmenorrheal. Other gynecological symptoms such as dysmenorrhea, chronic pelvic pain and infertility.

Diagnosis

The diagnosis of this condition is based on previous history of cesarean section and clinical symptoms (Fig. 16.21). US, hysteroscopy or (Fig. 16.22) MRI can clarify the suspition.

Treatment

Different treatments have been proposed and should be reserved for symptomatic patients. Medical treatment with of oral contraceptives reduces menstrual blood. The

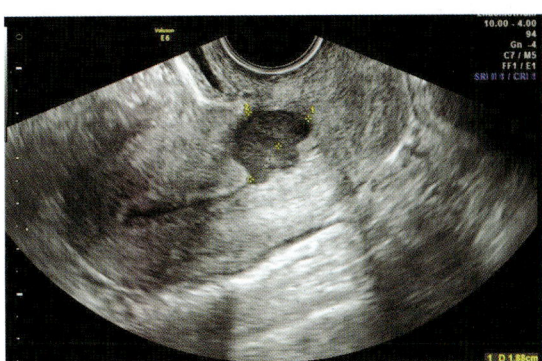

Fig. 16.21: USG showing isthmocele

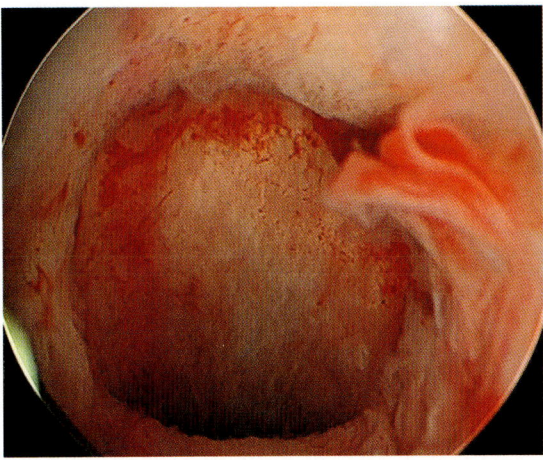

Fig. 16.22: Hysteroscopy isthmocele

published results on effectiveness are conflicting and there are no consistent studies about the use of the hormonal intrauterine device.

Surgical treatment allows for the correction of the defect. A reparative treatment can be done laparoscopically or a resectoscopy correction can be performed mainly to improve the symptoms. A vaginal repair technique has also been described.

Conclusion

Thus hysteroscopy plays a major role in treating infertility.

- Hysteroscopy has become are important tool in diagnosis as well as treatment and correction
- Office hysteroscopy is the most preferred technique.
- Office hysteroscopy see and treat completely fits in the philosophy of the uterus.

AUB and Hysteroscopy

Nitin Shah, Manorhita Gaikwad

INTRODUCTION

Abnormal uterine bleeding (AUB) can be defined as a state of abnormal bleeding with or without any clinically detectable organic, systemic and iatrogenic pathology. This phenomenon is further subdivided into categories depending on the variations in the normal menstrual cycle, which includes changes in regularity, frequency, volume and duration of menses, amount of blood loss, chronicity and reproductive status.

Very recently, the terminology "Abnormal Uterine Bleeding" was put forward to incorporate all kinds of abnormal gynecological bleedings. It included bleeding of organic or non-organic (endocrinal or idiopathic) causes.

It comprehensively encompasses the traditional terms of menorrhagia, poly-menorrhea, metrorrhagia, oligomenorrhea, hypomenorrhea and dysfunctional uterine bleeding (DUB).

Abnormal uterine bleeding is one of the most common clinical problems in gynecology. It accounts to approximately 33–35% of gynecological complaints. The proportion rises in peri- and postmenopausal women.

Apart from the obvious physical discomfort, women also report depression, anxiety, sexual discomfort when suffering from heavy menstrual bleeding. It creates a major impact on women's physical and mental well-being. From last decade, with the improvement and development of newer modalities, much wider range of diagnostic as well as therapeutic therapies have become available.

Previously the diagnostic modalities had always been comprised of simple methods like gynecological and speculum examinations. In later times, transvaginal or trans-abdominal ultrasound was the next tool for majority of the diagnostic investigations. It showed a low specificity and a poor sensitivity. For decades, dilatation and curettage (D&C) has been a key diagnostic procedure for AUB.

With the discovery of hysteroscopy, new avenues were opened for many diagnostic and therapeutic techniques. In this chapter we discuss the use of hysteroscopy in AUB.

CLASSIFICATION

In order to create an universally acceptable nomenclature for AUB, International Federation of Gynaecology and Obstetrics (FIGO) and American College of Obstetrician and Gynaecologists (ACOG) introduced a newer system of terminology.

The newer classification system for AUB is known by acronym PALM-COEIN (FIGO-2011) (Table 17.1).

Table 17.1: PALM-COEIN classification of AUB

Structural causes (PALM)		Non-structural causes (COEIN)	
Polyps	AUB-P	Coagulopathy	AUB-C
Adenomyosis	AUB-A	Ovulatory dysfunction	AUB-O
Leiomyomas	AUB-L	Endometrial (primary disorders of	AUB-E
• Submucosal	AUB-L SM	mechanisms regulating local	
• Other	AUB-LO	endometrial hemostasis)	
Malignancy and hyperplasia	AUB-M	Iatrogenic	AUB-I
		Not yet specified	AUB-N

The introduction of hysteroscopy opened new dimensions for evaluation of various causes of AUB. It has replaced the blind and traditional procedure of D&C, which had a high diagnostic failure rate. A therapeutic D&C could not suffice the benefit provided for the different causes mentioned in the above classification. Many of the causes like polyp, submucous fibroid or adenomyosis could not be explored, diagnosed and treated via this traditional method of treatment. Hysteroscopy provided a better vision along with the obvious diagnoses of various such lesions. With the enhancements in the hysteroscopic maneuvering techniques, different hysteroscopic operative methods came into existence and started playing a major role for minimally invasive surgeries. Now hysteroscopy has been accepted as the gold standard in evaluation of uterine cavity.

DIAGNOSTIC HYSTEROSCOPY

An ideal diagnostic test should be a non- or minimally invasive, easy to perform, easily acceptable, cost effective and with high sensitivity and specificity.

Diagnostic hysteroscopy though being increasingly employed for evaluation of AUB, it is still underutilized. Since the introduction of hysteroscopic techniques, the procedure has undergone significant modifications, contributing to an increase in surgeon's convenience and patient's compliance. Introduction of fiberoptics, reduction in the caliber of the endoscopes, use of simpler distending media

and availability of safer local infiltrative anesthetics have all contributed to an increasing utilization of this technique in evaluation of uterine cavity. More than 50% of all diagnostic hysteroscopies, are still performed in operation theatres (OT) due to previous nonavailability of smaller caliber endoscopes. Now, however, with the innovation of smaller caliber endoscopes, awareness of hysteroscopy as an OPD procedure is being increased.

Compared to ultrasound, hysteroscopy allows a direct visualization of endometrial cavity. It enhances the acuity of detection of any focal lesion. It simultaneously aids for the directed biopsy for any focal lesions in the same sitting thus eliminating the need for a separate procedure. Now hysteroscopy guided biopsy can be performed as an office procedure. It is the best choice for screening as well as diagnostic purposes.

Hysteroscopy is a safe, highly sensitive diagnostic procedure that provides useful information about the uterine cavity and represents ideal method in evaluation of patients with AUB. Endometrial biopsy improves the diagnostic accuracy of hysteroscopy in detecting endometrial pathology. Adequate diagnosis is crucial for selection of treatment of AUB, hence, enabling physicians to avoid unnecessary surgical interventions.

Office endometrial biopsy is a minimally invasive option for endometrial evaluation when at risk of malignancy. Detection rates of malignancy are higher in postmenopausal women than in premenopausal women. Most common cause for AUB in premenopausal women is polyps or submucous fibroids, whereas in postmenopausal women it is endometrial hyperplasia or endometrial atrophy. Reviewing the majority studies from the literature, it is seen that the sensitivity of hysteroscopy for detection of intrauterine pathology exceeds 80%. That validates hysteroscopy to be a diagnostic tool for detecting AUB.

Techniques for Diagnostic Hysteroscopy

Patients are subjected to hysteroscopic and histologic diagnosis in an outpatient department. Endometrial biopsy is carried out at the end of hysteroscopic examination. Reusable biopsy forceps or disposable techniques like Vabra aspiration, Perma or Novak curette are used for biopsy.

OPERATIVE HYSTEROSCOPY

"See and treat the pathology" is the common hysteroscopic clinical practice. It significantly reduces multiple OT visits, anesthesia risks as well as increases cost effectiveness. Submucous fibroid, polyp or malignant growths can be seen and steps can be taken to deal with them. This is especially useful when polyp/fibroid is small and can be missed on curettage. Negative hysteroscopy is of great value too. It enables gynecologists to render medical management and avoid a major surgery.

The main indication for hysteroscopy is menstrual irregularities followed by infertility. The incidences of annual hysteroscopic findings vary according to the age group and presentation. Perimenopausal menorrhagia is the most common indication. The indications also include intermenstrual or postcoital bleeding.

The main causes of abnormal uterine bleeding are:

a. Submucous myomas
b. Endometrial polyps
c. Endometrial atrophy
d. Endometrial hyperplasia
e. Post-pregnancy metrorrhagia.

Preparation of the Patient

As a preventive measure, intramuscular or sublingual atropine is given to prevent vagal reflexes.

Patient is placed in dorsolithotomy position. Careful cleaning of perineum including vagina and cervix is done after which the hysteroscope is introduced. In cases of heavy bleeding, the uterine cavity is distended with liquid medium with a continuous flow system. Curettage, if required, should be done after the hysteroscopic evaluation.

1. Submucosal and Intramural Myomas

In most cases, intrauterine myomas remain latent for a long time and manifest after age of 35. In approximately 80% of cases, they can more or less protrude into the cavity. They are rarely pedunculated intracavitary myomas and displacement into the cervix is very rare.

Hysteroscopic appearance usually shows a smooth surface with endometrial lining over the fibroid. If there is extensive progression in the cavity, it may result in endometrial compression giving rise to ulcerations and necrosis of the apex of the growth. At times, the submucous fibroids are multilobulated, pearly white in color and show one or more vessels on them (Fig. 17.1).

In an innovative technique introduced by Dr. Nitin Shah, a 5 mm laparoscopic tenaculum is introduced from the side of hysteroscope to bring out the partially resected submucous fibroid along with the capsule. This technique is also useful for bringing out foreign bodies, polyps, etc. (Figs 17.2 to 17.4).

2. Endometrial Polyp

Endometrial polyps are exophytic growths of the mucous linings of the endometrium. They differ in size, shape, number and appearances.

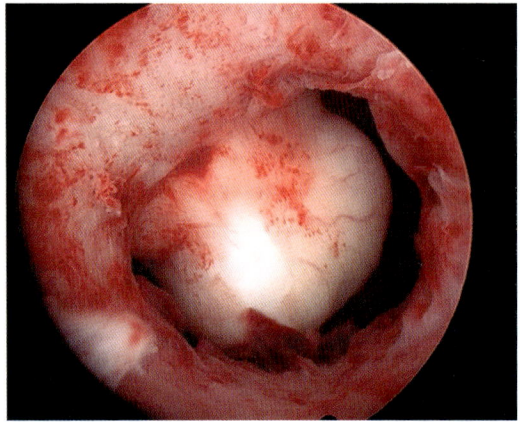

Fig. 17.1: Submucous myoma protruding inside the uterine cavity

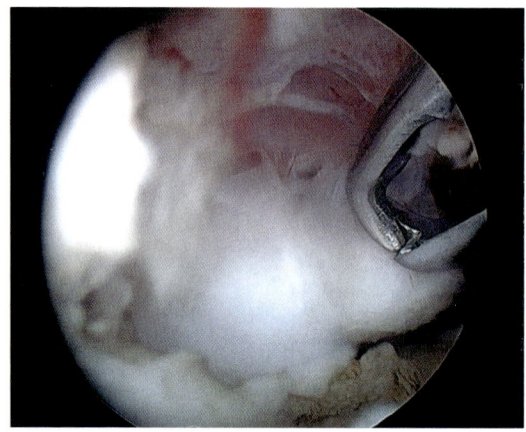

Fig. 17.4: Excision of partially resected myoma with the help of laparoscopic tenaculum

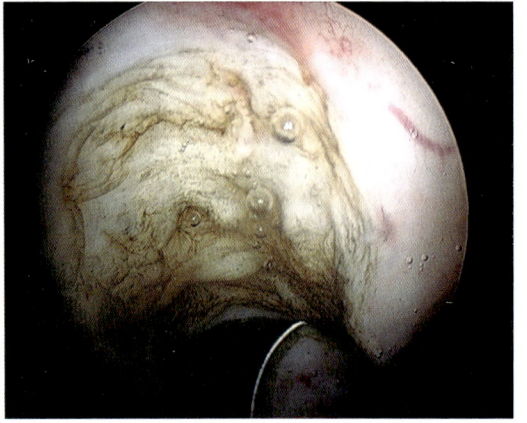

Fig. 17.2: Partial resection carried out with resectoscope

The surface epithelium of the polyp is smooth and similar to surrounding epithelium. They differ from pedunculated fibroids in the manner of surface epithelium and vascularity through the peduncle along with the surface of the growth. Polyps can be associated with glandular hyperplasia and can remain latent for a longer period of time. Curettage proved ineffective being a blind procedure. Hysteroscopic resection of polyp has delivered a great amount of convenience and efficiency (Fig. 17.5).

3. Endometrial Atrophy

This type of AUB is commonly seen in post-menopausal women. It may occur in reproductive

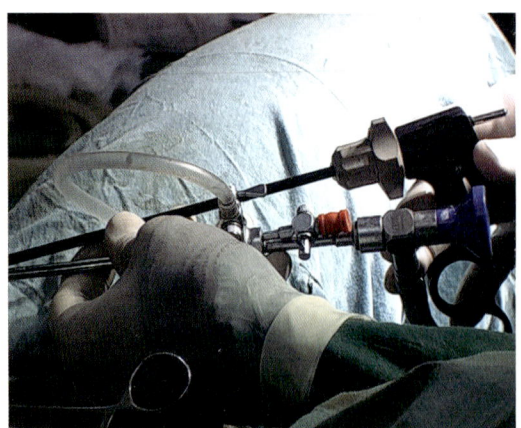

Fig.17.3: Insertion of laparoscopic tenaculum alongside the hysteroscope

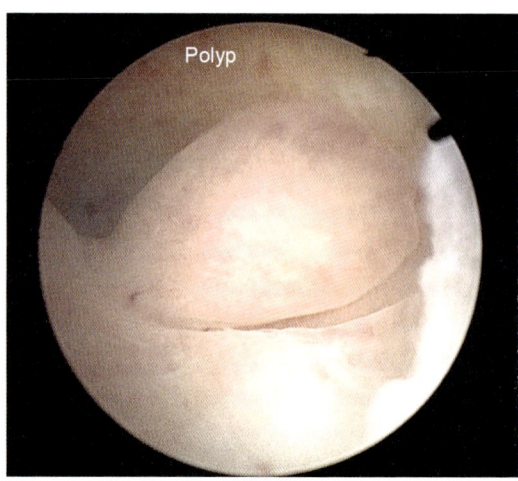

Polyp

Fig. 17.5: Endometrial polyp

period as a final involutionary state of a previous metropathia.

The bleeding occurs from the ruptured capillaries beneath the atrophic surface epithelium. The surface epithelium, near the onset of menopause, undergoes the climacteric changes. It becomes fragile and thin. The network of vascular capillaries and glandular structures close to the surface undergo morphological modifications leading to increased fragility of the stroma. Owing to this fragility, minor uterine bleeding occurs in 45% of postmenopausal women. The cause of endometrial atrophy may be due to total absence of estrogen or failure if uterine receptors to be responsive to estrogen.

The hysteroscopic picture shows thin endometrial mucosa. It is often transparent and reveals underlying vascular network. Often few petechiae are observed during the examination. In severe atrophy, the epithelium looks smooth and whitish without any significant vascular networks.

4. Endometrial Hyperplasia (Metropathia Hemorrhagica, Schroeder's Disease)

This type is commonly seen in premenopausal women. The cause may lie in ovaries or disturbances in rhythmic secretions of gonadotropins. There is variable amount of myohyperplasia with symmetrical enlargement of uterus to a size of about 8–10 weeks due to simultaneous myohypertrophy.

On hysteroscopy, the endometrium looks thick, congested and often polypoidal. There is intense glandular hyperplasia with marked disparity in sizes. Larger glands give appearance of "Swiss cheese" pattern. These glands are empty and are lined by columnar epithelium. A hysteroscopic biopsy can be taken during the procedure or by curettage after the hysteroscopy (Fig. 17.6).

5. Post-pregnancy Metrorrhagia

In cases of post-pregnancy or post-abortive metrorrhagia, hysteroscopy is advisable to

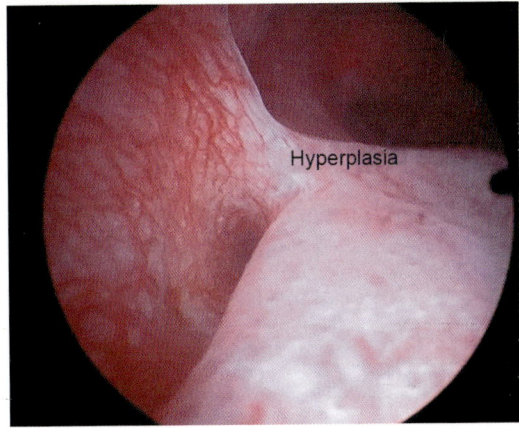

Fig. 17.6: Endometrial hyperplasia

confirm the removal of all abortive debris from the uterine cavity. Osseous metaplasia of endometrium is one of the complications of medical or surgical MTP giving rise to metrorrhagia and secondary infertility in later years (Figs 17.7 and 17.8). Removal of this metaplasia proves beneficial for the fertility. Laparoscopic tenaculum method was useful while removing osseous debris from the cavity.

FIRST-GENERATION ENDOMETRIAL ABLATION TECHNIQUES (FEAT)

First-generation or hysteroscopic methods of endometrial ablation include transcervical resection (TCRE), endometrial laser ablation (ELA), and rollerball ablation (RBA). A good learning curve and a mentoring expertise

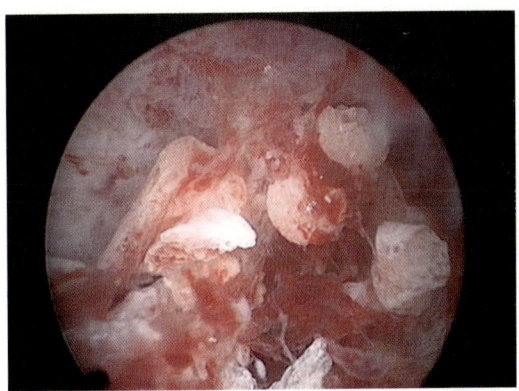

Fig. 17.7: Osseous metaplasia of the endometrium

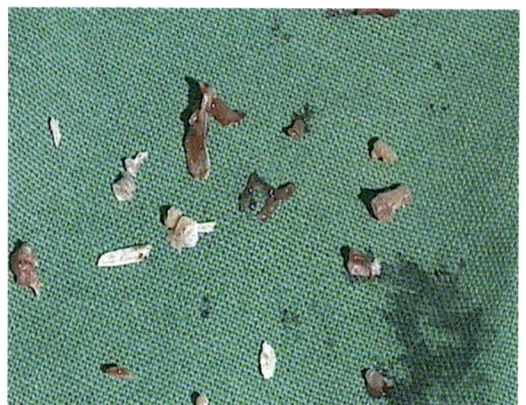

Fig. 17.8: Osseous debris removed hysteroscopically

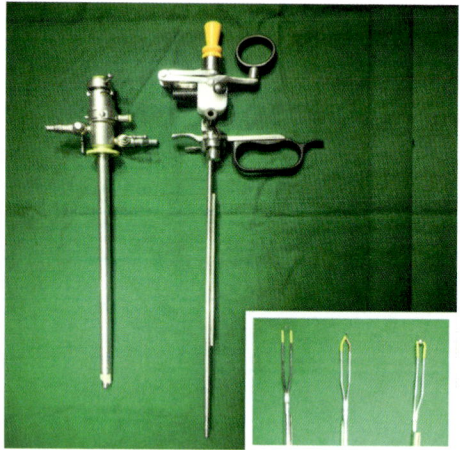

Fig. 17.9: Resectoscope assembly with electrode loops inset

helps one to master these techniques which prove very effective in hysteroscopic management of AUB.

Compared to hysterectomy, these treatments are associated with lower morbidity, shorter hospitalization, faster recovery and reduced treatment costs. As a result, the first-generation ablation techniques are recognised as "gold standard" ablation methods. It is employed as an elective alternative to hysterectomy or when hysterectomy is contraindicated.

A. Transcervical Resection (TCRE)

The advantage of TCRE is that the procedure is under vision and depth of resection ideally includes 2.5 to 3 mm of myometrium in which the endometrial glandular elements are found.

Procedure

The use of the loop-shaped electrode through a monopolar or more recently bipolar continuous flow resectoscope, produces efficient resection of the endometrium and the underlying superficial myometrium and is the only technique which provides tissue for histopathology (Fig. 17.9).

Depending on the energy source used, there are two types of the procedure.

1. *Monopolar resectoscope:* The energy flow used is monopolar while using this resectoscope. Because of its monopolar nature, non-conducting distension media like 1.5% of glycine is used. It has to be used carefully with strict monitoring of input and output. As glycine is hypotonic, it may cause fluid overload and dilutional hyponatremia.

2. *Bipolar resectoscope:* With the recent invention of bipolar resectoscope, many of the complications were eliminated and a better safety for the patient was advocated. The distension medium used is normal saline that was associated with less electrolyte disturbances than with electrolyte free solutions.

The resection carried out in TCRE is global including the cornual ends which give best results. TCRE certainly is a proven alternative to hysterectomy with higher satisfaction rates and better compliance.

Advantages

1. Suitable even for thicker endometrium.
2. Provides endometrial tissue for histology.
3. Other lesions like polyp or fibroids can be removed at the same time.
4. Lesser operating time, hospital stay and costs compared to hysterectomy.
5. Lesser intraoperative blood loss.

Disadvantages

1. Great risk for uterine perforation.
2. Greater operative skills are required.

3. Fluid overload syndrome (for monopolar resectoscope).

B. Hysteroscopic Laser Endometrial Ablation

The goal of these procedures is denudation of endometrium from the uterus by means of tissue destruction procedures like coagulation, vaporization and carbonization. A destruction up to a depth of 4–5 mm produces a therapeutic intrauterine synechiae (Asherman's syndrome) and scarring leading to oligomenorrhea or amenorrhea.

Laser energy suitable for hysteroscopic surgery must not be absorbed by water. It should be able to transmit through fibers. For these criteria, Nd: YAG is ideal for the intrauterine surgeries as it is a fiber laser with a tissue destruction up to the depth of 5–6 mm. The laser energy is delivered to the tissues via a 600 or 800 mm bare quartz fiber-guided through the operating hysteroscope. Power settings are usually between 40 and 80 W which gives a power density of 4000 to 6000 W/cm².

Advantages

1. Perforation less likely than resection.
2. Tissue coagulation to 5–6 mm.
3. Small fibroids or polyps can be vaporized.

Disadvantages

1. Slowest of all techniques.
2. Fluid overload syndrome.
3. Need for special laser safety procedures and guidelines.
4. Expensive investment and running cost.
5. No endometrial specimen for histology.

C. Hysteroscopic Rollerball Endometrial Ablation

Introduction of rollerball became popular after laser ablation because of its relative simplicity and cost advantage. It is safe, effective and quicker to perform. The concept of laser and rollerball differed only in the means of energy used. The energy used in rollerball is electro-surgical. The rollerball usually are in two sizes, small, i.e. 2.5 mm and large, i.e. 5 mm with respect to diameters. Electrocoagulation of the endometrium is done with the help of these electrodes.

Advantages

1. Easier and quicker to perform.
2. Less risk of uterine perforation, fluid absorption and hemorrhage.

Disadvantages

1. No endometrial specimen for histology.
2. Use of monopolar energy thus non-conducting media leading to fluid retention syndrome.

Overall, excessive surgical interventions were avoided after the introduction of FEAT (First-generation endometrial ablation techniques). A significant level of operating skills and training becomes absolute to produce better safety along with the better results. FEAT requires general anesthesia, exposing the patient to added complications. Nonetheless, the advantage of these procedures exceed far more than those of hysterectomies.

CONCLUSIONS

In about 60% of pre- and postmenopausal women with AUB, lesions are found with these advanced techniques nowadays. Submucosal myoma, endometrial polyp or hyperplasia are the most common lesions found in premenopausal women. Endometrial atrophy, polyp or malignancies are more commonly seen in postmenopausal women. Therefore hysteroscopy is a visionary diagnostic measure for detection of early malignant lesions in older women. However, hysteroscopic diagnosis always requires histopathological confirmation. In atrophic endometrium, hysteroscopy proves beneficial for avoiding biopsy to save the patient from hemorrhage. Hysteroscopy has given a great advantage of time and perception to the clinicians. Being gold standard, it has awarded the gynecological fraternity a great deal minimal access and a maximum benefit.

Hysteroscopy in Recurrent Pregnancy Loss

Richa Sharma, Rahul Manchanda, Nidhi Chandil

Recurrent pregnancy loss (RPL), also referred to as *recurrent miscarriage* or *habitual abortion*, is defined as 3 consecutive pregnancy losses prior to 20 weeks gestation and affects 2–5% of the couple. Approximately 15% of all pregnancies result in spontaneous loss and only 30% of all conceptions result in a live birth. Risk of abortion in subsequent pregnancies is 30% after 2 losses and 33% after 3 losses among patients without a history of a live birth. This strongly indicates a role for evaluation after just 2 losses in patients with no prior live births or an earlier evaluation may be further indicated if fetal cardiac activity was identified prior to a loss, woman older than 35 years and infertility.

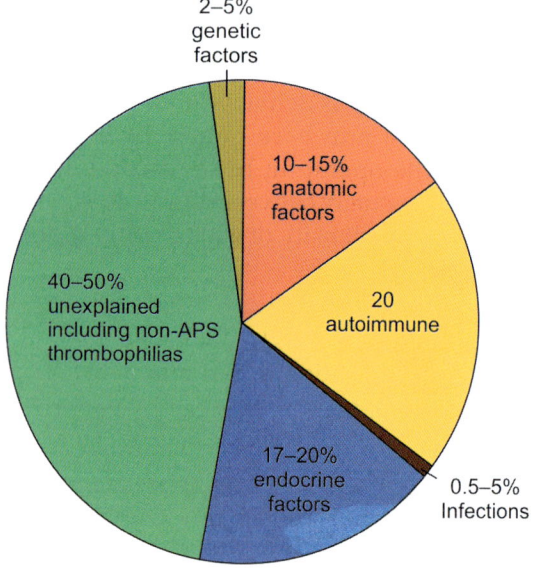

Fig. 18.1: Etiology of recurrent pregnancy loss

Etiology

Parental chromosomal abnormalities, untreated hypothyroidism, uncontrolled diabetes mellitus and endocrine disorders, certain uterine anatomic abnormalities, antiphospholipid antibody syndrome (APS heritable and/or acquired thrombophilias), immunologic abnormalities, infections, and environmental factors (Fig. 18.1).

Anatomic uterine abnormalities account for 10% to 15% of cases of RPL and cause miscarriage by interrupting the vasculature of the endometrium, prompting abnormal and inadequate placentation.

Acquired uterine abnormalities include endometrial polyps, myomas and intrauterine adhesions. Congenital uterine abnormalities (CUA) are the consequence of an abnormal development of the Müllerian ducts and are found in 8.4–12.6% of women with RPL, which is seven to eight times higher than the general population. CUAs include septate, bicornuate, unicornuate, didelphic, and arcuate uteri. Role of the arcuate uterus in causing RPL is unclear. Diagnostic evaluation for uterine anatomic anomalies should include office hysteroscopy.

Diagnosis

Intrauterine abnormalities may be visualized using various modalities, including hysterosalpingography (HSG), transvaginal sonography (TVS), sonohysterography (SHG), and hysteroscopy. HSG is very sensitive (98%) but has low specificity (34.9%). Transvaginal sonography is more specific (96.3%) and sensitive (100%) to HSG. SHG has a specificity of 87% and a lower sensitivity of 70% and 3D USG is helpful in the evaluation of IUAs, with sensitivity of 87% and specificity of 45%.

Hysteroscopy is considered the **"gold standard"** in the diagnosis of intrauterine abnormalities.

Hysteroscopy Procedure

With the invention of BETTOCCHI integrated office hysteroscope (BIOH), which has 30° telescope, 4 mm size with channel for semirigid 5 Fr operating instruments. "Vaginoscopic approach" or "no-touch technique" is recommended for the atramautic insertion of the hysteroscope and complete visualization of vagina, cervical canal, uterine cavity and 2–3 mm of proximal tubes. Grasping forceps and scissors are excellent for treating adhesions, smaller cervical polyps, and endometrial polyps but larger endometrial polyps, or thick lesions (e.g. submucous fibroids) are difficult to treat successfully using such miniature instruments and without cervical dilation. New generation of electrical generators, allowing the use of bipolar energy on miniaturized electrodes, has been presented (Autocon 400 II; Karl Storz Endoscopy, Tuttlingen, Germany). The main advantage of these instruments is that they are reusable, thereby reducing the costs of office operative procedures.

1. ENDOMETRIAL POLYP

The prevalence of endometrial polyps is 32% among infertile women and 2–3% among women with RPL. Small polyps (<2 cm) do not cause infertility but cause increased pregnancy loss (Fig. 18.2a–c).

Endometrial polyps can be effectively and safely treated with hysteroscopic polypectomy, with reduced recurrence rate (Fig. 18.3).

AAGL 2012 considers:

a. That the infertile women are more likely to be diagnosed with an endometrial polyp (Level B).

b. For the infertile patient with a polyp, surgical removal is recommended to allow natural conception or assisted reproductive technology a greater opportunity to be successful (Level A).

c. Increasing age is the most common risk factor for the presentation of an endometrial polyp (Level B).

d. Polyps may naturally regress in up to 25% of patients, with small polyps more likely to resolve spontaneously (Level A).

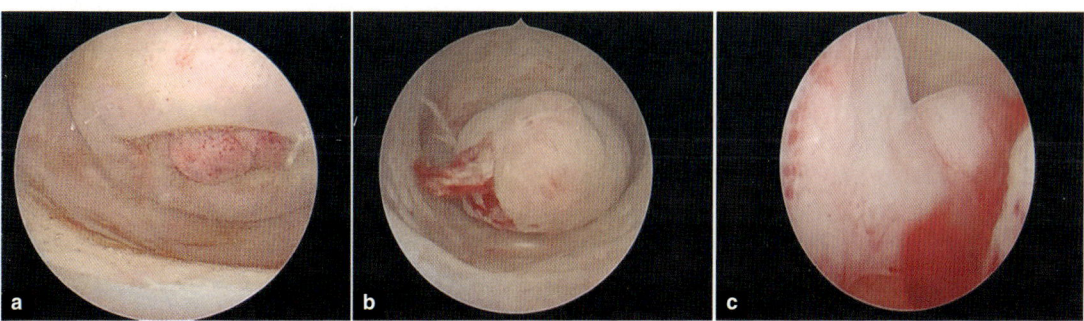

Fig. 18.2a to c: (a) Endometrial polyp protruding at the external os; (b) Single endometrial polyp; (c) Multiple endometrial polyp

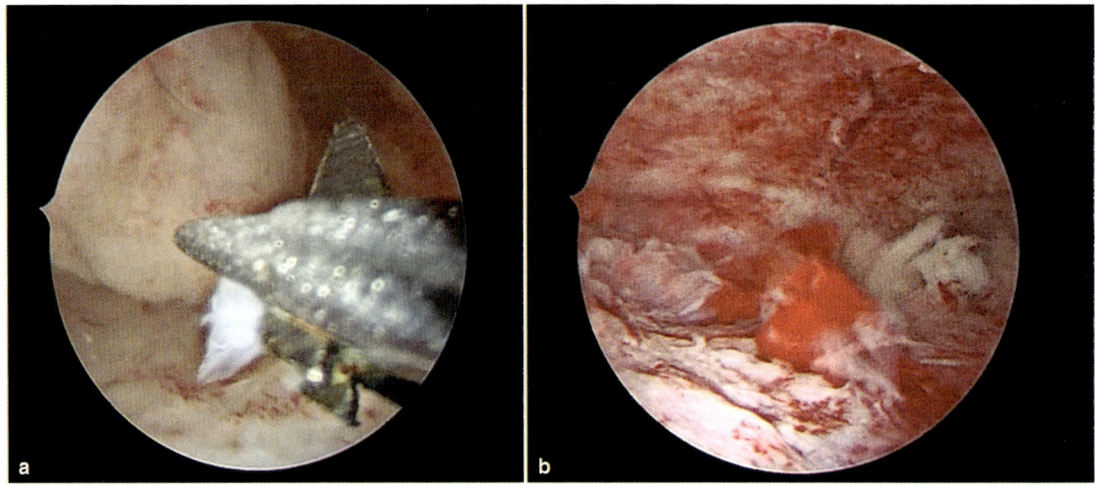

Fig. 18.3a and b: (a) Polypectomy with scissors; (b) Endometrium after polypectomy

Evidences in Support of Hysteroscopic Polypectomy

Jan Bosteels et al. Cochrane Database of Systematic Reviews Feb 2015.	Persistent endometrial polyps are likely to impair reproductive performance and that hysteroscopic polypectomy before IUI could be considered as an effective intervention
Pérez-Medina T, Hum Reprod. 2005 Jun; 20(6): 1632–5.	Hysteroscopic polypectomy is an effective measure for conception
Stamatellos I et al Arch Gynecol Obstet. 2008 May; 277(5):395–9.	Hysteroscopic polypectomy appears to improve fertility and increase pregnancy rates irrespective of the size or number of the polyps

2. SUBMUCOUS MYOMAS

Submucosal myomas are found in 4.5% of women with RPL (Fig. 18.4). Intramural fibroids larger than 5 cm, as well as sub-mucosal fibroids of any size, can cause RPL.

The mechanisms whereby submucous-myomas causes pregnancy loss probably could be due to the endometrium overlying submucous myomas and opposite the myoma shows glandular atrophy, which may impair implantation and nourishment of the developing embryo.

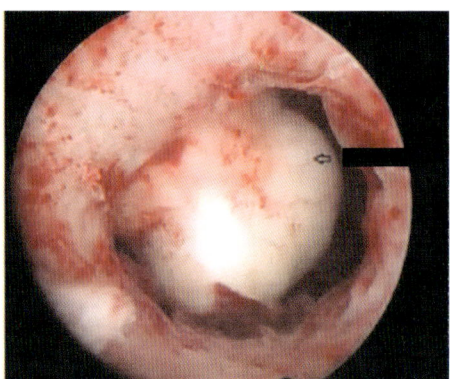

Fig. 18.4: Submucous myoma

The AAGL (2012) considers HSG less sensitive and specific when submucous myomas are concerned. Hysteroscopy revealed high sensibility, specificity, and accuracy in the diagnosis of submucous fibroids and a good correlation with histological diagnosis.

There are 3 basic methods for removing leiomyomas under hysteroscopic guidance: Morcellation, cutting with an electrosurgical loop or scissors and vaporization (Fig. 18.5a,b). When performing radiofrequency-based hysteroscopic myomectomy on RPL or infertile women, every effort should be made to minimize thermal damage to the tissue adjacent to the incision. Care must be taken to ensure the loop does not touch adjacent endometrium. The depth of thermal injury in

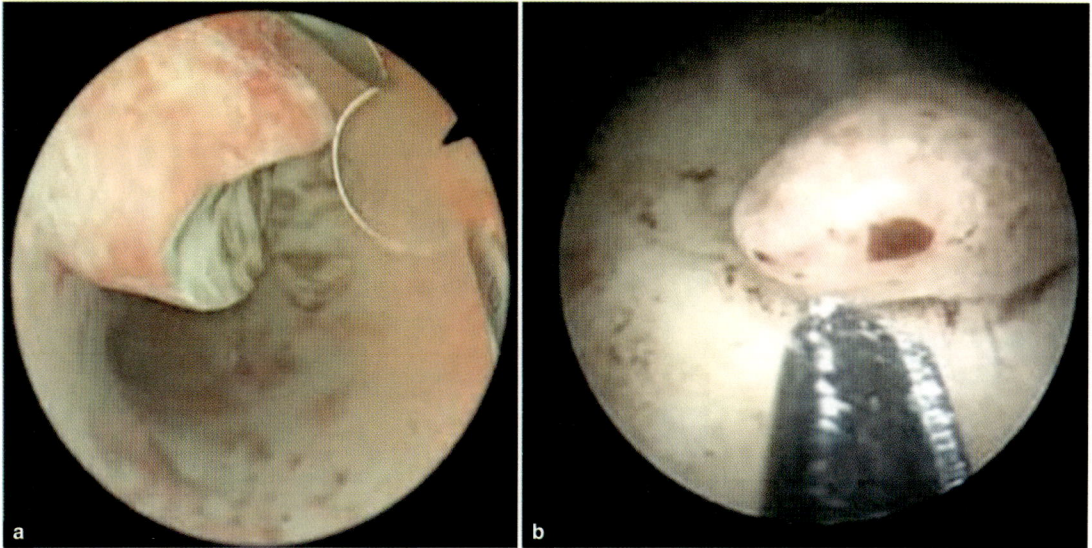

Fig. 18.5a and b: (a) Myomectomy by resectoscope; (b) Myomectomy by scissors

tissue is proportional to a number of factors including the voltage of the output and the exposure time. If the power setting is too low for the surface area of the electrode that is used, the electrode will drag in the tissue, thereby increasing the time of exposure and thus the depth of thermal injury.

According to the **ASRM (2008),** hysteroscopic myomectomy is indicated for intracavitary myomas and submucous myomas having at least 50% of their volume within the uterine cavity. In infertile women and those with recurrent pregnancy loss, myomectomy should be considered only after a thorough evaluation has been completed. Types 0, 1, and 2 up to 4–5 cm diameter can be effectively treated with hysteroscopic transcervical resectoscopic myomectomy (TCRM), with high success rates. However, type 2 myomas may require a multistaged procedures. Women with a normal uterine size and having less than 2 submucous myomas *vs* enlarged uterine size with more than 3 myomas may be at a risk of repeat surgery 9.7% and 35% respectively at 5 years. Myomectomy significantly improve live birth rates from 57% to 93%.

AAGL (2012) recommends that the for women desiring future fertility, an abdominal approach to submucous myomectomy should be considered when there are 3 or more submucous myomas or in other circumstances where hysteroscopic myomectomy might be anticipated to damage a large portion of the endometrial surface (Level B).

Postmyomectomy, 35–40% risk of intrauterine synechiae after multiple submucous myomectomies. In such cases, second look hysteroscopy and appropriate adhesiolysis should be considered.

Evidences in Support of Hysteroscopic Myomectomy

Pritts EA (2009) Meta-analysis	Fibroids with a submucosal component causes decreased clinical pregnancy and implantation rates and its removal, improves fertility
Shokeir T (2010) RCT	Fertility rates appeared to increase after hysteroscopic myomectomy of type 0 and type I myomas (P <0.05)

3. INTRAUTERINE ADHESIONS OR ASHERMAN'S SYNDROME

Wide spectrum of uterine syneche or adhesions exists in terms of severity and location. It could be thin, filmy, diffuse, broad

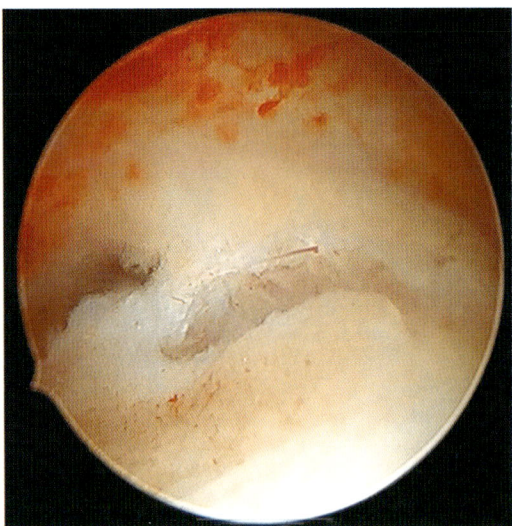

Fig. 18.6: Severe intrauterine adhesions obliterating the cavity

to dense, thick and fibrous bands that ultimately obliterates the cavity (Fig. 18.6). Adhesions may arise from endometrium, myometrium and connective tissue. Repeated pregnancy losses are observed in 14% of patients with intrauterine adhesions.

Various classifications are used but MEC classification based on the severity, is the most simple and applicable.

MEC (Manchanda's Endoscopic Centre) Classification of Asherman's Syndrome

Severity	Extent of adhesions
Grade 1 Mild	Less than 1/3rd of uterine cavity obliterated (flimsy/dense adhesions)
Grade 2 Moderate	1/3rd to 2/3rd of uterine cavity obliterated (flimsy/dense adhesions)
Grade 3 Severe	More than 2/3rd of uterine cavity obliterated (flimsy/dense adhesions)

AAGL Recommendation for Diagnosis of IUAs

1. Hysteroscopy is the most accurate method for diagnosis of IUAs and should be the investigation of choice when available (Level B).

2. If hysteroscopy is not available, HSG and hysterosonography are reasonable alternatives (Level B).

The main aim of intervention is to restore the volume and shape of the uterine cavity to normal and to facilitate communication between the cavity and both the cervical canal and the fallopian tubes along with prevention of recurrence of adhesions.

Hysteroscopic treatment enables lysis of IUAs under direct vision and with magnification. The uterine distention required for hysteroscopy may itself lyse mild adhesions, and blunt dissection using only the tip of the hysteroscope may further lyse adhesions. Mechanical division of adhesions by scissors and needle have best results. Monopolar and bipolar electrosurgical instruments and the Nd-YAG laser can also be used with the advantages of precise cutting and good hemostasis but may lead potential visceral damage if uterine perforation occurs (Fig. 18.7a–c). Myometrial scoring is another technique to create a uterine cavity in women with severe IUAs, 6–8 incisions of 4 mm depth are created in the myometrium using electrosurgery with a Collin's knife electrode. Anatomic success reported is 50–71%.

AAGL Guidelines for Treatment of IUAs

1. Direct visualization of the uterine cavity by hysteroscopy along with adhesiolysis is the treatment of choice for IUAs (Level B).

2. Extensive or dense adhesions must be treated by an expert hysteroscopist (Level C).

3. Because of the suppressive or inflammatory effect on the endometrium, neither progestin-releasing nor copper or T-shaped IUDs should be used after surgical division of intrauterine adhesions (Grade C).

4. Only limited data supports Foley catheter or an IUD after surgical lysis of IUAs. There exists the potential for increased infection rates, and neither technique can be recommended for routine use outside of clinical trials (Grade C).

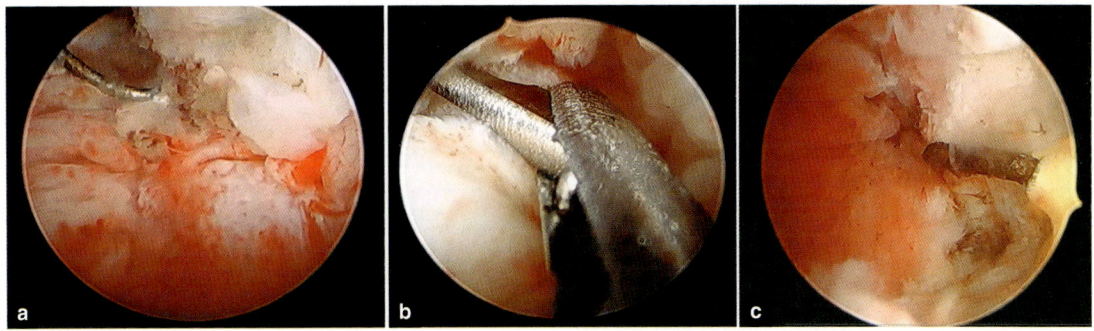

Fig. 18.7a to c: (a) Adhesiolysis by resectoscope; (b) Adhesiolysis by scissors; (c) Adhesiolysis by Collin's knife

5. Barriers such as hyaluronic acid and auto-cross-linked hyaluronic acid gel seem to reduce the risk of adhesion recurrence and may be of benefit after treatment of IUAs. At this time, their effect on post-treatment pregnancy rates is unknown, and they should not be used outside of rigorous research protocols (Grade A).
6. Postoperative hormone treatment using estrogen, with or without a progestin, may reduce recurrence of IUAs (Grade B).
7. Medications to improve vascular flow to the endometrium should not be used outside of rigorous research protocols (Grade C).
8. No evidence to support or refute the use of preoperative, intraoperative, or post-operative antibiotic therapy in surgical treatment of IUAs (Grade C).

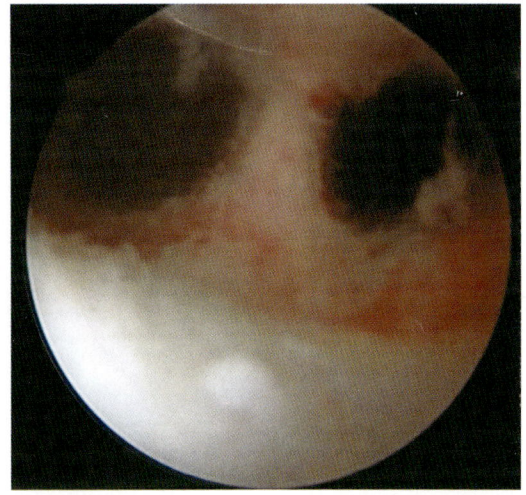

Fig. 18.8: Partial septum showing cat's eyes appearance

4. UTERINE SEPTUM

The uterine septum is the congenital uterine anomaly, which may be partial or complete, thick or thin (Fig. 18.8). Prevalence ranges between 1 and 2 per 1,000 to 15 per 1,000 women and its association with RPL is as high as 76%.

American Society for Reproductive Medicine (ASRM 2016) radiologically defines—*Normal/arcuate:* Depth from the interstitial line to the apex of the indentation is 90 degrees. *Septate:* Depth from the interstitial line to the apex of the indentation >1.5 cm and angle of the indentation (Fig. 18.9).

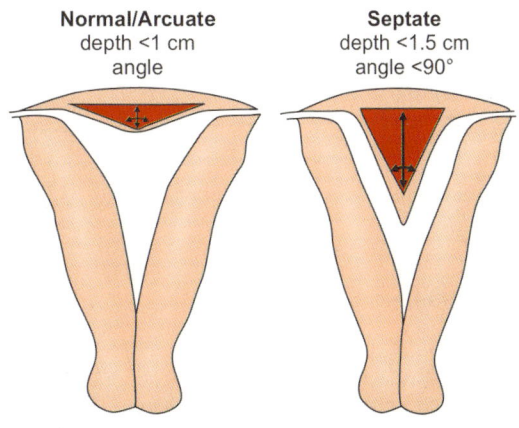

Fig. 18.9: Diagnosis of septate uterus—ASRM 2016

Gold standard method for diagnosing Müllerian anomalies is hysterolaparoscopy and the treatment is hysteroscopic metroplasty or hysteroscopic transcervical division or incision of the uterine septum using cold scissors, unipolar or bipolar cautery, laser, bipolar electrosurgical needle or resectoscope with an operating loop. Moving the hysteroscope from side to side and visualisation of both the ostia on a panoramic view from the level of internal os verifies completion of resection (Fig. 18.10a–d). Concurrent laparoscopy or transabdominal ultrasound decreases the risk of uterine perforation, and help in complete removal of the septum. After successful hysteroscopic septum, patients have near normal pregnancy outcomes, with term delivery rates of approximately 75% and live birth rates approximately 85%.

Principles of Metroplasty

1. To horizontally divide the septum rather than excise the septum

2. Fundal myometrium should be at least 1.5 cm in depth

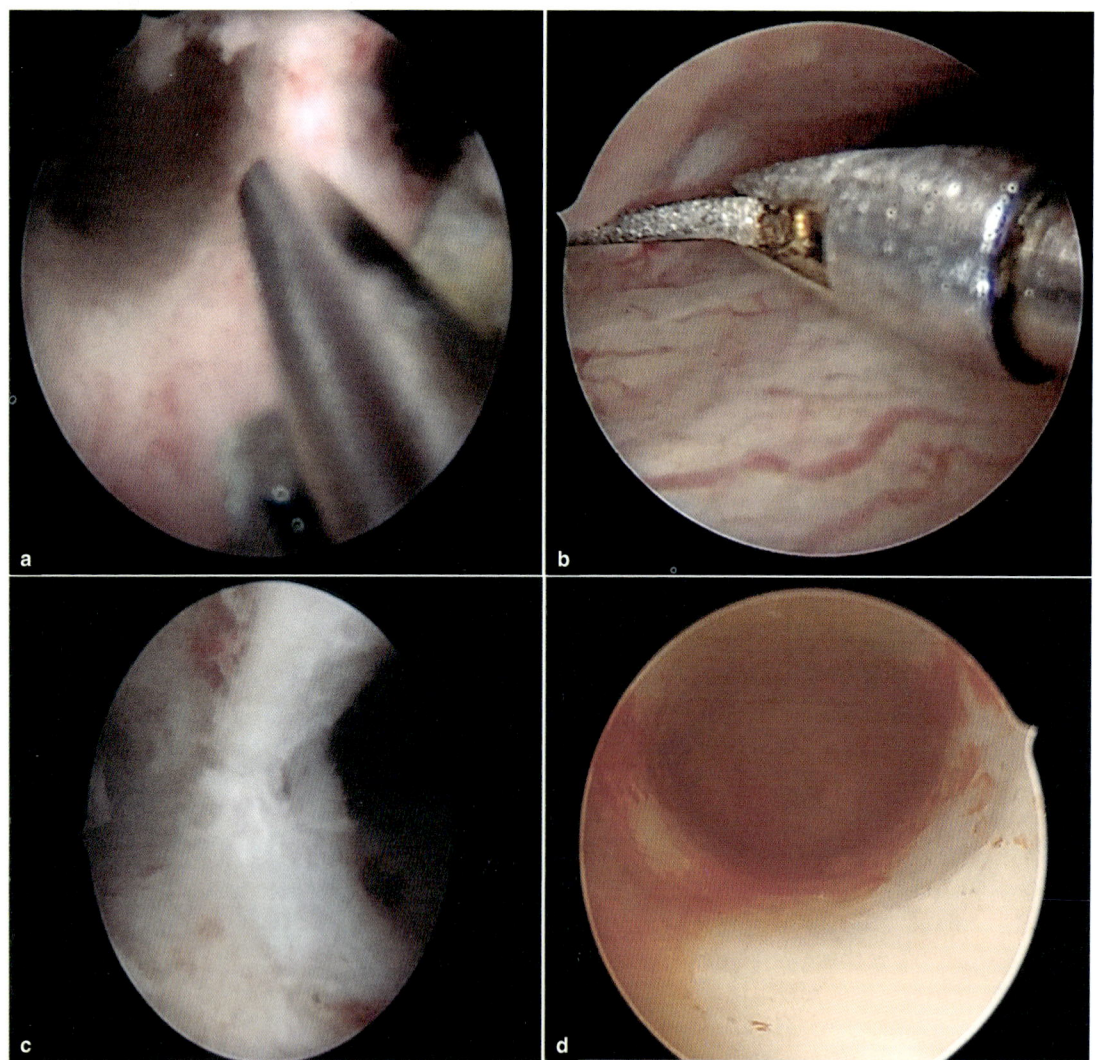

Fig. 18.10a to d: (a and b) Septoplasty with scissors; (c and d) Cavity restoration after septoplasty

3. Postsurgery, IUCD insertion for at least 3 months with estrogenisation is only recommended for wide or complete septa.

Evidences in Support of Hysteroscopic Metroplasty

National Institute for Health and Care Excellence (NICE) (2013) review of 2528 women (37 studies)	Women with septate uterus and a history of recurrent miscarriage or infertility reported a live birth rate of 60% after hysteroscopic metroplasty. 'Take home baby rate' increased from 9% before hysteroscopic metroplasty to 87% after the procedure.
ASRM 2016	Improvement in live-birth rates in women with a history of prior pregnancy loss, recurrent pregnancy loss, or infertility.
National Institute for Health and Care Excellence (NICE) (2017)	No evidence that hysteroscopic septum resection improves reproductive outcome in women with a septate uterus and outweighs the possible complications of the procedure.

5. UNICORNUATE UTERUS

Unicornuate uterus, which belongs to class II of AFS classification, and 13.3% associated with RPL (Fig. 18.11a,b). The reproductive outcome with unicornuate uterus is poor probably due to reduced capacity of the uterine cavity, with a possibility of live birth of 29.2%, prematurity 44%, 1st trimester miscarriages 24.3%, ectopic 4%, 2nd trimester miscarriage of 9.7% and intrauterine fetal death of 10.5%.

Currently the only acceptable surgical procedure is hysteroscopic transcervical uterine incision (TCUI), which rests on the principle of surgically expanding the uterine cavity.

Transcervical uterine incision procedure (TCUI) is done using hysteroscopic bipolar electroresectoscope to create new uterine fundus with a width of ≥2 cm . TCUI involves shallow transverse incision over the narrowed fundal part using a wire loop or needle electrode, followed by 4 cm long and 1 cm deep vertical incision over the lateral walls starting at fundal region but taper to stop at the level of the isthmus (Fig. 18.12a–d). Aim is to create an inverted triangular-shaped uterine cavity (Fig. 18.13).

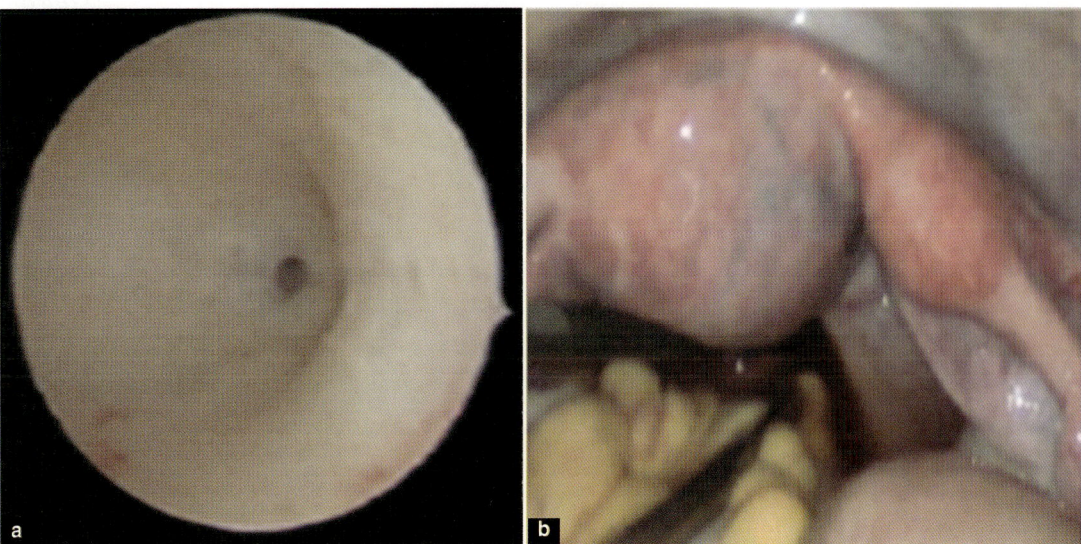

Fig. 18.11a and b: (a) Hysteroscopic view of unicornuate uterus with one ostia; (b) Laparoscopic view of unicornuate uterus with rudimentary

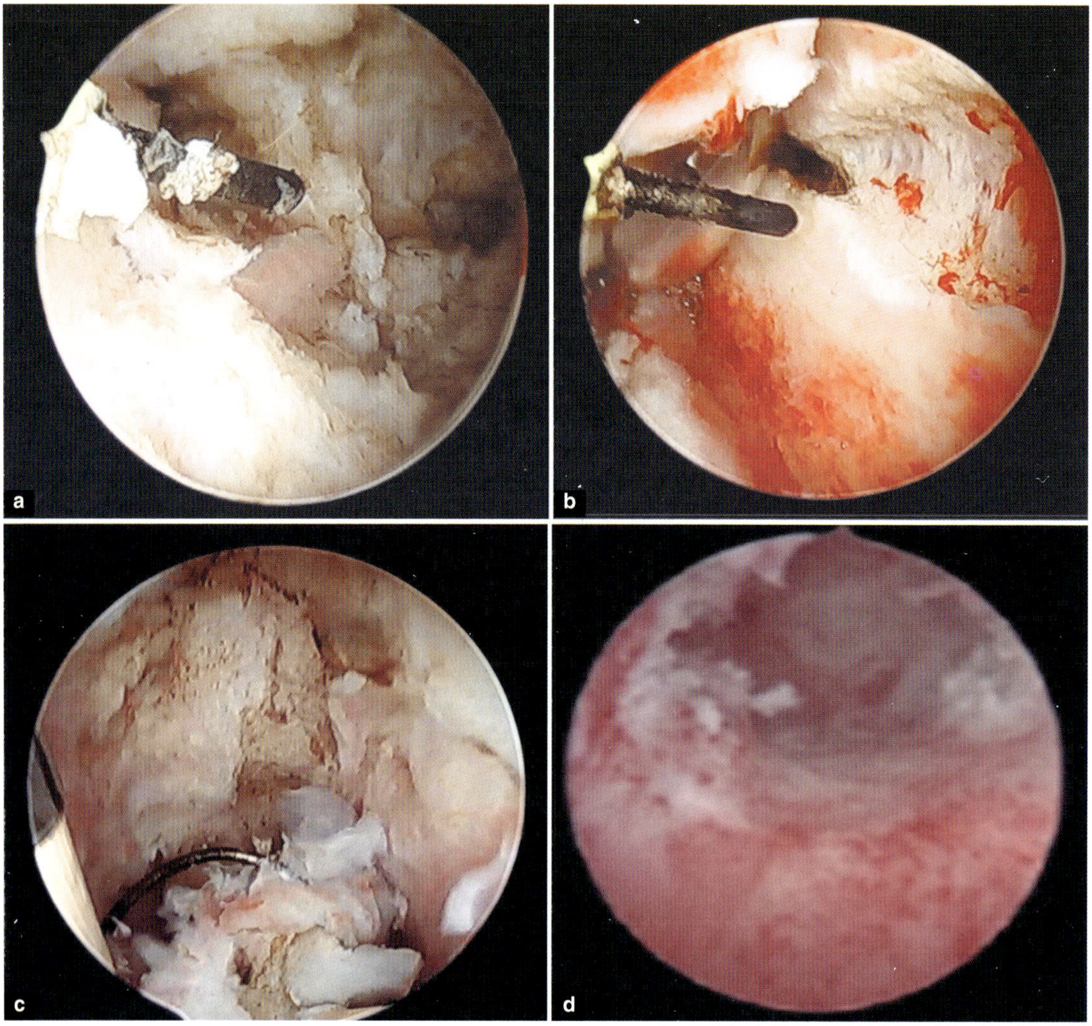

Fig, 8.12a to d: (a and b) TCUI with needle electrode; (c) TCUI with wire loop; (d) Cavity restoration after TCUI

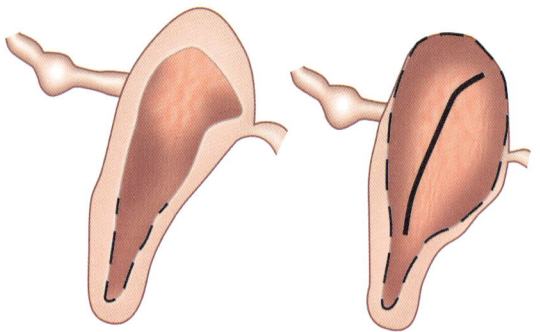

Fig. 18.13: Diagrammatic representation of TCUI

Evidences in Support of TCUI

Xia et al TCUI (33 cases) Chin Med J (Engl). 2017	20 patients conceived and 16 had live birth. Significant reduction in the first-trimester miscarriage rate, increase in term delivery, and live birth rates after TCUI
Mitha M, Manchanda R (India) 2 cases IJSS 2018	Both conceived, delivered vaginally and babies survived

Flowchart 18.1: Management

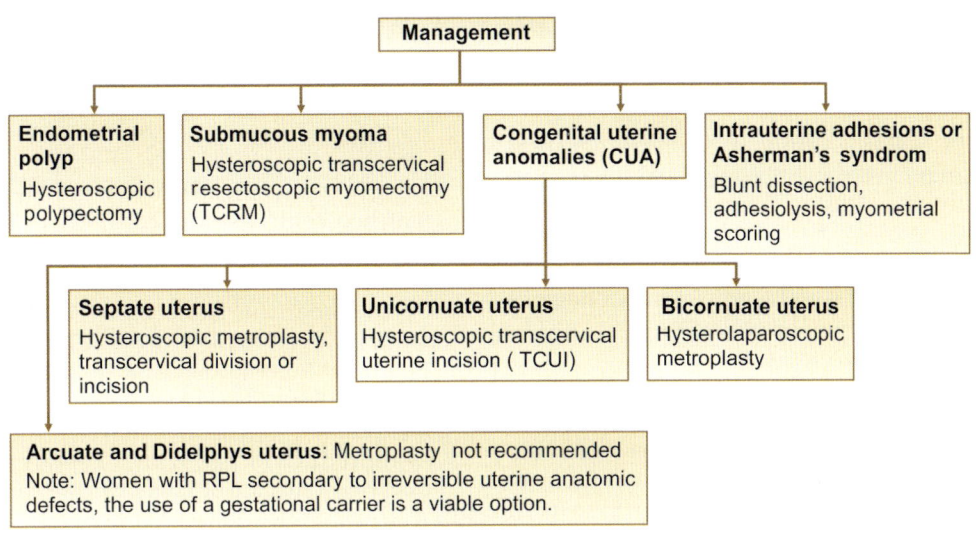

Management

Endometrial polyp	Submucous myoma	Congenital uterine anomalies (CUA)	Intrauterine adhesions or Asherman's syndrom
Hysteroscopic polypectomy	Hysteroscopic transcervical resectoscopic myomectomy (TCRM)		Blunt dissection, adhesiolysis, myometrial scoring

Septate uterus	Unicornuate uterus	Bicornuate uterus
Hysteroscopic metroplasty, transcervical division or incision	Hysteroscopic transcervical uterine incision (TCUI)	Hysterolaparoscopic metroplasty

Arcuate and Didelphys uterus: Metroplasty not recommended
Note: Women with RPL secondary to irreversible uterine anatomic defects, the use of a gestational carrier is a viable option.

Flowchart 18.2: Postsurgery care

Postsurgery care

General care

Specific care
(Corrected anomalies Asherman's adhesiolysis)

- Can resume normal daily activities, next day
- Avoid strenuous activity or sports for 1 week
- Non-steroidal anti-inflammatory drugs (NSAIDS) to control post-operative pain every 6 hours for the first 24 to 48 hours
- Avoid intercourse, douching, soaking in a tub or swimming as bacteria in the water can enter the uterus

Uterine cavity is healed by 2 months postoperatively, so waiting period of 2 months prior to conception is recommended

Antibiotic therapy: Broad spectrum

Adhesion prevention

Solid barriers : Insertion of an IUD without copper wire for 1 month or Foley's catheter for 3 to 10 days

Semi-solid barriers: Auto-cross-linked hyaluronic acid gel

To increase vascular flow to endometrium: Aspirin, nitroglycerine, and sildenafil citrate

Hormonal treatment

For Asherman's

Severity of adhesions	Conjugated estrogen (21 days)	Medroxy progesterone acetate (7 days)
Mild adhesions	0.625 mg BD	10 mg BD
Moderate adhesions	1.25 mg BD	10 mg BD
Severe adhesions	1.25 mg QID	10 mg BD

for CUA

Daily oral dose of 2.5 mg conjugated equine estrogen with or without opposing progestin for 2 or 3 months

References

1. Macklon NS, Geraedts JPM, Fauser BCJM. Conception to ongoing pregnancy: the "black box" of early pregnancy loss. Hum Reprod Update. 2002;8:333–343.

2. Holly B Ford, Danny J Schust. Recurrent Pregnancy Loss: Etiology, Diagnosis, and Therapy Rev Obstet Gynecol. 2009 Spring; 2(2): 76–83.

3. Management of Recurrent Early Pregnancy Loss. Washington, DC: The American College of Obstetricians and Gynecologists; 2001. ACOG Practice Bulletin No. 24).

4. Jan Bosteels Jenneke Kasius Steven Weyers Frank J Broekmans Ben Willem J Mol Thomas M D'Hooghe. Hysteroscopy for treating subfertility associated with suspected major uterine cavity abnormalities. Cochrane Database of Systematic Reviews 21 February 2015.

5. Pérez-Medina T, Bajo-Arenas J, Salazar F, Redondo T, Sanfrutos L, Alvarez P, Engels V. Endometrial polyps and their implication in the pregnancy rates of patients undergoing intrauterine insemination: a prospective, randomized study. Hum Reprod. 2005 Jun; 20(6):1632–5.

6. Stamatellos I, Apostolides A, Stamatopoulos P, Bontis J. Pregnancy rates after hysteroscopic polypectomy depending on the size or number of the polyps. Arch Gynecol Obstet. 2008 May; 277(5):395–9.

7. AAGL Practice Report: Practice Guidelines for the Diagnosis and Management of Submucous Leiomyomas. Journal of Minimally Invasive Gynecology, Vol 19, No 2, March/April 2012.

8. Pritts EA, Parker WH, Olive DL. Fibroids and infertility: An updated systematic review of the evidence. FertilSteril. 2009 Apr; 91(4):1215–23.

9. Shokeir T, El-Shafei M, Yousef H, Allam AF, SadekE. Submucous myomas and their implications in the pregnancy rates of patients with otherwise unexplained primary infertility undergoing hysteroscopic myomectomy: a randomized matched control study. FertilSteril. 2010 Jul; 94(2):724–9.

10. Uterine septum: A guideline. Practice Committee of the American Society for Reproductive Medicine. FertilSteril. 2016 Sep 1;106(3):530–40.

11. Judith FW Rikken, Claudia R Kowalik, Mark H Emanuel, Ben Willem J Mol, Fulco Van der Veen, Madelon van Wely. Septum resection for women of reproductive age with a septate uterus. Cochrane Database of Systematic Reviews 2017.

12. A MadhuMitha, Rahul Manchanda, Sandhya Deora Hysteroscopic Transcervical Uterine Incision/metroplasty—a Novel technique for Unicornuate Uterus–Presentation of two cases. International Journal of Scientific Research Volume-7 |Issue-2| February-2018.

13. En-Lan Xia, Tin-Chiu Li, Sze-Ngar Sylvia Choi, and Qiao-Yun Zhou. Reproductive Outcome of Transcervical Uterine Incision in Unicornuate Uterus. Chin Med J (Engl). 2017 Feb 5; 130(3): 256–261.

14. Sravani Chithra, CH Rahul Manchanda, Nidhi Jain, Anshika Lekhi. 2016. Role of Hysteroscopy in diagnosis of Asherman's Syndrome: A Retrospective Study. International Journal of Current Research Vol. 8, Issue, 05, pp. 31963–31970, May.

Hysteroscopy in Retained Products of Conception

Alonso Luis, Carugno Jose

INTRODUCTION

The terminology retained products of conception (RPOC) refers to the presence of placental and or fetal tissue that remains inside the uterine cavity after the end of the pregnancy. This residual tissue can occur after a spontaneous or induced termination of pregnancy at any gestational age. Other frequently used terminology to describe the retention of placenta or other decidual tissues within the uterus are "placental polyp", "retained placental fragment" and "residual trophoblastic tissue".

The first documented reference that exists in the literature describing the presence of gestational products retained inside the uterine cavity after pregnancy dates back to 1884 when Baer published a case of a patient with a "placental polyp" diagnosed 12 years after pregnancy. Subsequently there have been multiple case reports describing this unfortunate clinical scenario.

DEFINITION

RPOC is defined as the presence of placental and/or fetal tissue that remains inside the uterus after a spontaneous pregnancy loss (miscarriage), planned pregnancy termination, or preterm/term delivery. The presence of RPOC after a spontaneous pregnancy loss distinguishes an incomplete from a complete abortion.

It is estimated that the incidence of RPOC is approximately 0.5% after surgical abortions during the first trimester[1] being more common after medical abortion, increasing its incidence as the gestational age of the termination of pregnancy advances[2] (Fig. 19.1).

Pathogenesis

There are two theories proposed trying to explain the etiology of this condition. The Eastman and Hellman theory supporting that this retained tissue represents a form of abnormal placentation (placental accreta) that

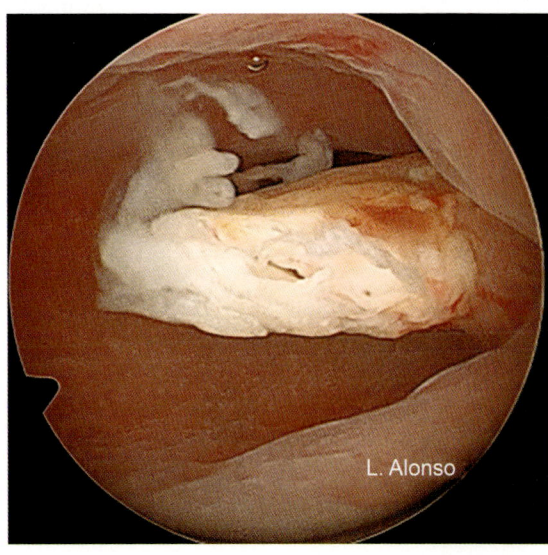

Fig. 19.1: Hysteroscopic view of RPOC

abnormally attaches to the uterine walls contributing to the difficulty of expulsion of the time of pregnancy termination.

The other theory is proposed by Ranney, favoring uterine atony produced at the fundic region and in the utero-tubal region that results in difficulty of expulsion of the retained tissue.

Although two theories have been postulated to try to explain why RPOC occurs, the ultimate cause is yet to be determined. Factors such as uterine contractility, the existence of associated malformations, advanced gestational age or pregnancies achieved through assisted reproduction techniques seem to play an important role in the development of this pathology.[3]

Clinical Symptoms

The symptoms can vary between patients related to the amount of tissue retained, the vascularization of the products and the length of time that has been retained. The main symptom is vaginal bleeding that can range from spotting to heavy vaginal bleeding that can result in acute anemia. Other frequent symptoms are uterine tenderness, pelvic pain and in cases of infection, fever. Significant uterine tenderness, heavy vaginal bleeding, cervical dilation, uterine enlargement, cervical motion tenderness or signs of systemic infection should prompt further evaluation for RPOC.

As a general rule, the presence of RPOC should be suspected in any case presenting with excessive bleeding that occurs after an abortion, miscarriage or delivery (both vaginal and by cesarean section).

Diagnosis

The accurate diagnosis of RPOC represents a challenge since it is considered normal to have some bleeding and discomfort or pain after the termination of a pregnancy, regardless of the week of gestation at which the termination occurs.

The gynecological examination reveals vaginal bleeding coming from the uterine cavity that, as we have mentioned previously, can vary in quantity from mild to massive bleeding. Occasionally, blood clots or debris can be seen protruding through a dilated external cervical os.[4] The bimanual examination helps us to determine the uterine size that is frequently large.

The determination of serologic levels of β-hCG usually has a limited value since it is usually maintained > 5 IU for a few days after the end of pregnancy. It can persist elevated depending on the hormonal activity of the retained products that occasionally does not have hormonal activity.

The presence of RPOC in the uterine cavity is not necessarily associated with positive values of β-hCG in blood. There will only be presence of elevated β-hCG (>5 IU) in blood in cases in which the persistent tissue has hormonal activity, which makes measurement of β-hCG in blood not clinically useful in the diagnosis of this pathology.

Without a doubt, ultrasound is the main imaging modality for the diagnosis of RPOC. The visualization of a mass inside the endometrial cavity is the most important finding in the ultrasonographic diagnosis of RPOC and the absence of debris inside the uterine cavity with the visualization of a thin endometrial stripe excludes this pathology with a predictive value of 100%[5] (Fig. 19.2).

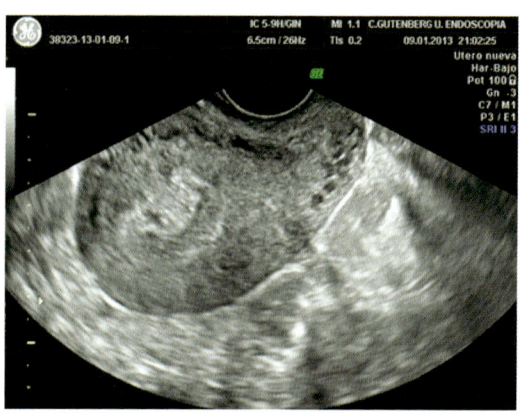

Fig. 19.2: USG showing RPOC

After the delivery of a viable fetus or an abortion, the endometrium undergoes a series of changes that are part of the mechanism of evacuation of the uterus, after this initial period of bleeding, the endometrium is visualized as a linear echogenic structure at 8 weeks postpartum of a viable fetus and between 1 and 2 weeks postabortion.[6] A retrospective study comparing the appearance of the endometrium in patients who underwent evacuation of retained tissue established that an endometrial thickness of 13 mm or greater as the best diagnostic criteria to diagnose the presence of RPOC.[7]

The absence of an intracavitary mass after 8 weeks postpartum or 2 weeks postabortion, rules out the presence of RPOC while an endometrial thickness greater than 13 mm, is considered as a pathognomonic diagnostic criterion for the ecographic diagnosis of this entity.

Occasionally, the retained products have high vascularization, with the use of Doppler technology, this vascularization can be appreciated not only in the retained material but also affecting the implantation area. Some authors argue that the implantation area remains highly vascularized during the postpartum and postabortion period of uterine involution.[5]

Hysteroscopy is considered the gold standard for the diagnosis of intrauterine pathology including gestational retained products. The hysteroscopic appearance of this pathology varies depending on the involution, vascularization and the degree of necrosis of the trophoblastic retained tissue, which results in no single hysteroscopic pattern. This is because the retained tissue undergoes a process of involution over time that makes changes in their macroscopic appearance, so it is important to know the different macroscopic aspects that this pathology presents.

The Gutenberg classification correlates the different ultrasound patterns with the hysteroscopic appearance of RPOC, which allows to anticipate the complexity and degree of difficulty that may be encountered at the time of uterine evacuation.[8]

This classification distinguishes four different patterns of ultrasound characteristics, based on the sonographic appearance of the intracavitary retained products, the intracavitary and myometrial vascularity of the implantation zone. The ultrasound classification distinguishes (Table 19.1):

- **Type 0:** The presence of a bright echogenic intrauterine mass (white), homogeneous and completely avascular.
- **Type I:** Heterogeneous echographic pattern with different echoes and minimally vascularization at intracavitary level.
- **Type II:** Heterogeneous echographic pattern with different echoes and highly vascularized at intracavitary level.
- **Type III:** Heterogeneous echographic pattern with different echoes and highly vascularized areas at both intracavitary and myometrial levels of the implantation zone.

The Gutenberg classification differentiates four ultrasound patterns that are based on retained tissue echogenicity as well as vascularization at both the intracavitary and the myometrial levels. The tissue sonographic

Table 19.1: Gutenberg classification of ultrasonographic patterns of retained products of conception

Type	Intrauterine echogenic mass	Intracavitary vascularization	Myometrial vascularization
Type 0	Homogeneous	No	No
Type I	Heterogeneous	Minimal	No
Type II	Heterogeneous	Highly	No
Type III	Heterogeneous	Highly	Present

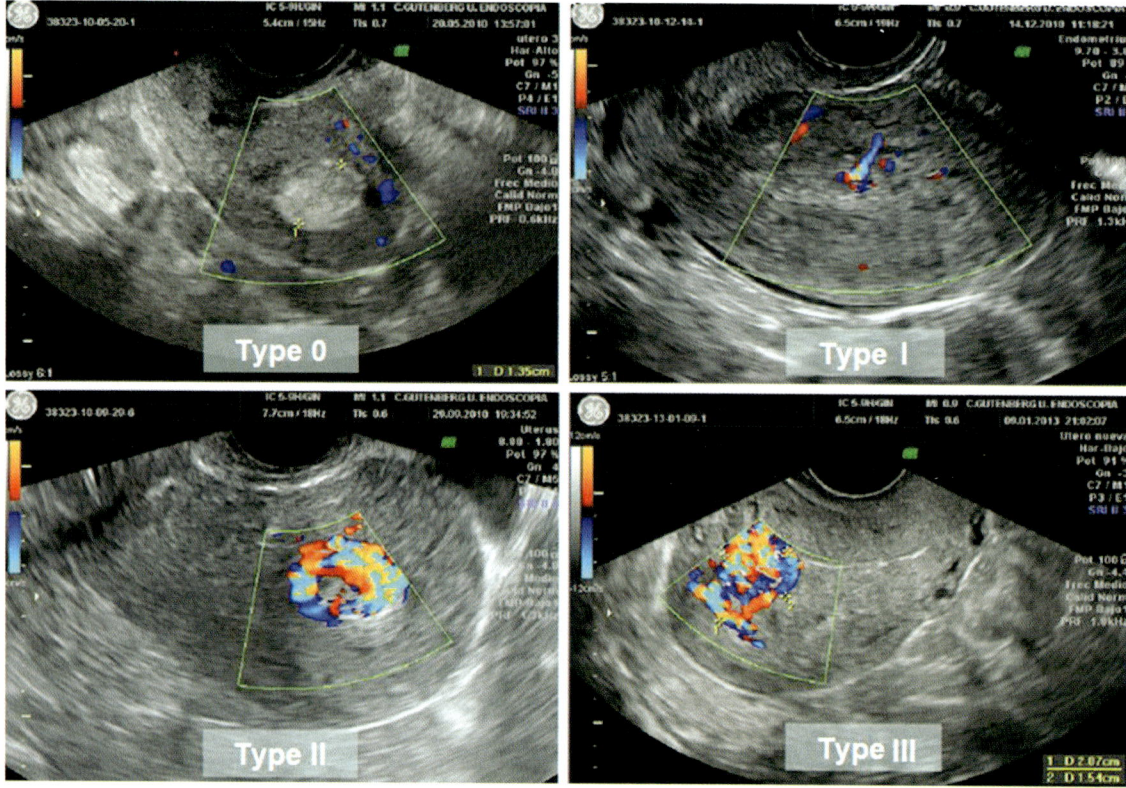

Fig. 19.3: Sonographic appearance of various forms of RPOC

appearance can undergo variations over time due to degenerative tissue modifications (Fig. 19.3).

The echographic patterns above referred have a direct correlation with the hysteroscopic patterns observed in these patients. Thus, the Gutenberg classification also distinguishes four hysteroscopic patterns (Table 19.2):

- **Type 0:** An intracavitary whitish mass is observed in which virtually no structure is defined.

- **Type I:** Chorionic villi are appreciated, well-defined but whitish due to the scarce vascularization of this tissue.
- **Type II:** Vascularized chorionic villi are observed, modifying the color making them reddish.
- **Type III:** The aspect of the chorionic villi is similar to the hysteroscopic pattern of type II, the difference is in the area of implantation of the tissue that presents vascular dilatations, aneurysms and AV shunts.

Table 19.2: Gutenberg classification of hysteroscopic patterns of retained products of conception

Type	Chorionic villi structure	Vascularity	Attachment
Type 0	Not defined	Normal	Loose
Type I	Well-defined avascular (white)	Normal	Focally
Type II	Well-defined vascular (red)	Mild vascular dilatation	Focally some loose and dense attachment
Type III	Well-defined vascular (red)	Severe vascular dilatation, aneurysms and AV shunt	Densely attached

The hysteroscopic patterns are very diverse and have been classified in four types that vary according to the process of involution experienced by the retained products. Except in type 0, in which no known structures are identified, the rest of the types show the presence of identified chorionic villi with different degrees of vascularization (Fig. 19.4).

The definitive diagnosis is established by the identification of chorionic villi in the pathology study of the retained tissue material. These chorionic villi can have a normal structure or present hyaline or necrotic degeneration giving place to the so-called "ghost villi".

Treatment

The treatment is generally dictated by the patient's hemodynamic condition, the gestational age that resulted in RPOC, the amount of product retained and the experience of the physician dealing with the condition.

a. Expectant Management

Expectant management could be considered in women with RPOC clinically stable with no evidence of infection. The reported success rates range from 50 to 85 percent at one to two weeks of follow-up, and up to 90 percent when subjects are followed for six weeks. There is no need to use antibiotic prophylaxis.

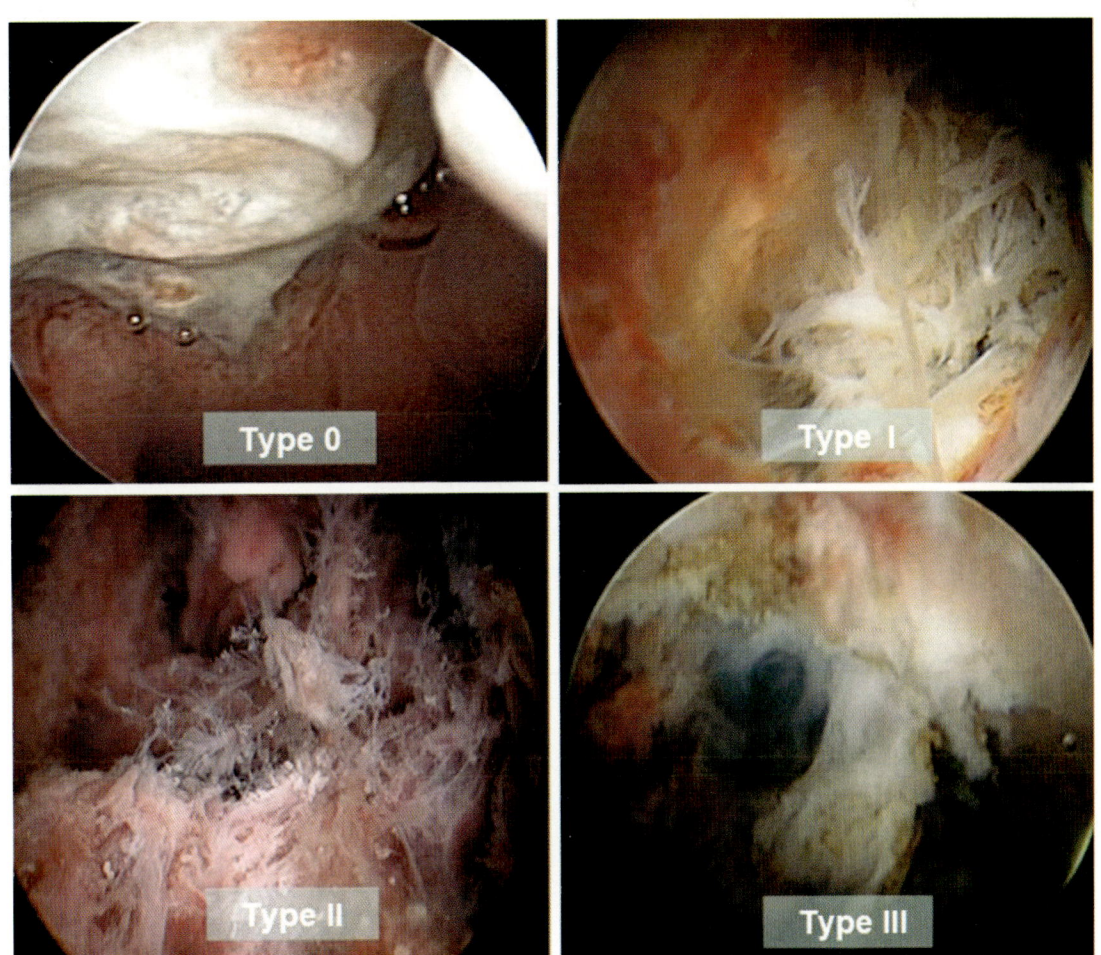

Fig. 19.4: Four types of hysteroscopic patterns

Patients should be counseled about signs and symptoms of infection and treated with antibiotics and surgical evacuation if they develop clinical sign or symptoms of endometritis.[9]

b. Medical Management

Different medical treatments have been described to facilitate the evacuation of RPOC. Misoprostol is one of the most widely used medications and has been shown to be effective in more than 90% of incomplete first trimester abortions. It is a safe and effective drug; the recommended dose for the treatment of incomplete abortions is 600 micrograms orally.[10] The advantages of misoprostol over other drugs (including prostaglandin E2) are safety, low incidence of side effects, low cost, and availability. The risks of complications or side effects are low.

It is reasonable to consider medical management in any stable patient with RPOC. Nonsurgical management may be indicated for women who wish to avoid the risks of a surgical procedure, particularly if they have had prior uterine evacuation and are concerned about uterine injury or synechiae. No trials have evaluated the use of prophylactic antibiotics in non-infected patients undergoing medically-induced evacuation of RPOC. Similarly to patients managed expectantly, women should be counseled about signs and symptoms of infection, and treated promptly with antibiotics if endometritis is suspected.

c. Surgical Management

The physical evacuation of RPOC through the technique of dilatation of the cervical canal and uterine curettage, either with fenestrated sharp curette or by suction with aspiration cannula, continues to be the most widely evacuation method used in clinical practice. Due to the focal nature of the pathology and that uterine curettage is a blind technique, there is risk of incomplete uterine evacuation, which has been reported as high as 20.8% after performing conventional curettage.[11] Moreover, this technique, when performed blindly,

can produce not only an incomplete evacuation but increases the possibility of injury to surrounding healthy endometrial tissue. We must always remember that the RPOC is a focal process. Also, performing a uterine curettage can damage the basal layer of the endometrium favoring the development of intrauterine adhesions or even Asherman's syndrome. The incidence of uterine adhesions in women who undergo repeated curettage for the evacuation of RPOC is reported at 40%, of which the majority (75%) correspond to grade III–IV intracavitary adhesions.[12]

The first report describing the use of the hysteroscope to treat this pathology was in 1984 when Tchabo used the hysteroscope for direct visualization to locate the implantation area of the retained products, extracting them later with hysteroscopoic graspers.[13] Subsequently Goldenberg used the resectoscope with a cutting blade to extract the retained gestational tissue under direct vision, using the handle as a curette and thus avoiding to injury the surrounding healthy tissue.[14]

The extraction of the remains under direct vision allows a greater precision, avoiding the injury of healthy tissue and thus decreasing the possibility of intrauterine adhesion formation. In addition, this technique allows a complete evacuation under direct visualization, so that an incomplete evacuation is extremely unlikely (Fig. 19.5).

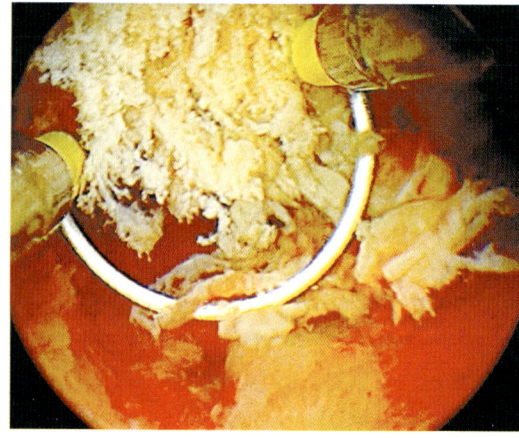

Fig. 19.5: Management of RPOC with resectoscope

Different instruments have been used for the hysteroscopic extraction of the retained gestational products. From the simple use of hysteroscopic scissors and forceps to the latest intrauterine morcellators, which allow an easier removal of residual tissue. It is important to take into account some factors that can increase the difficulty of this technique. In hemodynamically stable patient, there are two very important factors to consider. The size of the remains and especially the vascularization of the tissue and the implantation zone. The limitations in terms of size can be comparable to those use for hysteroscopic myomectomy, so that accumulations of debris over 5 cm in diameter can be difficult to remove in its entirety in a single procedure.

When hysteroscopy is performed in patients with RPOC there is usually also blood and blood clots inside the uterine cavity, so it is advisable to irrigate the uterine cavity suctioning the intrauterine blood and clots to improve intrauterine visualization allowing to identify the area of implantation of the retained products.

The other important factor to consider is the vascularization of the RPOC. Taking advantage of the Gutenberg classification, we can affirm that type 0 and type I RPOC can be extracted easily encountering only minimal bleeding, allowing the safe use of both mechanical (hysteroscopic scissors and grasper), or resectoscope using the loop as a curette or hysteroscopic morcellators.

In cases with increased vascularization (type II), it is frequently needed to perform selective coagulation of the base of the implantation area, since the bleeding that occurs after detaching the tissue from the uterine wall can be copious. Finally, patients with RPOC with profuse vascularization also in the myometrium (type III) require much more careful management, since there are arteriovenous communications and vascular dilatations in the area of implantation that can lead to massive bleeding.

It is important to perform a thorough evaluation of the patient, including ultrasound Doppler evaluation of the uterus before proceeding to evacuate the uterus. The vascularization of the retained tissue as well as the underlying myometrium is the most important factor that can determine the difficulty of the surgery as well as the possibility of associated surgical complications such as profuse uterine bleeding and uterine perforation.

Some authors prefer to delay the surgical intervention in cases of increased vascularization of the retained tissue (type II and type III) since a decrease in vascularization has been observed in both the placental tissue and the underlying myometrium when the intervention is postponed, this decrease in time-dependent vascularization correlates with less bleeding during the surgical procedure.[15]

We strongly recommend performing a second-look diagnostic hysteroscopy between 1 and 2 months after the initial evacuation of the products to ensure the integrity of the endometrial cavity and the absence of intrauterine adhesion formation.

CONCLUSION

Hysteroscopic evacuation of RPOC is a feasible, safe, and effective technique that prevents injury to surrounding healthy endometrium, which clearly reduces the possibility of complications such as intrauterine adhesion formation or incomplete evacuation of products of conception. There are different tools and techniques for removal of RPOC, their use depends on the availability and physician's experience. Any hysteroscopic technique is useful for the extraction of intrauterine retained products of conception, although in cases where there is high vascularization, we recommend the use of the resectoscope provided with energy that allows to selectively cauterize the blood vessels when needed. Special care should be taken with type III RPOC cases, since bleeding can be profuse, increasing the chance of severe complications.

References

1. Hakim-Elahi E, Tovell H, Burnhill M. Complications of first-trimester abortion: a report of 170,000 cases. Obstet Gynecol 1990;76:129–35.

2. Kahn JG, Becker BJ, MacIsaa L, Amory JK, Neuhaus J, Olkin I, et al. The efficacy of medical abortion: A meta-analysis. Contraception. 2000;61(1):29–40.

3. Baba T, Endo T, Ikeda K, Shimizu A, Morishita M, Kuno Y, et al. Assisted reproductive technique increases the risk of placental polyp. Gynecological endocrinology: The official journal of the International Society of Gynecological Endocrinology. 2013;29(6):611–4.

4. Hatada Y. An unexpected case of placental polyp with villi devoid of cytotrophoblastic cells. Journal of obstetrics and gynaecology: the journal of the Institute of Obstetrics and Gynaecology. 2004;24(2):193–4.

5. Durfee SM, Frates MC, Luong A, Benson CB. The sonographic and color Doppler features of retained products of conception. Journal of ultrasound in medicine: official journal of the American Institute of Ultrasound in Medicine. 2005;24(9):1181–6; quiz 8–9.

6. Bar-Hava I, Ashkenazi S, Orvieto R, et al. Spectrum of normal intrauterine cavity sonographic findings after first-trimester abortion. J Ultrasound Med 2001;20:1277.

7. Ustunyurt E, Kaymak O, Iskender C, Ustunyurt OB, Celik C, Danisman N. Role of transvaginal sonography in the diagnosis of retained products of conception. Archives of gynecology and obstetrics. 2008;277(2):151–4.

8. Tinelli A, Alonso L, Haimovich S. Hysteroscopy. Springer International Publishing; 2018.

9. Nanda K, Peloggia A, Grimes D, et al. Expectant care versus surgical treatment for miscarriage. Cochrane Database Syst Rev 2006; CD003518.

10. Blum J, Winikoff B, Gemzell-Danielsson K, Ho PC, Schiavon R, Weeks A. Treatment of incomplete abortion and miscarriage with misoprostol. International journal of gynaecology and obstetrics: the official organ of the International Federation of Gynaecology and Obstetrics. 2007;99 Suppl 2:S186–9.

11. Cohen SB, Kalter-Ferber A, Weisz BS, Zalel Y, Seidman DS, Mashiach S, et al. Hysteroscopy may be the method of choice for management of residual trophoblastic tissue. The Journal of the American Association of Gynecologic Laparoscopists. 2001;8(2):199–202.

12. Westendorp IC, Ankum WM, Mol BW, Vonk J. Prevalence of Asherman's syndrome after secondary removal of placental remnants or a repeat curettage for incomplete abortion. Human reproduction. 1998;13(12):3347–50.

13. Tchabo JG. Use of contact hysteroscopy in evaluating postpartum bleeding and incomplete abortion. The journal of reproductive medicine. 1984;29(10):749–51.

14. Goldenberg M, Schiff E, Achiron R, Lipitz S, Mashiach S. Managing residual trophoblastic tissue. Hysteroscopy for directing curettage. The journal of reproductive medicine. 1997; 42(1):26–8.

15. Hiraki K, Khan KN, Kitajima M, Fujishita A, Masuzaki H. Uterine preservation surgery for placental polyp. The journal of obstetrics and gynaecology research. 2014;40(1):89–95.

Hysteroscopy: Special Concern

Misplaced IUCD: Treating with Hysteroscopy

Haresh Vaghasia, Neha Lalla

INTRODUCTION

Intrauterine contraceptive device (IUCD) is one of the most preferred methods of contraception, especially in developing countries because of its safety, efficacy, easy to administer, longevity, affordability and reversibility.[1]

The first used IUCD was introduced in Germany by Ernst Grafenberg in 1920s. Approximately 150 million women worldwide use IUCD, most commonly in the form of copper IUD, and is second only to female sterilization as the most common form of contraception. Worldwide 13.6% couples use IUCD for birth control, however only 3.3% women use IUCD in India.[2]

Generally it is well tolerated and has very few unfavorable issues; one of which is displaced or lost IUCD. The prevalence of displaced IUCD is 3.6%.[3]

Types of IUCD Displacement

Displacement of IUCD can be classified as follows:

- Primary and secondary—depending upon the time of displacement.
- Partial or complete perforation—depending upon the degree of displacement ranges from embedment in the myometrium to complete transuterine perforation with a migration of the IUCD into the peritoneal cavity.[4]

Primary displacement occurs at the time of insertion, due to various factors as listed.

1. Anatomical Factors

- Atrophic uterus with small cavity in dysmorphic or contracture uteri in conditions like congenital infantalis uterus, PID, tuberculosis, etc.
- Enlarged uterine cavity in case of postpartum or post-abortal insertion.[5]
- Distorted uterine structure due to fibroids, adenomyosis, adhesions or anomalies.[5]
- Insertion in patients with history of previous LSCS displacement may occur in isthmocele or in the weak scar sulcus.

Displacement of IUCD may occur during direct insertion in weak uterine defect/false passage/scar causing partial or complete perforation without much realization as scar tissue being devoid of innervation is insensitive to pain.

2. Technical Factors

- Insertion by the hands of inadequately trained staff personnel.
- Use of inappropriate instruments.

Secondary displacement occurs at a later date, most commonly within first year of insertion due to various factors like:

1. Spontaneous expulsion

2. Fragmentation of device
3. Abnormal displacement due to excessive uterine contractions during menstruation or scarring within the uterine cavity, e.g. isthmocele, previous perforation.
4. Incidental pregnancy
5. Secondary uterine perforation.

Partial displacement or an embedded IUCD is a situation where there is an abnormally positioned IUCD within the endometrium or myometrium; however without an extension through the serosa. An IUCD can become embedded in the wall of the uterus or within the cervix. It may occur in up to 18% of females with an IUCD and is more common in females with smaller fundal endometrial diameters.

Complete perforation with migration of IUCD is a situation where IUCD is away from the endometrium or myometrium with an extension through the serosa perforating the uterus. The incidence rate is reported at ~2 in 1000.[6]

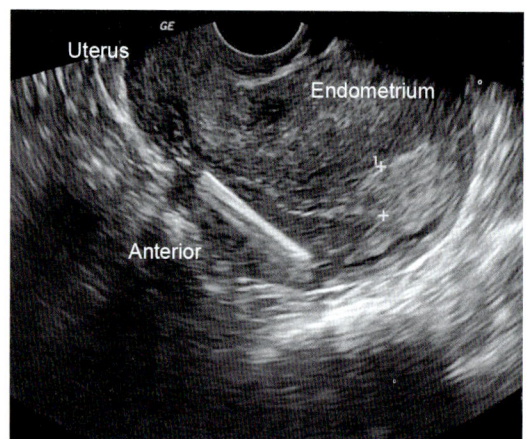

Fig. 20.1: IUCD partly in the false passage (same patient as Figs 20.7 to 20.11)

Clinical Presentation

Patient may present as various combination of the above mentioned classifications, although most patients are asymptomatic and the diagnosis is made either on routine follow-up or with concurrent gynecological conditions and in all cases, the IUCD 'strings' will be missing at direct speculum inspection. Some patients, however, may present with non-specific abdominopelvic pain depending upon the degree of displacement or perforation of uterine wall, infection and associated complications. Other presenting symptoms are irregular vaginal bleeding, abnormal discharge, recurrent UTI and dyspareunia. Peritoneal sepsis is a rare presentation.

Investigation

A transvaginal ultrasound plays key role in diagnosis and is recommended first-line investigation in all women with missing thread.[7] On USG TVS, the IUCD may appear eccentrically positioned in the endometrial

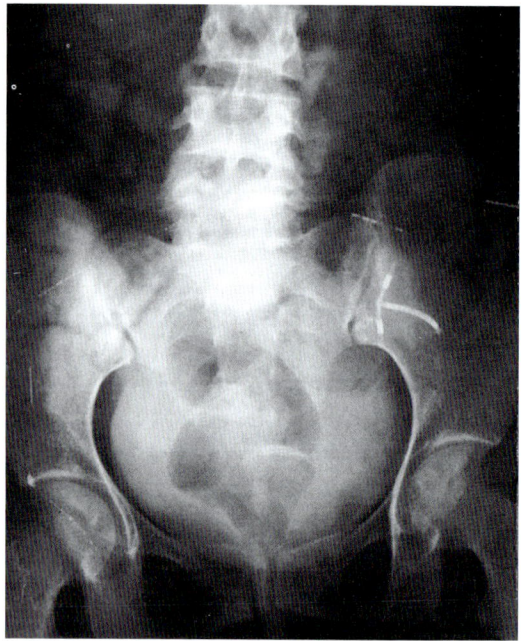

Fig. 20.2: IUCD in the pelvic cavity

cavity or may appear completely separate and away from the endometrium towards the myometrium (Fig. 20.1). However, in case of failure to visualize the IUCD on ultrasound scan, plain radiograph of abdomen and pelvis. AP and lateral views shall be performed preferably with an uterine sound within the uterine cavity as a marker as a second-line investigation. An IUCD lying lateral to midline on X-ray may suggest the diagnosis

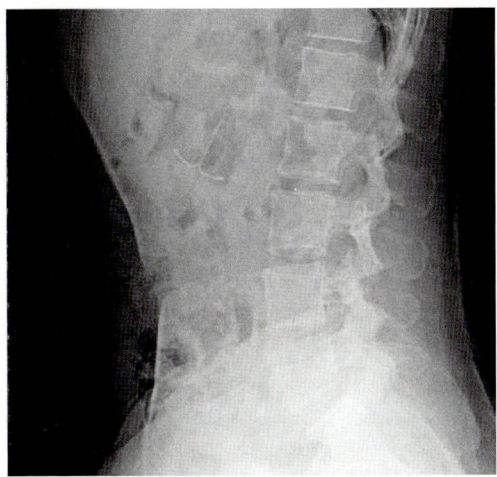

Fig. 20.3: IUCD in the abdominal cavity

of displaced or perforated IUCD (Figs 20.2 and 20.3). CT scan can be used in complex cases where visceral involvement or surgical complexity is suspected.

Treatment: Removal of Displaced IUCD

Misplaced or perforated IUDs should be removed even if considered innocuous, World Health Organization (WHO) has recommended removal of dislocated IUCD as soon as possible irrespective of their type and location.[8] Spontaneous IUD expulsion must be ruled out, when not proven on one modality of investigation. The expulsion rates for copper IUD vary from 1.8% within 2 years to 5% within 36 months.[9] Before deciding on the best method for removal it is necessary to know the type of displacement and the location of the ectopic IUCD.

Irrespective of the symptoms, IUCD must be removed as soon as possible for following reasons;
- To prevent further displacement and probable damage.
- Delay in removal may increase the complexity of the procedure with subsequent increase risk of complications. Numerous studies have shown that the perforated copper IUCDs causes severe peritoneal and omental reaction often than plastic devices.[10]

- All of the above can alter the future outcome.

Hysteroscopy is the "gold standard" for diagnosing and treating-locating, removing IUD. The principle of surgery is "see and treat" as with any other pathology.

Factors attributing complexity to the IUCD removal by hysteroscopy are:
- History of previous uterine surgeries
- Duration of the displacement or loss of thread
- Type of displacement of IUCD.

Surgical plan includes cervical ripening in postmenstrual phase when endometrium is thin allowing good vision, availability of concurrent USG and laparoscopy if needed.

Procedure

The approach can be either with office hysteroscope or conventional operative hysteroscopy. Office hysteroscopy has many advantages, a few of them are as follows: It is a simple, safe, effective, quick, well tolerated, cost-effective, avoidance of anesthesia, hospitalization, etc. Also the office procedure is psychologically well accepted because insertion of the IUCD does not require anesthesia.

While selecting office procedure one must pay attention to reduce the patient's discomfort. Few ideas which would help in a successful outcome are:
- Appropriate preoperative counselling.
- To plan the steps of the procedure before starting the procedure.
- Maintain office ambience peaceful and reassuring.

During the Procedure

- To keep the intrauterine pressure as low as possible ~60 mmHg.
- Avoid disturbing the myometrium by steady and gradual movements.

Office hysteroscopy is far more rewarding as patient appreciates the outcome after watching it herself. The success rate of the office procedure is very good. However, if one fails to remove IUCD in office set up, it still helps the further management. As first step, it helps in determining the complexity of the procedure depending upon the findings.

Technique

Office procedure by rule is carried out by vaginoscopic approach without application of speculum or vulsellum. After the vaginal distension, the cervix is identified and external cervical os is generally noted in posterior fornix. The instrument is then negotiated gently into the endocervical canal and one must observe for any signs of IUCD string or fragments. In case of presence of IUCD in the cervical canal, one must show patience and not to pull IUCD hastily in attempt to remove it out. However, try negotiating the scope in the cavity and trace IUCD completely, note and document the displacement in relation to cavity. This method ensures the successful and safe outcome by removing the complete IUCD without much discomfort to the patient.

Depending upon the displacement type the procedure may be simple or complex and requires varying degree of skills and technical application.

Simple Procedure

In cases of partial IUCD displacement the IUCD may be found loosely lying in the cavity either coiled or inverted with or without presence of the string (Figs 20.4 to 20.6). In the cases where string is still attached, to test the brittleness of the thread, a grasper is used to hold the string and a gentle tug is given. If the thread is strong enough, it will not break. This is the simplest of all cases and one should not attempt holding on to the IUCD limbs as that requires stronger grip and may deteriorate the grasper. Once string is drawn out of the cervix it can be held with convention artery forceps and removed gently.

In case if the thread is absent or friable any attempt to draw it out would be futile. Here,

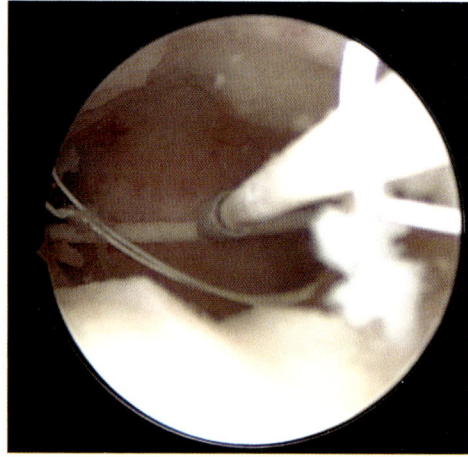

Fig. 20.4: IUCD with string inverted

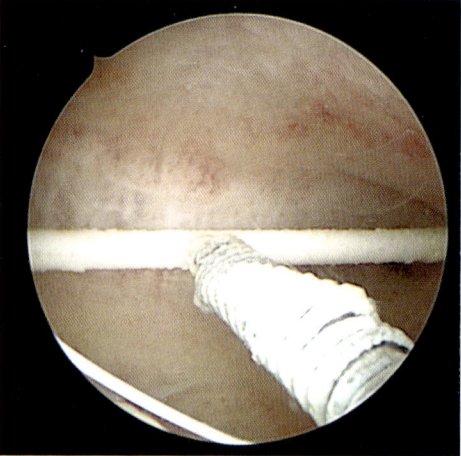

Fig. 20.5: IUCD with string inverted

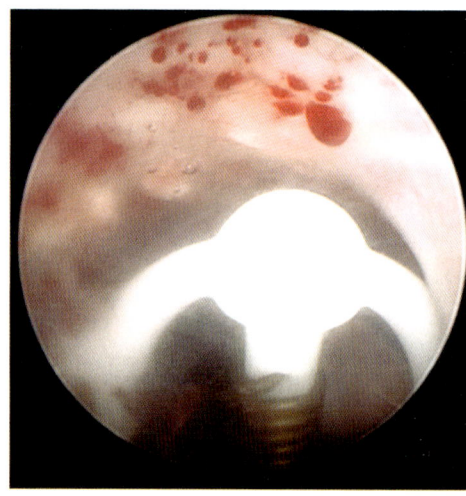

Fig. 20.6: Inverted IUCD with string inverted

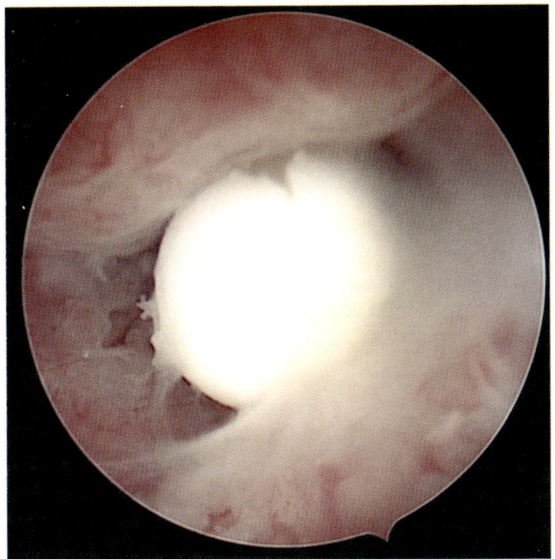

Fig. 20.7: IUCD with missing string (same patient as in Fig. 20.1)

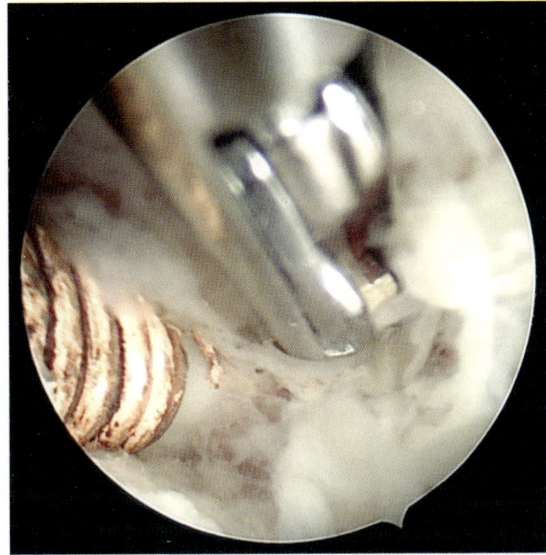

Fig. 20.8: Blunt dissection to release the IUCD

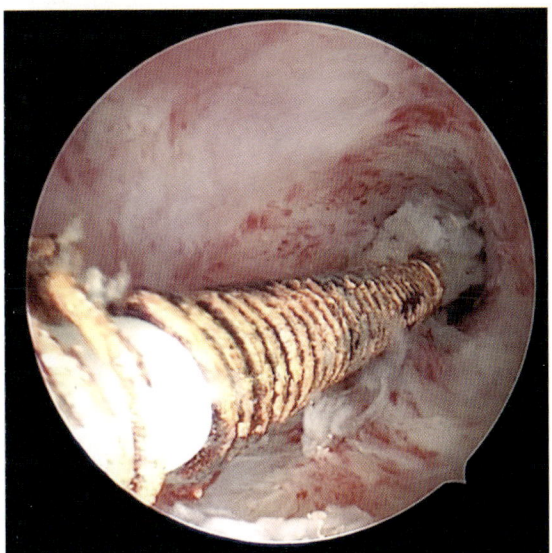

Fig. 20.9: IUCD with folded horizontal limbs (same patient as in Fig. 20.1)

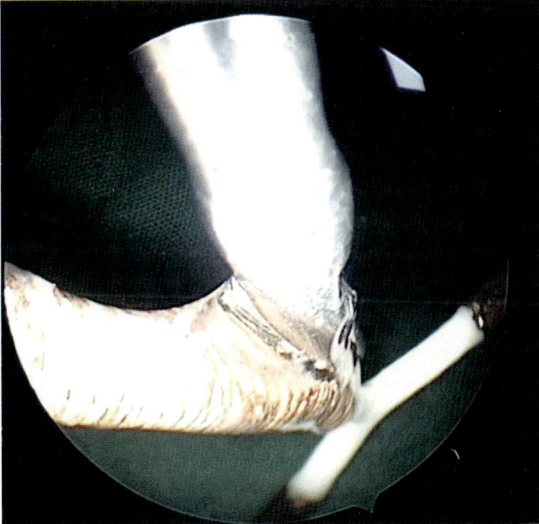

Fig. 20.10: IUCD retrieved completely

if the IUCD is free; the vertical limb can be grasped and gently withdrawn out under vision. The cases with coiled IUCD may require more than few attempts for extraction. The metal may be fragile and may fragment on handling, hence gripping the metal free part of the limb with a small knob generally makes extraction easy.

Complex Procedure

In complicated or complex cases, the IUCD may be found to have various degrees of displacement with other associated complexity, viz. presence of adhesion, fragmentation, coiling and limb embedment in wall or ostium (Figs 20.7 to 20.10).

The basic principle of extraction is to try and lower the grade of complexity by removing

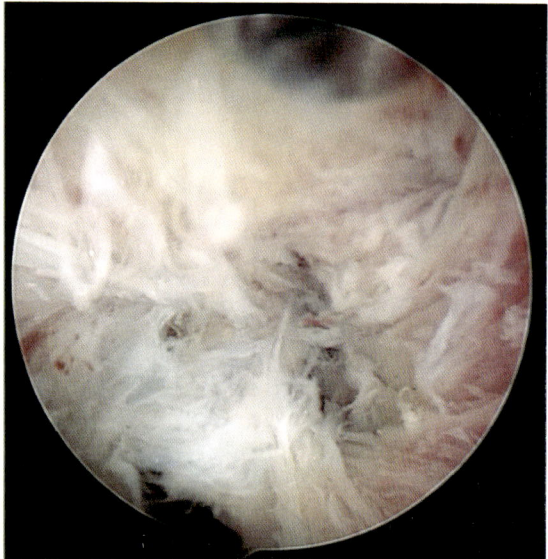

Fig. 20.11: False passage (in the center) where IUCD was displaced and internal os (at 7 o'clock position)

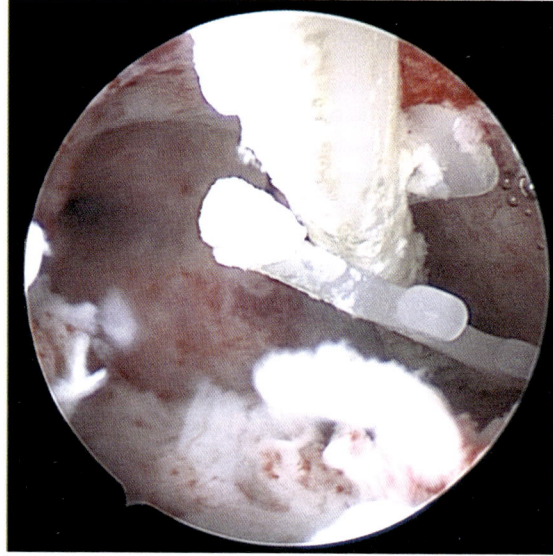

Fig. 20.12a: Multiload IUCD in one cornua with calcification and fins embedded

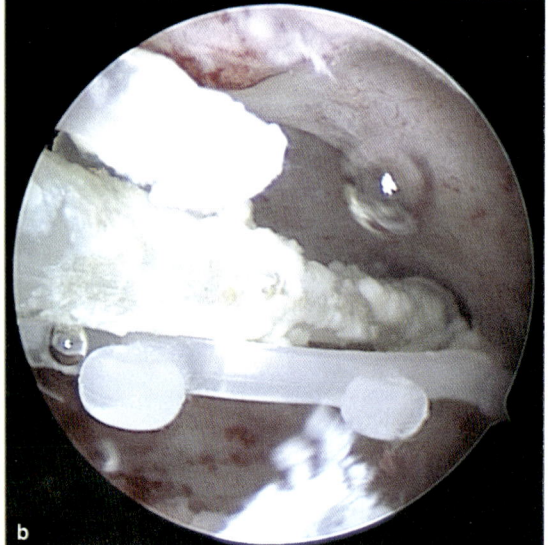

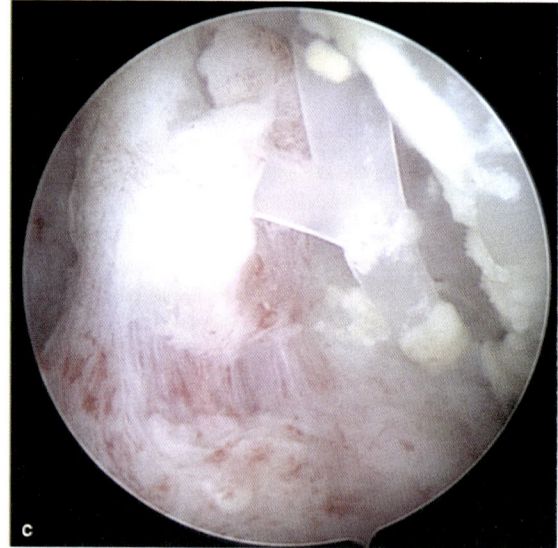

Fig. 20.12b and c: Multiload IUCD in one cornua with calcification and fins embedded

addition factors; like adhesion by adhesiolysis, extricating the embedded limbs off the walls in case of embedded IUCD to free the IUCD (Figs 20.11 and 20.12). Once free, IUCD can be extracted as in simple procedure technique.

Some practical tips which may help operator in accomplishing the task are as follows:

Follow all principles of hysteroscopy, viz. work close to the area of embedment or adhesion, remain oriented by intermittent panoramic view to avoid false passage, follow normal debris and secretion.

To easily locate the residual or missing fragments and completely embedded IUCD, lower the IU pressure and follow the white areas and post-patient in post-menstrual phase.

Small and frequent rotational tugs would aid release of the IUCD with much ease and preventing bleeding.

Always start with blunt dissection using grasper and in case of intense fibrosis use scissors.

Avoid using energy in false passages and deep embedment. Tiny fragments if pose potential risk of perforation may be left behind without much consequences.

After removal, the cavity is reviewed to check any leftover fragments of the IUCD, bleeding, and resultant defects in the endometrial cavity. In cases with deep embedment of IUCD office procedure may not be tolerated and patient may require anesthesia. Sometimes concomitant laparoscopy is very helpful to rule out adhesion with other organs and degree of perforation. This patient may have excessive bleeding at the end due to myometrial cuts, the active bleeders may be coagulated and stopped using bipolar instrument. However, oozing may stop or controlled by tamponade using intrauterine Foleys' catheter no. 8–10 F with 3–4 cc of distilled water instillation.

The cases with complete or near complete perforation must be excluded from hysteroscopic management. However, a basic hysteroscopy in these cases helps planning the extraction at laparoscopy or laparotomy.

CONCLUSION

85 million women worldwide use IUCDs.[11] The incidence of displaced IUCD is higher than documented. Hysteroscopy proves to be gold standard, safe and efficacious in diagnosis and treatment in most cases except the complex or complete perforations.[6] Office hysteroscopy proves superior in making precise quick diagnosis and appropriate treatment.

References

1. Barsual M, Sharma N, Sangwan K. Three hundred and twenty four cases of misplaced IUCD: a five years study. Trop Doct 2003;33:11–12.

2. International Institute for Population Sciences (IIPS), 2010. District level Household and Facility Survey (DLHS-3), 2007-08 : India. Mumbai: IIPS.

3. Niger J Med. 2009 Jul-Sep;18(3):303-5. Missing IUCD string: prevalence, diagnosis and retrieval in Nnewi, Nigeria. Ikechebelu JI1, Onwusulu DN.

4. Boortz HE, Margolis DJ, Ragavendra N, et al. Migration of intrauterine devices: radiologic findings and implications for patient care. Radiographics. 2012;32 (2): 335-52. doi:10.1148/rg.322115068-Pubmed citation.

5. Amirbekian S, Hooley RJ. Ultrasound Evaluation of Pelvic Pain. Radiol. Clin. North Am 2014;52 (6): 1215–35.

6. Harrison-Woolrych M, Ashton J, Coulter D. Uterine perforation on intrauterine device insertion: Is the incidence higher than previously reported?. Contraception 2003;67 (1): 53–6.

7. Caliskan E, Oztürk N, Dilbaz BO, et al. Analysis of risk factors associated with uterine perforation by intrauterine devices. Eur J Contracept Reprod Health Care 2004;8 (3): 150–5.

8. WHO; Mechanism of action, safety and efficacy of intrauterine devices, WHO Technical Report. Geneva; Switzerland, 1987;753.

9. Buckley CH. The pathology of intrauterine contraceptive devices. Current Top Pathol 1994; 86:307–30.

10. McKenna PJ, Mylotte MJ. Laparoscopic removal of translocated intrauterine contraceptive devices, Br J Obstet Gynaecol 1982 Feb;89(2): 163–5.

11. Reinprayoon D. Intrauterine contraception. Curr Opin Obstet Gynecol 1992 Aug;4(4):527–30.

Endometrial Ablation: Role of Hysteroscopy

Rajesh V Darade, Maryam Iqbal, Yousaf Latif Khan, Vinati Kishor Maniar

INTRODUCTION

Endometrial ablation is a minimally invasive gynecological surgical treatment for women with heavy menstrual bleeding who have completed childbearing. It involves the surgical destruction of the endometrium when it is destroyed or resected at the level of the basalis, which is approximately 4 to 6 mm deep, depending upon the stage of the menstrual cycle.

Hysterectomy has traditionally been regarded as the definitive surgical treatment for heavy menstrual bleeding but in spite of a 100% success rate (complete cessation of menstruation) and high levels of satisfaction, it is still a major surgical procedure with possibility of physical complications and also social and economic costs. In the mid-1980s, endometrial ablation techniques with the purpose of removing the entire thickness of the endometrium was introduced as a less invasive surgical alternative to hysterectomy. These led to a rapid decrease in the number of hysterectomies performed.

GENERAL CONCEPTS OF ENDOMETRIAL ABLATION

The endometrium has a great power of re-generation and the basal glands are believed to be the primary foci for endometrial regrowth. To suppress menstruation successfully it is essential to remove the full thickness of this lining, including the deep basal glands together with the superficial myometrium.

PATIENT SELECTION FOR ENDOMETRIAL ABLATION

General Criteria

- No desire for child bearing.
- Documented diagnosis of menorrhagia for benign causes.
- Anatomically normal uterine cavity.
- No obstructive intracavitary uterine pathology.
- Menorrhagia affecting quality of life with failed medical treatment.

Exclusion Criteria

- Desire for future pregnancy.
- Premalignant changes in the genital tract.
- Intrauterine devices in place.
- Congenital uterine abnormalities.
- Active genital or urinary tract infections at the time of procedure.
- Anatomic weakness of myometrium (previous classical incision of cesarean section or transmural myomectomy).

Endometrial ablation is also **relatively contraindicated** in women who are postmenopausal, have congenital uterine anomalies (e.g. bicornuate uterus), have a uterine cavity length that is greater than 10 to 12 cm, or have severe myometrial thinning.

Acute retro or ante flexion or retro or ante version of the uterus are not contraindications to endometrial ablation. In women with these uterine characteristics, incomplete ablation may result if the fundus cannot be reached with a non-resectoscopic ablation device. Thus, resectoscopic ablation may be preferable in this population.

Special Considerations

It is suggested not to perform endometrial ablation in women who are at an increased risk of endometrial cancer like women who are taking *tamoxifen* or have Lynch syndrome.

Women with a preoperative ultrasound suggestive of *adenomyosis* had a 1.7-fold increased risk of subsequent hysterectomy or repeat endometrial ablation.

Nulliparity is not a contraindication to endometrial ablation. *Grand multiparity* appears to be a risk factor for treatment failure.

Endometrial resection should be avoided in women who have a *bleeding disorder* or are taking *anticoagulants*.

PREOPERATIVE EVALUATION

Informed consent: Women who are considering endometrial ablation should be counseled about other medical, interventional radiologic, and surgical options for treatment. It is important to advise women that a successful result is most likely to be a reduction in the volume of uterine bleeding, and amenorrhea is not guaranteed. In addition, endometrial ablation does not regulate bleeding in women with irregular patterns. The risks of persistent or recurrent heavy uterine bleeding and of surgical complications should be reviewed. This discussion should be documented on the surgical consent form and in the medical record.

Evaluation: Preoperative evaluation, including perioperative risk assessment, is the same for endometrial ablation as for hysteroscopy. Pregnancy testing is performed; cervical cultures are appropriate if cervicitis is suspected.

Uterine evaluation

Endometrial sampling: Endometrial sampling is performed in all women prior to endometrial ablation to exclude endometrial hyperplasia or cancer. Ideally, this should be performed with enough time to receive the results and cancel the procedure, if neoplasia is found. However, if sampling has not yet been performed by the day of the procedure, it should be done just prior to the ablation.

Assessment of the uterus: The uterine cavity should be assessed for the presence of intracavitary myomas, endometrial polyps, or other abnormalities (e.g. uterine septum) that may interfere with endometrial ablation. Some lesions can be removed hysteroscopically on the day of the procedure prior to performing the ablation. Women with a history of transmural uterine surgery (e.g. cesarean delivery, myomectomy) should be evaluated for myometrial thinning.

Saline infusion sonography (SIS) or office hysteroscopy can be used to assess the uterine cavity. TVS alone can identify uterine lesions but does not define the contour of the cavity. Alternatively, office hysteroscopy may be combined with transvaginal ultrasound (TVUS).

In women with a large uterus on pelvic examination (>10 weeks size), it is prudent to sound the uterus to assess cavity depth prior to planning an endometrial ablation.

PREOPERATIVE PREPARATION

Cervical preparation is the same as for hysteroscopy.

Endometrial preparation with hormonal agents is used by most surgeons prior to resectoscopic ablation (with the exception of endomyometrial resection) and is also advised by the manufacturers of most non-resectoscopic ablation devices the goal of endometrial preparation is to thin the endometrium to facilitate tissue destruction.

Hormonal suppression with a gonadotropin-releasing hormone (GnRH) agonist (e.g. intramuscular leuprolide 3.75 mg/month) is the most commonly used method of endometrial preparation prior to endometrial ablation. Hormonal pretreatment should be initiated 30 to 60 days prior to the procedure. However, due to the expense, side effects, and delay of surgery, we choose to use ablation techniques that do not require GnRH agonist preoperative thinning (e.g. radiofrequency ablation).

The effectiveness of other hormonal agents for endometrial preparation prior to endometrial ablation is uncertain. Use of progestins (e.g. oral medroxyprogesterone acetate (MPA) 15 mg daily) instead of GnRH agonists offers the advantage of fewer adverse effects (e.g. menopausal symptoms).

There are few data regarding endometrial preparation with estrogen-progestin contraceptives or GnRH antagonists. Non-hormonal methods of preparation include: performing the procedure during the follicular phase of the menstrual cycle and uterine curettage.

TECHNIQUES

A large number of techniques have been developed to 'ablate' the lining of the endometrium.

The **first generation techniques** (laser, transcervical resection of the endometrium using monopolar and bipolar resectoscopes, roller ball) require visualization of the uterus with a hysteroscope and, although safe, require proper fluid monitoring, and depend on operator skill for success.

Over the past decade, a **second generation** of non-hysteroscopic techniques have become dominant, these are technically easier, thereby safer, involve shorter hospital stays and can be performed under local anesthesia.

The first generation ablation techniques have been traditionally acknowledged as the **"gold standard"**. Hence, the methods of endometrial destruction can be classified as:

Hysteroscopic procedures (resection methods): Direct hysteroscopic vision or first-generation techniques. These include monopolar and bipolar loop resection, roller ball ablation and Holmium lasers.

Blind ablation techniques (coagulation methods): Second-generation methods. These include the thermal balloons, cryoablation, microwave ablation radiofrequency and the hydrothermo ablator.

THE FIRST GENERATION ABLATION TECHNIQUES (HYSTEROSCOPIC PROCEDURES)

The endometrium is removed under direct hysteroscopic view either by excision with an electrosurgical loop or by ablating the endometrium with laser or radio-frequency (RF) to produce necrosis of the full thickness of the endometrium. DeCherney and Polan performed the first TCRE with a urologic loop electrode.

NEODYMIUM YAG LASER

The neodymium YAG laser delivers energy through an optical fiber via a specially adapted endoscope, which has a fluid inlet and outlet and a working channel. The activated fiber 600 μm in diameter is methodically drawn over the entire endometrial surface to achieve destruction down to the level of the superficial myometrium. Laser generators are big and expensive and required special training and handling. Use of this technique is confined to centers with laser facilities.

ENDOMETRIAL RESECTION (MONOPOLAR AND BIPOLAR)/TRANSCERVICAL RESECTION OF ENDOMETRIUM (TCRE)

The diathermy loop is used to shave of endometrium up to 7 mm wide and 3–4 mm deep (Figs 21.1 and 21.2).

Instrument Set-up for Resection

The initial descriptions for resection were by using the instruments used for the urological procedures. The electrosurgical generators used monopolar or bipolar. Depending on the type of generator used, the irrigating fluid changes.

Monopolar Resection

This is the traditional resection using the monopolar electrosurgical generator. The current flows from the resectoscope loop through the patient's body and exits through the patient plate or neutral electrode back to the generator. A larger and longer path through the patient's body is traversed. The contact of the patient plate should be larger than 25 cm to avoid exit site burns. The irrigation has to be non-electrolytic (nonconductive) like 1.5% glycine or mannitol 5%. These fluids do not cause dispersion of the current. The active electrode being much smaller than the return electrode, generation of heat is maximum at the active electrode. Generation of the heat at the tissue interface is responsible for effects like desiccation, coagulation and vaporization.

Bipolar Resection

The generators available for bipolar resection is an addition to the armamentarium in the past decade. The active and return electrode are in close proximity and hence the shorter path of current flow through the patients body. The irrigation fluids used for the procedure are electrolytic (conductive) in nature and no patient plate is required. The return path can be through the other stem of the loop, through a special return electrode designed on the loop or through the sheath of the resectoscope. The tissue destruction effects are due to the production of high energy plasma at the tip of the active electrode (plasma kinetic technology). This high energy plasma is seen as an orange glow called the 'corona'.

Advantages of the bipolar technology
- Greater margin of safety as the TURP syndrome produced due to glycine absorption in monopolar resections does not occur. Although the fluid absorption is the same, the hyponatremia does not occur. The hypo-osmolar effects of glycine and hyper ammonemia due to glycine metabolism are obviated.
- There is better hemostasis as the depth of coagulative effect is more.
- Tissue charring is much less compared to the monopolar technology.
- Visibility is better as the refractive index of saline is closer to water than glycine.
- Patients with pacemakers do not get cautery interference.
- The loop has self-cleaning properties as the plasma corona cleans away the tissue and debris sticking to the loop.

INSTRUMENT CART FOR TCRE

An endoscopy cart must carry various electrical devices that have a stable, non-variable power supply, which is properly electrically grounded. The cart carries the following equipment:
- Medical grade monitor for displaying the endovision camera images. Dedicated HD monitors with high resolution are now available.
- Light source like the xenon or LED light.
- Endovision camera. These may be single or three chip. Now HD cameras are becoming more popular.
- Electrosurgical unit, either monopolar or bipolar. The newer bipolar units have the option of switching over to the monopolar technology if desired.

- A pump or hysteromet for distension of the uterine cavity. These are preferred over the routine pressure bags.

The instrument trolley should have the resectoscopy unit (i.e. the resectoscope sheath, working element, telescope), light cable, high frequency cord and the proper loops required for resection. Routine gynecology instruments like the speculum, tenaculum and a set of Hagar's dilators should be available.

Anesthesia regional anesthesia (spinal or epidural) is the preferred anesthesia. However, the procedure can also be performed under general anesthesia or paracervical block with deep sedation.

Cervical dilation: This is done usually mechanically using the Hegars dilators. Cervical dilation may be difficult in nulliparous women, prior cesarean sections and cervical stenosis. Misoprostol, a synthetic prostaglandin El analogue (200–400 microgram 6 hours before the procedure) may be administered orally or intra-vaginally for cervical ripening.

Fluid absorption: This needs to be monitored closely as the risk of absorption and the resultant volume overload is poorly tolerated by elderly patients and patients with poor left ventricular function. Monitoring the inflow and the outflow can readily do this. Ideally in each case, a maximum allowable fluid absorption limit (MAFA limit) should be calculated. This is done by the formula MAFA limit = 17.6 mL/kg. Adhering to this limit does not let the hyponatremia go beyond 10 mEq/L.

Operative Procedure

The resectoscope is inserted in the uterus as atraumatically as possible. The dilatation should be gentle so that the visibility inside the uterine cavity is pristine. The irrigation pump helps in distending the uterine cavity. The degree of distension can be adjusted by altering the outflow channel. Partially closing the channel distends the cavity. Irrigation pressure of 100–110 mmHg and flow rate setting of 200–400 ml/min on the pump gives adequate visibility inside the uterine cavity. The electrosurgical generator is set to a pure cut mode of 80–90 watts and coagulation to 50–60 watts. It is prudent to check the settings with the settings chart provided with the machine.

The resection can be performed in either of the following ways:

- **Fundus first:** Where the resection is begun near the cornu. Either a circumferential resection at tubal ostium or proceeding cornu to cornu.
- **Walls first:** Strips are taken from the anterior, posterior and lateral walls and the intervening ridges are then smoothened by taking additional chips. The four cardinal strips are removed separately and can be helpful in localizing and lateralizing the pathology.

The chips should be at least 3 mm deep. The superficial 1–2 mm of myometrium should be included to ensure a complete ablation of the deep basal glands of the endometrium. The resection should end at the internal os. Chips collecting inside can obscure the view.

Adequate hemostasis should be confirmed prior to the termination of the procedure. The 3 mm ball electrode is useful to run over the resected area to achieve deeper coagulation and hemostasis.

Technological Advances

- The bipolar technology by Olympus has the 'mushroom or button electrode,' which vaporizes the endometrium similar to a laser. The technique is relatively easy to master, but does not provide tissue or histological examination
- The small resectoscope: System 22 by Schoelly. The standard resectoscope is 26 F and sometimes difficult to insert in patients with cervical stenosis. The system 22 is a complete resectoscope set with the outer sheath size of 22 E. The telescope is 2.3 mm. This set has its own working element and

loops. The resultant chip size is proportionately smaller and hence the procedure takes a longer time.

Complications of TCRE

Immediate Complications

- **Fluid overload and TUR syndrome:** Hyponatremia fluid overload and glycine toxicity are the hallmark of this syndrome. Strict monitoring of the inflow and outflow is mandatory. The resection time should be limited in patients with prior low sodium levels. Administration of furosemide and saline to tackle fluid overload should be a standard practice.
- **Cervical trauma:** Ecto- or endocervical lacerations.
- **Uterine perforations and rupture:** The incidence is less than 2%. These occur half the time on insertion of the scope and in half the patients during the resection. Uterine rupture occurs only if there is gross myometrial thinning and occurs at the site of previous scars. Perforation should he immediately suspected when the endometrial cavity collapses around the hysteroscope creating a compromised view of the uterine cavity.
- **Bleeding (0.8–4%):** This can occur intraoperatively or postoperatively. Intraoperative bleeding can be tackled using the roller ball with coagulation setting of 30–40 Watts. Sometimes, the control of bleeding may be done by inserting specially designed balloons. The balloon is placed in the uterine cavity and inflated to tamponade the uterine wall. A 8 or 10 no. Foley's catheter may used for the same purpose. The balloon should be kept in place for 6–8 hrs and then partially deflated for 6 hrs. Delayed postoperative bleeding may occur.
- **Infection:** Incidence is less than 1% and can he avoided with giving proper broad-spectrum antibiotic cover.
- **Air embolism:** The sources of the air are gaseous products of resection or room air. Steep Trendelenburg position should be avoided and gas bubbles should be sucked out. Careful dilation prevents opening of the venous channels and avoids this problem.
- **Postablation tubal sterilization syndrome:** Some women who have undergone tubal ligation prior to endometrial ablation experience cyclic or intermittent pelvic pain. The proposed etiologies of this are: (1) bleeding from active endometrium that is trapped in the uterine cornua and/or (2) uterine contracture and intrauterine scarring. The incidence of this complication is as high as 10% in some reports.

Late Complications

Cervical stenosis can lead to hematometra. This is seen in 1–2% cases.

ROLLERBALL ENDOMETRIAL ABLATION

Hysteroscopic resection required different, newer surgical skills, which made the procedure technically challenging. In the late 1980s, rollerball endometrial ablation was introduced as an easier to perform alternative to endometrial resection. The same basic equipment was used, the only difference being that the energy was delivered through a ball electrode rather than a loop, dispersing the current over a wider area. The ball is drawn methodically over the entire endometrial surface achieving destruction to a depth of 4–5 mm. The 3 mm diameter of the ball electrode enables the procedure to be quicker than the laser or resection loop. The ball is also good fit for the uterine cornu making it potentially safer than the loop.

Advantages claimed for the loop over roller ball include the ability to deal with polyps or fibroids and its effectiveness for thicker, unprepared endometrium. The removed chips also provided a specimen for histological examination.

A combined technique evolved in which the ball electrode was used for the fundus and cornu, and loop resection was carried out for the remainder of the endometrium.

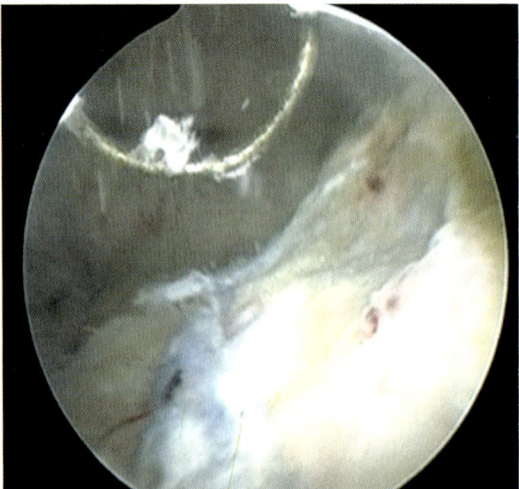

Fig. 21.1: Ablation with loop

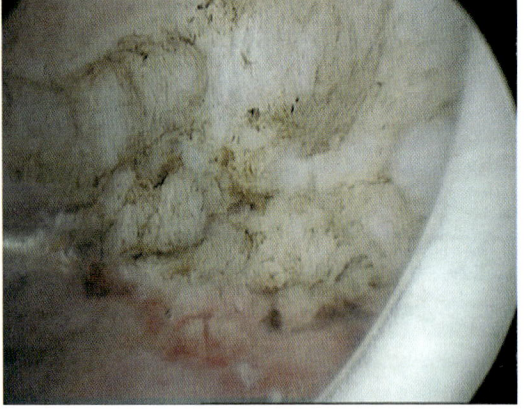

Fig. 21.2: Ablation in process

Outcome

Varies with age of the patient and length of time from when the procedure was performed.

Subsequent surgery
- The overall rate of subsequent surgery following all types of endometrial ablation ranges from 17 to 25%.
- Women who are less than 45 years old at the time of endometrial ablation appear to be at a higher risk of treatment failure than older women. The risk of subsequent hysterectomy or repeat ablation was two-fold in women less than 45 years old versus those 45 years or older (54 versus 27 percent in one study).

- Long-term failure of endometrial ablation may be up to 40% of women who undergo endometrial ablation under the age of 40.

Non-resectoscopic versus resectoscopic ablation: Non-resectoscopic and resectoscopic endometrial ablation result in comparable rates of amenorrhea and patient satisfaction. Resectoscopic endometrial ablation is associated with more frequent use of general anesthesia, a longer operative duration, and an increased risk of some surgical complications (e.g. irrigation fluid overload). Technical skill requirements are another potential barrier to the use of resectoscopic ablation, since, currently, many surgeons are less experienced with these techniques. Resectoscopic techniques are less costly per procedure than non-resectoscopic ablation.

Improvement in bleeding symptoms: Women may experience irregular bleeding following endometrial ablation, so the success of the procedure cannot be determined until 8 to 12 weeks postoperatively. Most women with successful ablation will have a reduction in uterine blood and 50% have amenorrhea. Many women have improvement in dysmenorrhea.

Patient satisfaction: Patient satisfaction rates were high for both types of ablation at one year (91 versus 88%, or 1.2, 95% CI 0.9–1.7)

Complication rates: The following perioperative complications were significantly less likely following non-resectoscopic compared with resectoscopic ablation: Irrigation fluid overload (0 versus 0.3%, OR 0.2, 95% CI 0.04–0.8), hematometra (0.9 versus 2.4%, OR 0.3, 95% CI 0.1–0.9), and cervical laceration (0.2 versus 2.2%, OR 0.2, 95% CI 0.1–0.6).[81] In addition, the rate of uterine perforation was lower, though this was not statistically significant (0.3 versus 1.3%, OR 0.3, 95% CI 0.1–1.0).

Cost: Non-resectoscopic endometrial ablation devices are generally more expensive than the resectoscopic instruments used for rollerball ablation or wire loop resection. In addition, non-resectoscopic procedures are more commonly performed under local anesthesia and/or in an office setting, which have lower procedural costs.

Follow-up

Routine postoperative care

- Patient is advised avoiding intercourse, tub bathing, and use of tampons for a week.
- Women can resume work 2 to 3 days following the procedure.
- Most patients need NSAIDs for 2 to 7 days post-procedure.

The most common post-operative side effects of endometrial ablation are cramping and vaginal discharge. Light vaginal bleeding or pink-tinged discharge is often present for two to three days. Uterine cramping may persist for 24 to 72 hours. Most women can resume normal activities in one to three days.

Counsel patients to contact if they have severe or persistent pelvic pain or vaginal bleeding or low grade fever or foul smelling discharge. Patients must be counseled about the need for contraception.

Tips and Tricks

- Treatments should only include the endometrium and avoid treating the cervix, to minimize the development of central hematometra. Treat only the lower uterine segment.
- Comprehensive prep imaging with saline infusion sonography, hysteroscopy, or MRI. Do not rely on endometrial biopsy alone without imaging. It is important to exclude intracavitary pathology such as endometrial polyps, intracavitary fibroids, endometrial hyperplasia or malignancy.

- Counsel patients regarding the need for lifelong contraception as ablation is not a method of contraception.

Pregnancies have been reported up to one decade after endometrial ablation can be complicated and associated with prematurity, postpartum hemorrhage, retained products of conception, ectopic pregnancy, and death.

- Re-evaluate the patient who presents months or years later after ablation with pain, even in the absence of menstruation as patients may develop central uterine hematometra, cervical stenosis, retrograde endometriosis, or cornual hematometra, and present with chronic or cyclical pain. Evaluate with pelvic imaging such as TVS or MRI.
- Recurrence of heavy menses after endometrial ablation, should be offered conservation medical therapy or minimally invasive hysterectomy. Avoid offering a repeat endometrial ablation, as serious complications have been reported in patients who have been treated with another endometrial ablation including: Uterine perforation, hemorrhage, excessive fluid absorption, and genital tract burns.

Bibliography

1. DeCherney AH, Polan ML. Hysteroscopic management of intrauterine lesion and intractable uterine bleeding. Obstet Gynecol 1983;61:392–397.
2. Fawaz E, et al. Resectoscopic surgery may be an alternative to hysterectomy in high risk women with atypical endometrial hyperplasia. Journal of Minimally Invasive Gynecology 2007;14:68–73.
3. https://www.ncbi.nlm.nih.gov/pubmed/9093249
4. Magos AL, et al. Transcervical resection of endometrium in women with menorrhagia. Br Med J 1989;298:1209–1212.
5. www.ncbi.nlm.nih.gov/m/pubmed/1495687/

Hysteroscopic Markers in Endometrial Tuberculosis

Alka Kumar, Atul Kumar

Genital tuberculosis is a major cause of infertility in developing countries. Tripathi and Tripathi stated that genital tuberculosis is mostly a secondary manisfestation of primary TB, the most common primary site being the lungs.[1] They reported that the genital tract is vulnerable to this disease after puberty, and most cases occur during the child bearing period.

Genital tuberculosis (GTB) is a disease of no symptoms or masquerades as other gynecological conditions. Most of the times, TB is diagnosed while evaluation of infertile patient. In genital tuberculosis, tubal and endometrial involvements are so common that spontaneous pregnancy is practically not possible. Hysteroscopy has become instrumental in real sense in diagnosing and treating endometrial tuberculosis.

The mode of spread is usually hematogenous or lymphatic and occasionally occurs by the way of direct contiguity with intra-abdominal or peritoneal focus.[4,5] The focus in the lungs often heal and the lesion may lie dormant in the genital tract to reactivate in later life. The term extrapulmonary tuberculosis (EPTB) is used to describe isolated occurrence of TB at sites other than lung. It is estimated that 5–13% of all pulmonary TB patients develops genital involvement.

Endometrial tuberculosis tends to manifest as infertility and or lower abdominal pain. Endometrial tuberculosis may have severe reproductive consequences on fertility in spontaneous as well as *in vitro* fertilization cycles. The consequences of GTB are infertility: It is the commonest presentation of GTB (40–80%) among genital TB cases responsible for both primary and secondary infertility.

- Blockage of tubes, tuberculous endosalpingitis, perisalpingitis, causing loss of tubal functions, adhesions, and TO masses
- Ovarian affection causing anovulation, ovarian abscess, and destruction
- Tubercular endometritis causing
  - Synechiae
  - Granular ulcerative lesions
  - Ostial fibrosis
  - Obliteration of endometrial cavity.
  - Changes in immunocompetent LGL (large granular lymphocytes) in endometrium results in inflammation which disturbs the cytokine balance because of TH 1 dominance resulting in inhibition of trophoblast invasion and implantation failure in miscarriage.

Reproductive failure: Conception is difficult in the presence of genital tuberculosis and when it occurs, it is complicated by abortion or an extrauterine location which results in ectopic pregnancy.

Tubercular endometritis: This is a type of chronic endometrial inflammation which affects the receptivity of endometrium. So even a good quality embryo fails to implant because of inherent problems within the endometrium. In GTB, endometrial receptivity is affected in three ways: (a) Adverse impact on immunophysiologic "markers" or molecules; these molecules are essential to make the endometrium receptive for embryonic implantation. (b) Disordered vascularization of the endometrium by immunomodulatory mechanism causing vascular thrombus formation, activation of antiphospholipid antibodies, reduction of subendometrial blood flow by tubercular involvement of the basal layer of endometrium through hematogenous spread via basal endometrial artery. (c) Atrophy of endometrium and synechiae formation.

Being a paucibacillary disease, demonstration of *Mycobacterium tuberculosis* is not possible in all cases. Various blood tests, non-specific tests, serological (e.g. PCR), sono-radiological investigations like USG, HSG, and MRI tried to diagnose this disease.

Ultrasonography (USG): USG has a very limited role in diagnosis of endometrial TB. But some findings on transvaginal sonography (TVS) raise the suspicion of TB. The findings can be endometrial synechiae, fluid collection in endometrial cavity, irregular endometrium, less or no endometrial growth in response to growing follicle in ovulation study. Doppler studies may show low uterine artery perfusion and high resistive index at the time of hCG trigger and embryo transfer.[13]

Hysterosalpingography (HSG): It is a very useful procedure for evaluating the internal architecture of the uterine cavity. In cases of intrauterine synechiae, it helps in knowing the contour, irregularity of the uterine cavity. Previous hysterosalpingography really guides us in very bad cases of uterine synechiae while performing hysteroscopy.

- In endometrial TB, the synechiae and intrauterine adhesions are characteristically irregular, angulated, and stellate-shaped with well-demarcated borders.
- Unilateral scarring may cause obliterations of uterine cavity on one side giving rise to a pseudounicornuate uterus.
- Scarring in TB may result in conversion of triangular uterine cavity into a T-shaped cavity. An asymmetric small sized uterine cavity is usually due to TB.[2,3]

Many past studies have considered fluid hysteroscopy to be a reliable and useful examination for investigating endometrial tuberculosis.[6–13]

Hysteroscopy is a useful modality in diagnosing endometrial tuberculosis. Classical hysteroscopic findings of endometrial tuberculosis is a rough dirty looking bizzare pale endometrium with gland openings not seen and with with overlying whitish deposits[6–10,12,13] and adhesions (Fig. 22.1). However, all of these signs may not be seen in the same case or their intensity may vary. In order to reach to a diagnosis all the markers of tuberculosis have to be carefully evaluated. Whitish deposits are the most pathognomic of tuberculosis however they may not be always be seen especially since the superficial layer of the endometrium sheds every 28 days and along with the

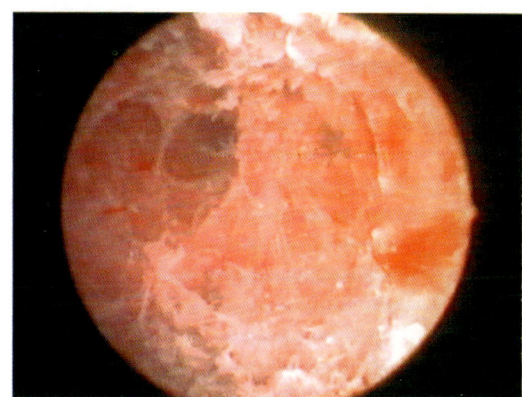

Fig. 22.1: A bizzare pale scarred thin dirty-looking endometrium with whitish deposits and flimsy adhesions, and with no endometrial gland openings visible

endometrium the said deposits also shed.[14] Hence the best time for conducting hysteroscopic examination is in the premenstrual phase so that any overlying deposits are not missed out. A classical endometrial deposit under high magnification is seen in Fig. 22.2. Large tubercles are also often seen (Fig. 22.3). The confirmation of diagnosis of tuberculosis was made by PCR and BACTEC culture.

The hysteroscopic markers of endometrial TB are:

1. Bizare endometrial architecture
2. Tubercular deposits (microscopic to large macroscopic structures)
3. ILL defined endometrial gland openings
4. Adhesions/synechiae

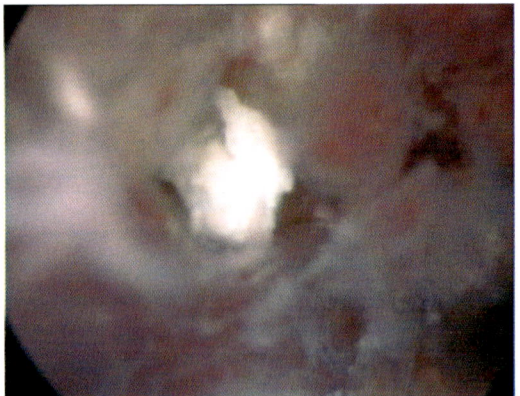

Fig. 22.2: A solitary endometrial tubercular deposit seen under high magnification

Endometrial scarring is one of the pathognomic features in endometrial tuberculosis especially if whitish deposits overlying the endometrium are also seen. Endocervical scarring is also frequently seen in endometrial tuberculosis.

In endometrial tuberculosis intraluminal adhesions in the interstitial part of the fallopian tube can often viewed at hysteroscopy by placing the microhysteroscope tip very close to the tubal orifice and viewing with a source magnification of 25X.[8]

At times the whitish deposits do not overly the endometrium and instead they are anchored to flimsy adhesions by being impregnated in the same[9] (Fig. 22.4). These flimsy adhesions are not shed with menstruation hence the impregnated deposits are seen even in the postmenstrual phase.

In some cases, the whitish deposits are not seen over the endometrium at hysteroscopy. Such deposits are seen after vital staining with methylene blue dye. In such cases, the hysteroscope is removed and chromopertubation is done with methylene blue dye, followed by reintroduction of the hysteroscope. Glistening white, highly reflective deposit situated are observed against the background of a dark blue-stained endometrium resembling a "starry sky" appearance[9] (Fig. 22.5). We have observed the starry sky appearance and used

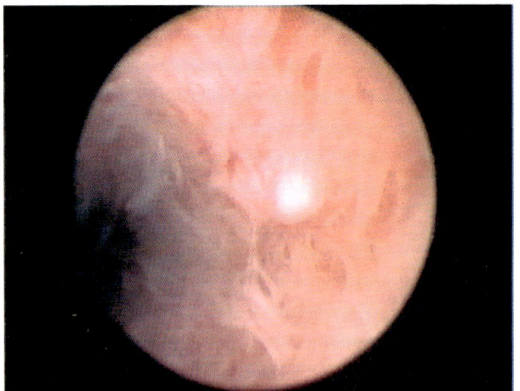

Fig. 22.3: A whitish tubercle is present over the scarred left lateral wall of the endocervical canal

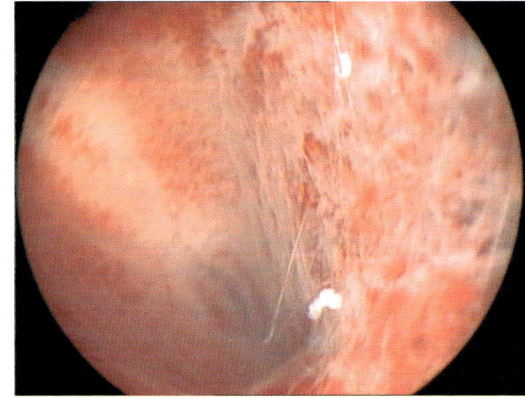

Fig. 22.4: Tubercular deposits impregnated over flimsy adhesions

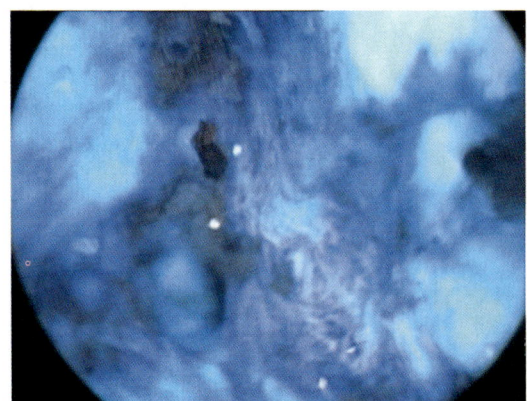

Fig. 22.5: Starry sky appearance over the anterior uterine cavity wall

it to diagnose endometrial tuberculosis on multiple occasions over a 21-year period. It appears that the methylene blue dye is not taken up by the caseous tubercular deposit but is taken up by the surrounding endometrium. The unstained caseous deposit reflects white light in contrast to the surrounding dark blue endometrium, thereby giving a starry sky appearance.

At times panoramic hysteroscopy with 1X magnification using a conventional telescope (27005 BA; Karl Storz GmbH and Co., Tuttlingen, Germany) reveals an endometrium unremarkable except for subtle scarring, which could also be overlooked. The endometrium is next visualized using a Hamou Micro-Hysteroscope II (26157 BT; Karl Storz)[8,11] in the panoramic view at 20X at-source magnification, which reveals a rough-looking endometrium as though it had been sprinkled with a coarse whitish powder. The endometrial surface is bumpy, with diffusely scattered small conical papillary projections, and no endometrial glands are observed.[11] Herein the term 'at source magnification' relates to the magnification provided by the telescope and not by the video mechanism of the telescope.

Hysteroscopic visualization of the endometrium after antitubercular therapy often shows an improvement in the mucosal morphology. A closer visualization at increased magnification is helpful in demonstrating the remnants of a healing tubercular pathology after antitubercular therapy.[10] Relook hysteroscopy after anti-tubercular therapy guides the surgeon towards prognosis and results of anti tubercular therapy.

References

1. Tripathi SN, Tripathi SN. Endometrial tuberculosis. J Indian Med Assoc, 85:136, 1987.
2. Jahromi BN, Rarsanezhad ME, Ghane-Shirazi R. Female genital tuberculosis and infertility. Int J Obstet Gynecol. 2001;75:269–72.
3. A. Tinelli et al. (eds.), Hysteroscopy. PP665–676.
4. Schaefer G. Female genital tuberculosis. Clin Obstet Gynecol. 19:223, 1976.
5. Siegler AM, Kontppoulous V. Female genital tuberculosis and the role of hysterosalpingography. Semin Roentgenol. 14:295, 1979.
6. Kumar A, Kumar A. Endometrial tuberculosis. J Am Assoc Gynecol Laparosc 2004;11:2.
7. Kumar A, Kumar A. Unusual appearing tubercular deposits at hysteroscopy. J Minim Invasive Gynecol 2004;14:144.
8. Kumar A. Kumar A. Intraluminal tubal adhesions. Fertil Steril. 2008; 89(2): 434–5.
9. Kumar A, Kumar A. Hysteroscopic findings of starry sky appearance and impregnated cobwebs in endometrial tuberculosis. International Journal of Gynecology and Obstetrics 126 (2014) 280–1.
10. Kumar A. Kumar A. Relook hysteroscopy after antitubercular therapy. Fertil Steril. 2008; 89(3):701–2.
11. Kumar A. Kumar A. Surface architecture in endometrial tuberculosis. Article in press. JMIG.
12. Kumar A, Kumar A. Endometrial tuberculosis in a unicornuate uterus with a rudimentary horn. Article in press. JMIG
13. Cicinelli, et al. Tubercular Endometritis: A Rare Condition Reliably Detectable with Fluid Hysteroscopy JMIG. 2008; 15(6):752.
14. Sherman ME, Mazur MT, Kurman RJ. Benign diseases of the endometrium. In: Kurman RJ, editor. Blaustein's Pathology of the Female Genital Tract. New York: Springer; 2002.

Hysteroscopy in the Menopause

Nagendra Sardeshpande, Abhishek Chandavarkar

INTRODUCTION

The premenopause is a phase of gradual transition in a woman's life occurring during the late fourth and early fifth decade (47–55 years) and is characterized by gradual waning of ovarian function leading to hypoestrogenism and disruption of the ovulatory cycle and imbalances in the hypothalamo-pituitary-ovarian axis. Due to estrogen-progesterone and other endocrine–autocrine and paracrine dysfunction, this phase is characterized by changes in the endometrium. This is followed by complete cessation of ovarian function resulting in menopause and atrophy of the endometrium and uterine tissue (Figs 23.1 and 23.2).

Typically, the perimenopause is characterized by luteal phase insufficiency and endometrial defects due to insufficient progesterone production by the ageing ovarian follicles. Overexposure to estrogen due to anovulation can lead to hyperplasia and abnormal uterine bleeding. In the later part of the perimenopause, especially in women with prolonged anovulation, obesity, hypertension and hypothyroidism, abnormal uterine bleeding can be the manifestation of endometrial cancer.

Hysteroscopy has revolutionised the field of evaluation and therapy within the uterine cavity over the last few decades. This has been

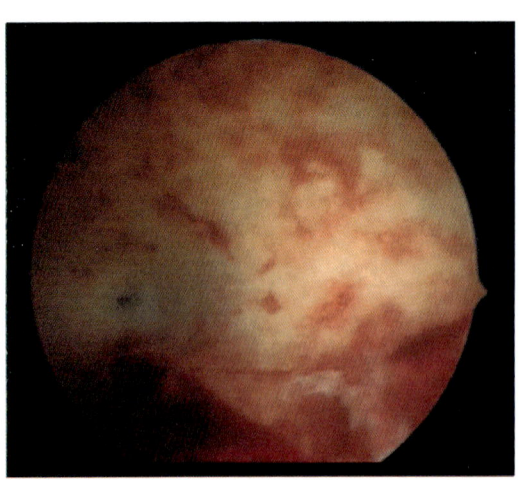

Fig. 23.1: Bald endometrium

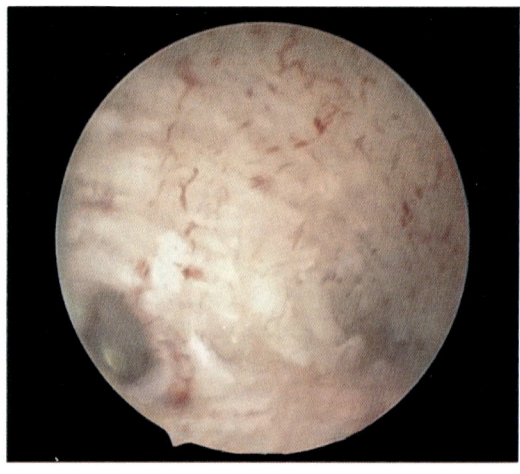

Fig. 23.2: Postmenopausal atrophic endometrium

due to increasing experience and familiarity of gynecologists with the procedure, increased awareness about minimally invasive surgery among patients and improved instrumentation.

INDICATIONS FOR HYSTEROSCOPY IN THE PERIMENOPAUSE

The classic and commonest indication for hysteroscopy in the perimenopause and menopause is abnormal uterine bleeding.[1] Of course, a good transvaginal ultrasound is mandatory prior to proceeding with any invasive procedure.[2] Ultrasound can reveal a thickened endometrium or space occupying lesions with the cavity or fluid within the endometrial cavity which can be further evaluated by hysteroscopy. Hysteroscopy can accurately help differentiate between endometrial polyps, hyperplasia and endometrial cancer with 90–95% sensitivity and specificity.[1] Hyperplasia will appear as diffuse thickening of the endometrium and may contain cystic space (cystic glandular hyperplasia) (Fig. 23.3a to d). Endometrial polyps appear as delicate pinkish lesions with a thin or thick pedicle with a vascular supply passing through the pedicle (Figs 23.4 and 23.5). Submucous fibroids are firm, globular and whitish in appearance and may be bosselated (Fig. 23.6). Endometrial

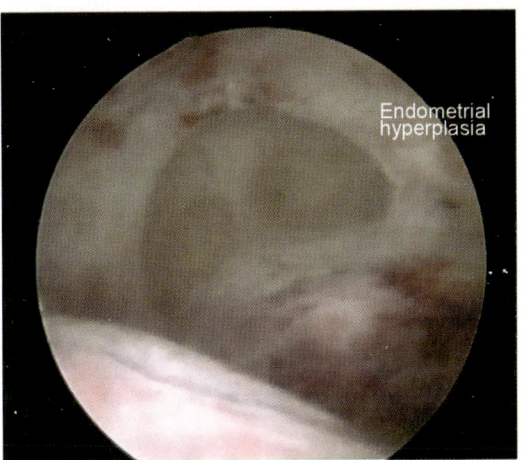

Fig. 23.3a: Endometrial hyperplasia

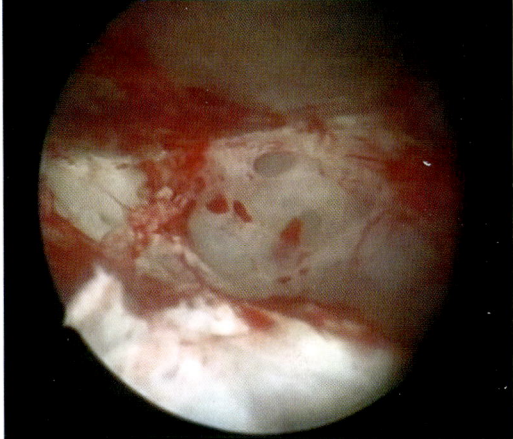

Fig. 23.3b: Cystic glandular hyperplasia

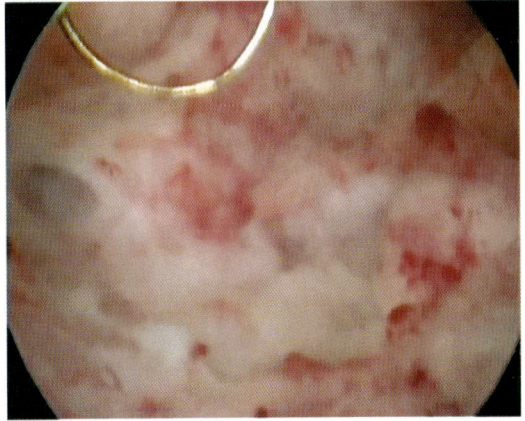

Fig. 23.3c: Swiss cheese hyperplasia of the endometrium

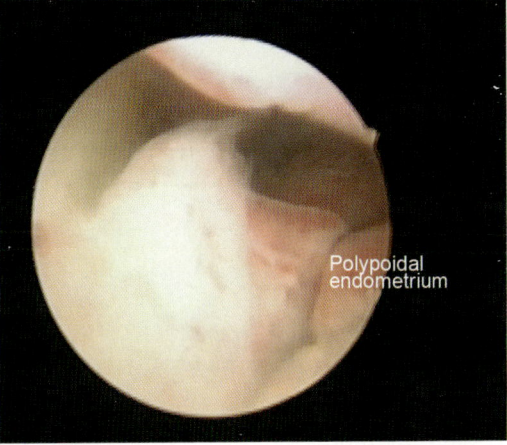

Fig. 23.3d: Polypoidal endometrium

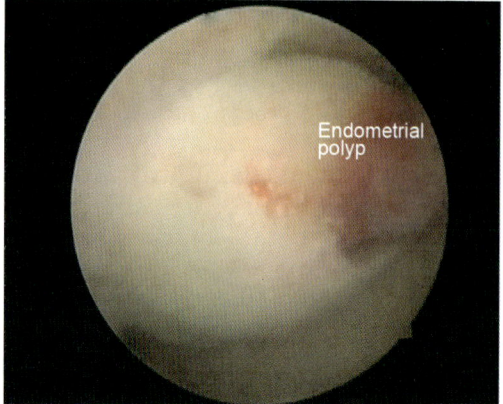

Fig. 23.4: Endometrial polyp hysteroscopy

cancer usually appears as a focus of thickened or polypoidal endometrial with diffuse aberrant vascularization (Fig. 23.7a to d). However, sometimes endometrial sarcomas may mimic the appearance of a submucous fibroid (Fig. 23.8). Women in the perimenopause may present with foul smelling vaginal discharge due to pyometra (Fig. 23.9a to c). Pyometra can be due to cervical stenosis or a manifestation of endometrial or cervical cancer. At the end, a targeted biopsy of these lesions with a hysteroscopic scissors or a grasping forceps helps resolve the diagnosis.[3,4]

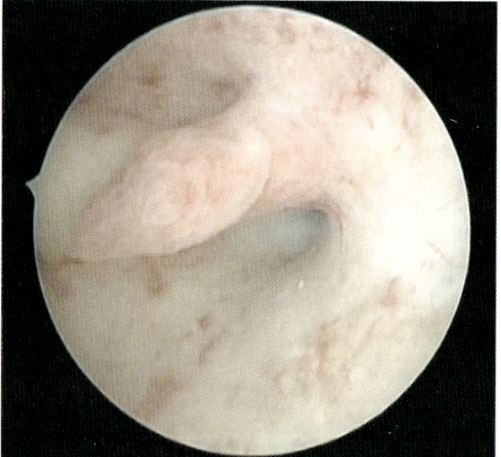

Fig. 23.5: Endometrial polyp with atrophic endometrium

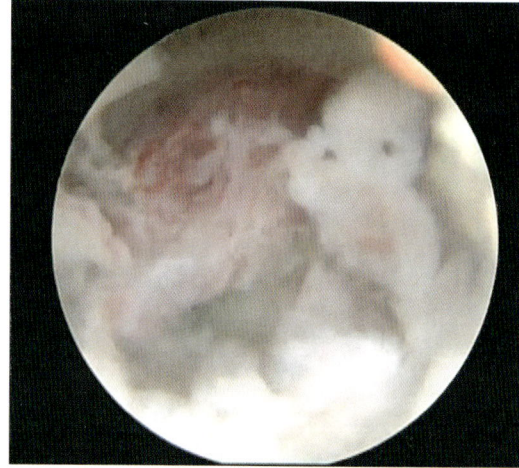

Fig. 23.7a: Endometrial carcinoma

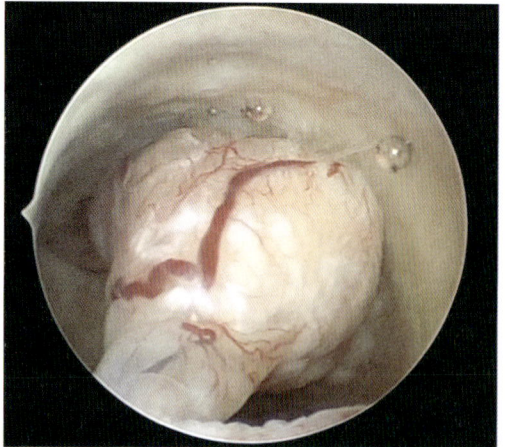

Fig. 23.6: Submucous fibroid in a menopausal woman

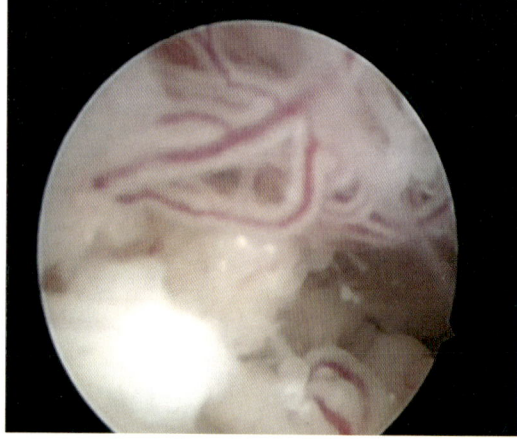

Fig. 23.7b: Aberrant vasculature in diffuse endometrial cancer

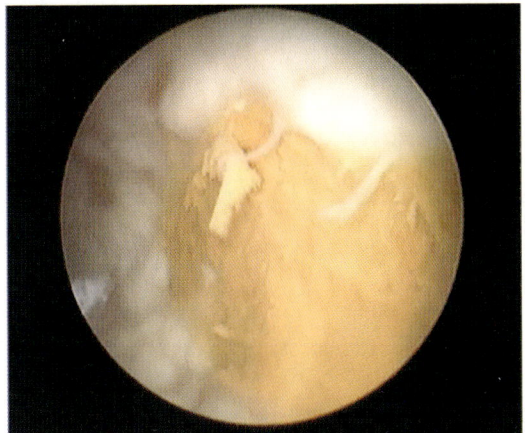

Fig. 23.7c: Endometrial cancer with ulceration

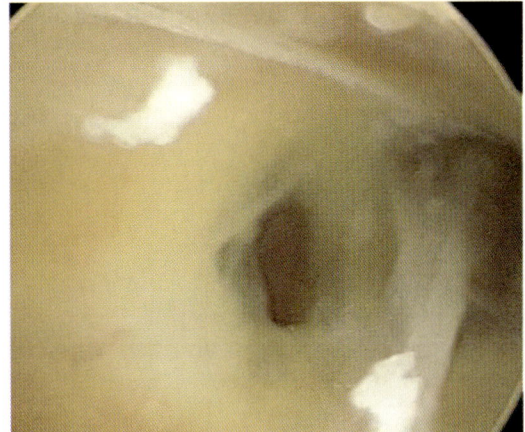

Fig. 23.9a: Pyometra

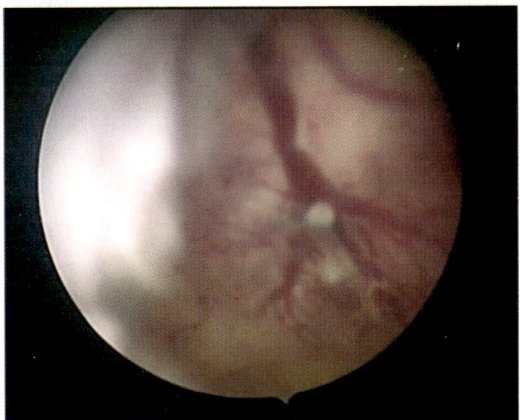

Fig. 23.7d: Neovascularization in early endometrial cancer

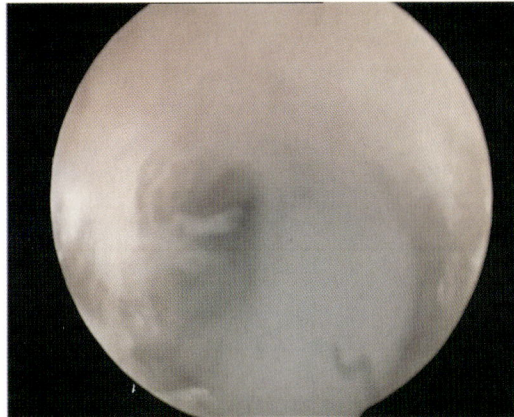

Fig. 23.9b: Pyometra in a menopausal uterus

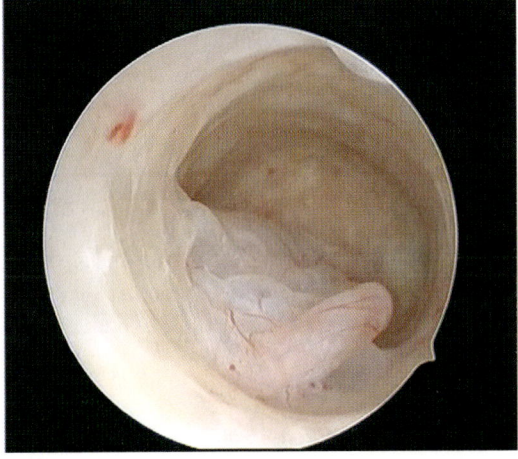

Fig. 23.8: Endometrial sarcoma presenting as a postmenopausal mass

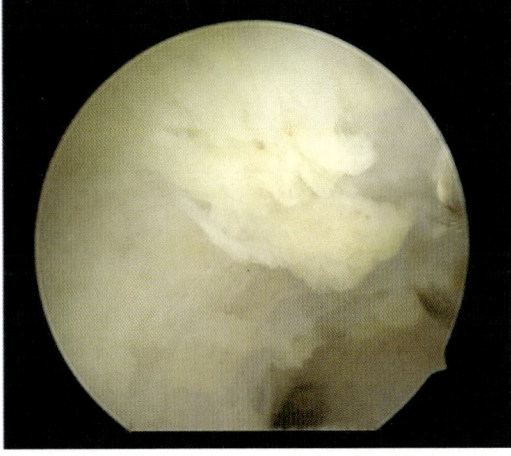

Fig. 23.9c: Pus flakes in the endometrium in a menopausal woman who is to undergo IVF

The other indication for a hysteroscopy in the perimenopause and menopause is as a preventive therapy. Any ultrasound showing an endometrial thickness of 5 mm or more requires evaluation. Hysteroscopy along with an endometrial biopsy helps rule out or confirm endometrial pathology and decide future definitive therapy.[3]

A number of women in the menopause or perimenopause require infertility therapy in the form of ART. Evaluation of the cavity to rule out congenital (Müllerian anomalies) or acquired pathology (fibroids, polyps or hyperplasia) is mandatory before proceeding with embryo transfer into the cavity (Figs 23.10 and 23.11). However, recents studies have refuted the benefit of a routine hysteroscopy prior to ART. This is understandable since high quality ultrasound can rule out abnormalities in the cavity leaving hysteroscopic evaluation and therapy only for those cavities showing abnormalities on ultrasound.

The last group of women requiring hysteroscopy in the perimenopause and menopause are those with unusual situations. These include an unexpected pregnancy with retained products of conception following medical termination of pregnancy or a spontaneous abortion (Figs 23.12 and 23.13). Women with

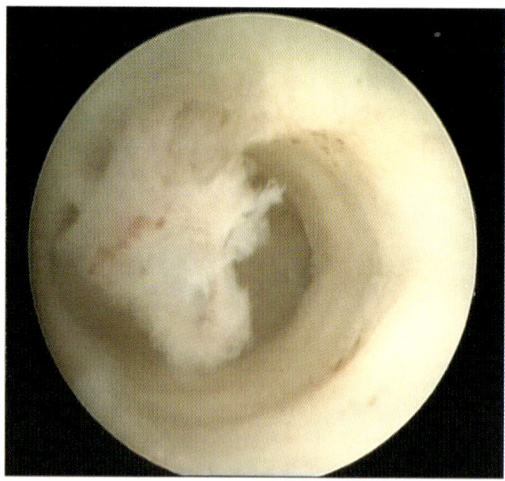

Fig. 23.11: Narrow T-shaped uterus in a perimenopausal woman set to undergo IVF

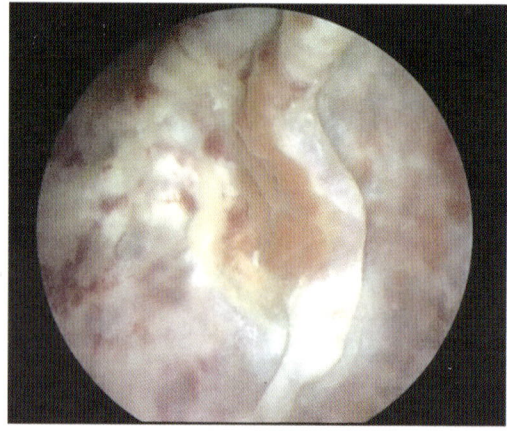

Fig. 23.12: Old retained products of conception

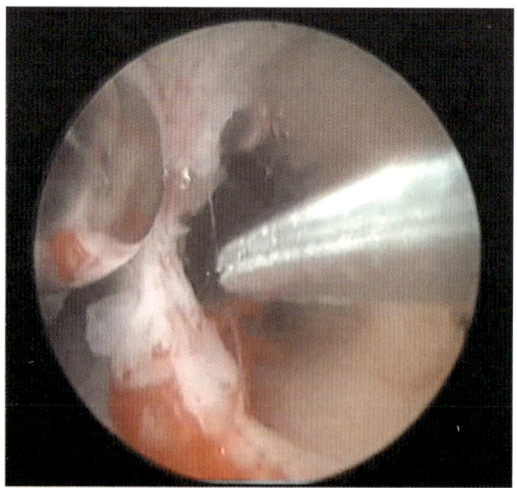

Fig. 23.10: A large uterine septum with scanty endometrium in spite of estrogen priming

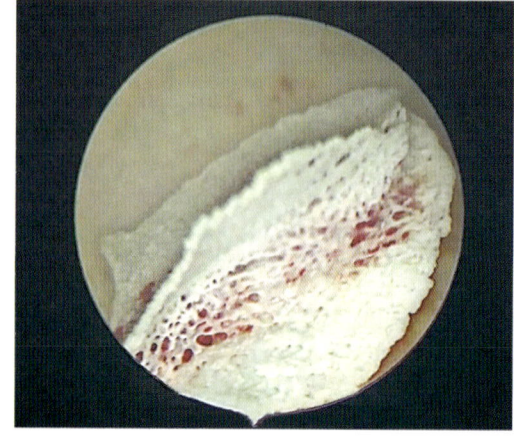

Fig. 23.13: Old fetal cartilage or osseous metaplasia in a menopausal woman

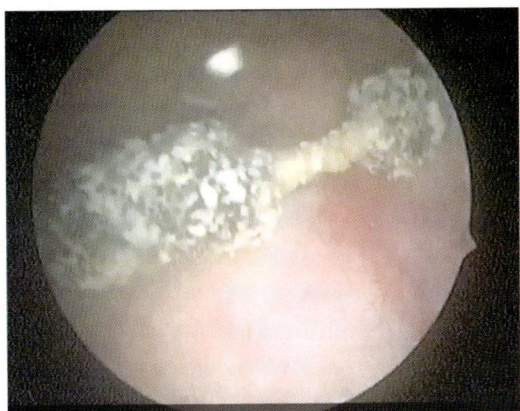

Fig. 23.14: Cu T perforated into the bladder 15 years earlier presenting in a menopausal woman with recurrent urinary tract infection with intravesical calcification seen on ultrasound

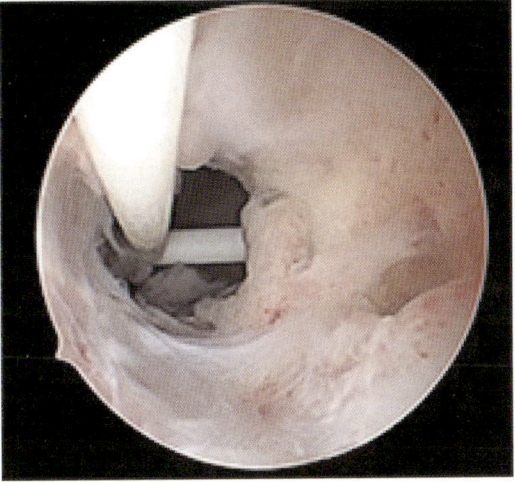

Fig. 23.15: Embedded missing Cu T in a perimeno-pausal woman

a foreign body such as a forgotten IUD may present with chronic pain or leucorrhea leading to unexpected detection of the foreign body (Figs 23.14 and 23.15).[3]

THERAPEUTIC HYSTEROSCOPY IN THE PERIMENOPAUSE

Today is the field of minimally invasive surgery. More and more women are demanding conservation of the uterus in the presence of benign pathology. Hysteroscopic evaluation of the cavity in the presence of abnormal uterine bleeding may reveal isolated solitary benign polyps or submucous fibroids without any other pathology in the myometrium or adnexae.

Simple resection of the submucous fibroids or polyps can result in a complete cure (Figs 23.16 to 23.21).[5]

Treatment of congenital uterine pathology such as a septum or T-shaped uterus or acquired pathology such as endometrial polyps or fibroids improves results of ART. Hence, operative hysteroscopy in menopausal women definitely improve ART results in this group. Preoperative priming of the endo-metrium with estrogen therapy for a few

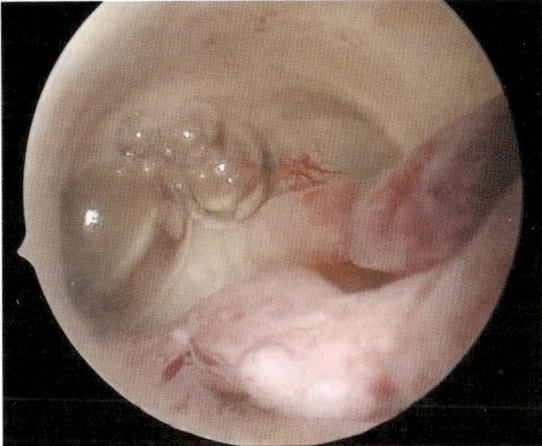

Fig. 23.16: Multiple endometrial polyps in a setting of atrophic endometrium

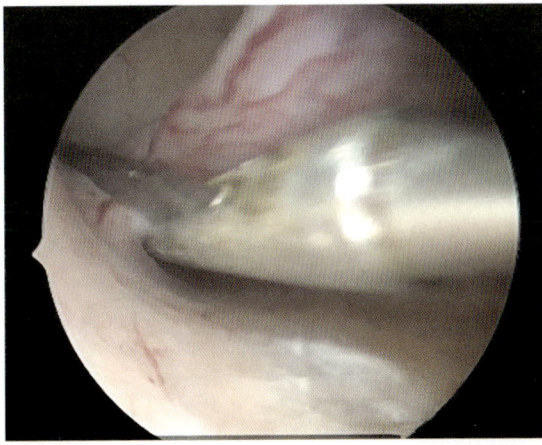

Fig. 23.17: Polypectomy with hysteroscopic scissors

weeks before performing metroplasty may help in rapid regeneration of the endometrium over the operated area within the uterine cavity.[6]

TCRE (transcervical resection of the endometrium) is a much maligned procedure

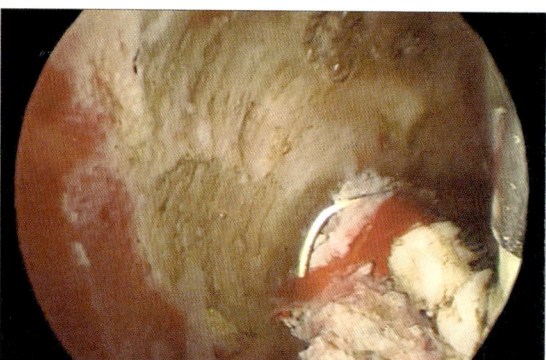

Fig. 23.21: Myomectomy completed. Note the circular myometrial fibers

partly because of inadequate experience on part of the gynecologists and wrong selection of the patients. The patients have to be explained regarding the benefits and limitations of the procedure. It should be avoided in the setting of multiple uterine fibroids, endometrial hyperplasia or adnexal pathology. With proper selection, patient satisfaction rates range from 70 to 90% and reduction in bleeding or amenorrhea is in the range of 80–85%. This also reduces the incidence of hysterectomy in women in the absence of extra-endometrial pathology. The reoperation and hysterectomy rates following TCRE is in the range of 15–20%. TCRE can also be used in the presence of small submucous fibroids without any significant increase in reoperation rates. Important steps in performing a successful TCRE include using a roller ball and vaportrode to ablate deeper endometrium and pockets of adenomyosis after resecting the endometrium till myometrium is visible using a loop electrode (Fig. 23.22a to c). Recent studies have also shown the efficacy of combining TCRE with a LNG IUD insertion especially with adenomyosis and hyperplasia without atypia.[7]

TECHNICAL MINUTIAE OF HYSTEROSCOPY IN THE PERIMENOPAUSE

Menopause is accompanied by atrophy of the endometrium and myometrium. This leads to

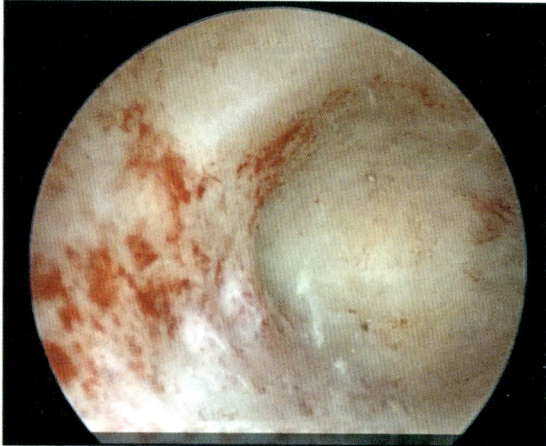

Fig. 23.18: Polypectomy completed

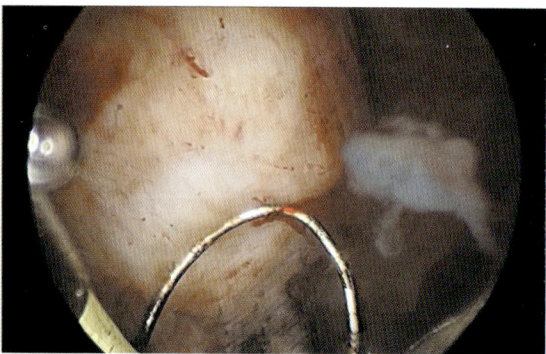

Fig. 23.19: A large submucous myoma in a post-menopausal woman

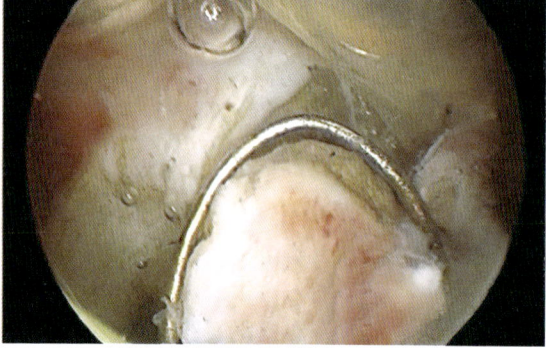

Fig. 23.20: Myoma resection with loop electrode

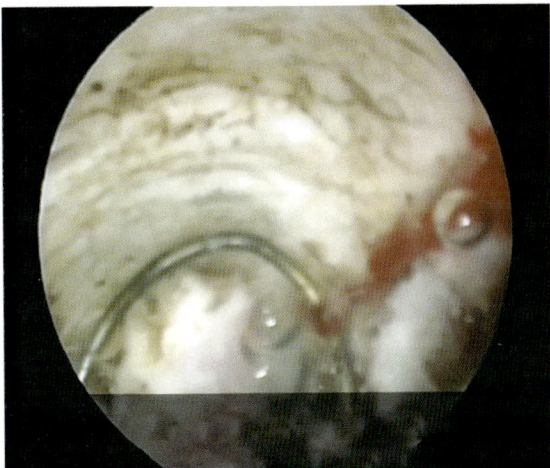

Fig. 23.22a: Note the depth of excision of endometrium in TCRE with exposure of underlying myometrium

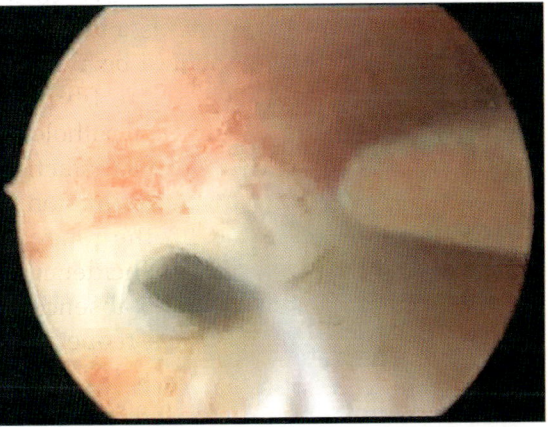

Fig. 23.22b: Adenomyotic crypt

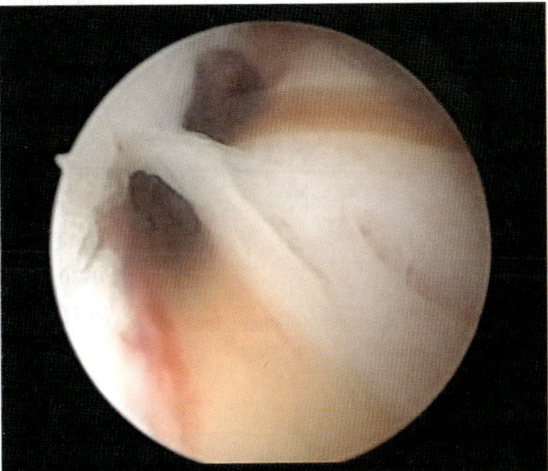

Fig. 23.22c: Endocervical adenomyotic crypt

a smaller volume uterine cavity. The cervix is often devoid of lubricating cervical mucus and stenotic. This can lead to difficulties in negotiating the cervical canal and entering the endometrial cavity (Fig. 23.23). The risk of perforation through the cervix or fundus in higher. Using smaller diameter 2–3 mm hysteroscopes or integrated systems (BIOS) along with higher fluid pressure during cervical entry and gradual entry through the cervical canal under hysteroscopic vision helps reduce the risk of perforation. Vagino-scopic approach without holding the cervix with a vulsellum reduces patient discomfort and allows hysteroscopy to be performed as an outpatient procedure with no anesthesia and minimal or no sedation.[8] Preoperative oral or sublingual misoprostol 200–400 micrograms 4–6 hours prior to the procedure helps softening the cervix and facilitates cervical entry.[9]

Operative hysteroscopy can also be per-formed using smaller operating sheaths and resectoscopes allowing easier manipulation in the narrow uterine cavity.

Fluid monitoring is extremely important especially in menopausal women. The thin atrophic endometrium allows rapid absorp-tion of fluid into the vascular system. Also

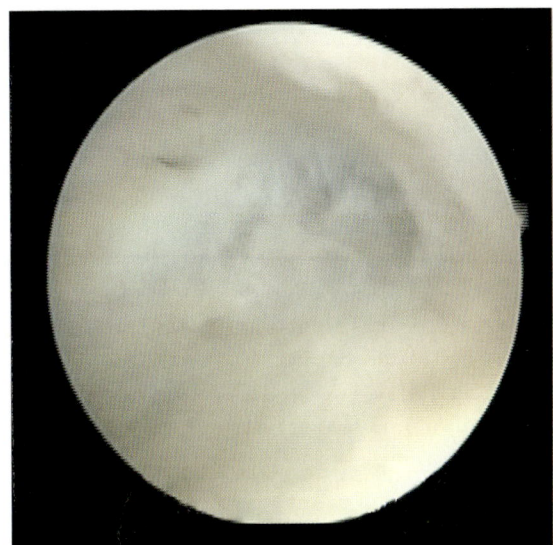

Fig. 23.23: Severe cervical stenosis

menopausal women may have cardiac issue and hypertension or diabetes making them more susceptible to complications such as pulmonary edema due to rapid hemodynamic changes and alteration in electrolyte balance. Hence, using dynamic pressure just adequate for visualization by manipulating the inflow and outflow channels prevents overdistention and rapid fluid absorption. On the other hand because of the atrophic nature of tissue and reduced vascularity, bleeding interfering with surgery is less of a problem in this group of women.

One concern of hysteroscopy in menopausal women with abnormal uterine bleeding is the spread of endometrial cancer cells through the fallopian tubes into the peritoneal cavity leading to upstaging of the cancer. Studies have shown the presence of endometrial cancer cells in peritoneal fluid and peritoneal lavage fluid after hysteroscopy. However, its clinical significance is poorly understood and studies do not show any evidence of worsened prognosis. However, given the concern, it is always wiser to use low pressures of 40–60 mm Hg during the initial phase of diagnostic hysteroscopy till one can view the lesion and have a reasonable idea of the pathology.[10]

CONCLUSION

Hysteroscopy is an integral aspect of the diagnostic and therapeutic armamentarium in gynecology. Its role in perimenopausal and menopausal women cannot be overestimated not only as a diagnostic and therapeutic procedure but also as a preventive procedure especially in and era where there is increased concern over the alarming increase in hysterectomies especially in women with essentially normal uteri. Hence, it is imperative that women all over the world and especially those in developing countries are made aware of the benefits and limitation of this procedure and gynecologists incorporate this essential tool as an integral part of their practice to provide the best possible therapeutic options to women.

References

1. Bronz L, *et al.* Hysteroscopy in the assessment of postmenopausal bleeding. Kochi OR (ed): Hysteroscopy—State-of-the-Art Contrib Gynecol Obstet. BSEL, Karger, 2000, vol 20; 51–9.
2. Boudaya F, *et al.* The contribution of ultrasound in the exploration of postmenopausal menorrhagias. Pan Afr Med J, Jan 2016; 24: 175.
3. Bettochi S, *et al.* Hysteroscopy and menopause: past and future. Curr Opin Obstet Gynecol, Aug 2005; 17 (4): 366–75.
4. Costa L, *et al.* Hysteroscopy in menopause: analysis of the technique and accuracy of the method. Rev Bras GinecolObstet, Oct 2008; 30 (10): 524–30.
5. Cornitescu F, *et al.* Clinical, histopathological and therapeutic considerations in non-neoplastic abnormal bleeding in menopause transition. Rom J Morphol Embryol. Jan 2011; 52 (3): 759–65.
6. Grigore M, *et al.* Comparative study of hysteroscopy and 3D ultrasound for diagnosis of uterine cavity abnormalities. Rev Med Chir Soc Med Nat Iasi. Oct 2016; 120 (4): 866–73.
7. Zheng J, *et al.* Comparison of combined transcervical resection of the endometrium and levonorgestrel containing intrauterine system treatment versus levonorgestrel containing intrauterine system alone in women with adenomyosis: A prospective clinical trial. J Reprod Med, Aug 2013; 58: 285–90.
8. Cooper N, *et al.* Vaginoscopic approach to outpatient hysteroscopy: a systematic review of the effect of pain. BJOG, 2017; 117: 532–9.
9. Ganer H, *et al.* Different routes of misoprostol for same day cervical priming prior to operative hysteroscopy: a randomized blinded trial. JMIG, March 2017; 24 (3): 455–60.
10. Kovacs P. Does hysteroscopy worsen endometrial cancer? AJOG, 2012; 207: 71 e1–e5.

Application of Hysteroscopy in Endometrial Precancerous Lesions and Endometrial Cancer

Xiang Xue, Jinyan Zhao, Shan Xu

With the development of minimally invasive techniques, the advantages of hysteroscopy in the diagnosis and treatment of malignant endometrial cancer have become increasingly prominent. Hysteroscopy, especially hysteroscopic lesions localized biopsy, is considered as the "gold standard" for the diagnosis of endometrial lesions. Dilation and curettage (D&C) with hysteroscopic guidance is recommended over D&C alone for its higher accuracy and superior diagnostic yield.[1] Hysteroscopy, although not required, is recommended with directed D&C to include any discrete lesions as well as the background endometrium. Hysteroscopic resection can be used as a safe option for young women with fertility needs to improve response and recurrence rates in the early endometrial carcinoma or precancerous lesions. In recent years, hysteroscopic resection combined with oral progesterone therapy has been considered as an alternative treatment method for early-stage endometrial cancer, since it allows the patients to regain fertility in a short period.

1. THE APPLICATION OF HYSTEROSCOPY IN THE DIAGNOSIS OF ENDOMETRIAL PRECANCEROUS LESIONS AND ENDOMETRIAL CANCER

A. The Characteristics of Endometrial Cancer and the Diagnostic Advantages of Hysteroscopy

i. *Specific Hysteroscopic Features for Malignant Endometrial Cancer*

Hysteroscopy allows doctors to see the entire uterine cavity and to biopsy targeted spots simultaneously in an outpatient setting. It is a safe examination with low incidence of complications. Endometrial malignancy under hysteroscopy is characterized by whitish or cyanosis; necrosis, hemorrhage, and calcification. The surface shows atypical vascularization, more specifically, irregular ramifications, blurred outlines, inconsistency vascular axis and irregular or ulcerated surface. Most tumours share the same characteristics, namely friable and susceptible to bleed.

The specific hysteroscopic features for an endometrial malignancy (Fig. 24.1a to g):

  a. Pale anterior wall with tubercle;

  b. Abnormal hyperplasia tissue, atypical blood vessel formation;

  c. Cauliflower-like growth and papillomatous;

  d. Thickened areas with irregular surfaces;

  e. "Bridge-like" area accompanied by irregular blood vessels;

  f. Friable, surface irregularities;

  g. Gray lumps;

ii. *The Advantage of Hysteroscopy Diagnosis*

For the diagnosis of uterine abnormalities, especially the focal ones, hysteroscopy with

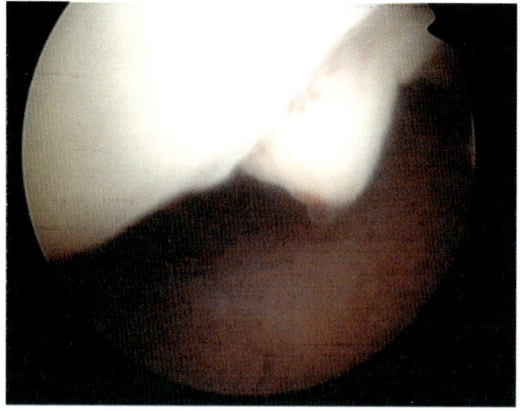

Fig. 24.1a: Pale anterior wall with tubercle

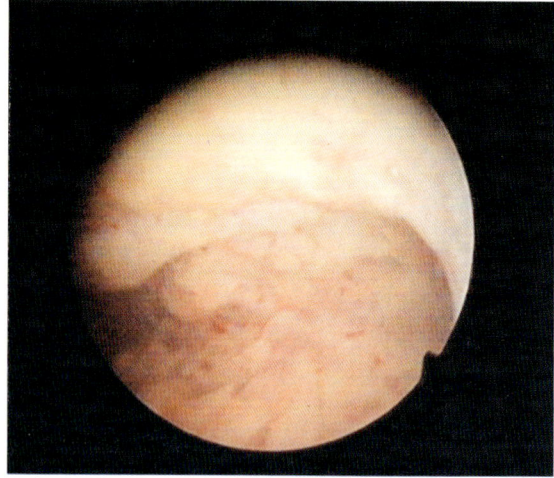

Fig. 24.1d: Thickened areas with irregular surfaces

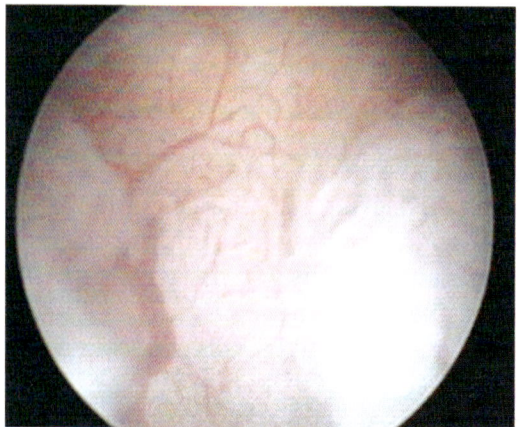

Fig. 24.1b: Abnormal hyperplasia tissue, atypical blood vessel formation

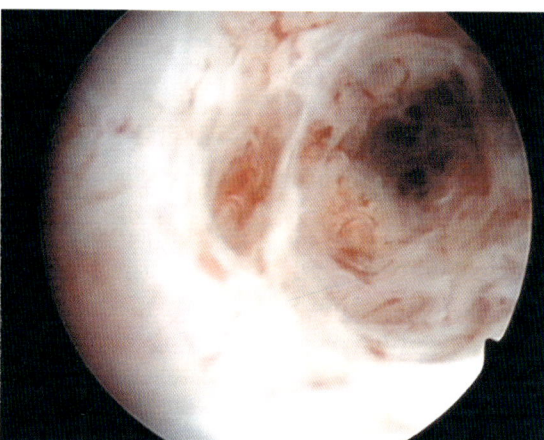

Fig. 24.1e: "Bridge-like" area accompanied by irregular blood vessels

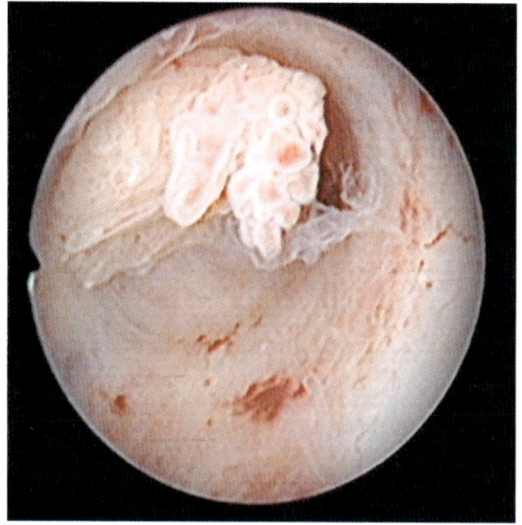

Fig. 24.1c: Cauliflower-like growth and papillomatous

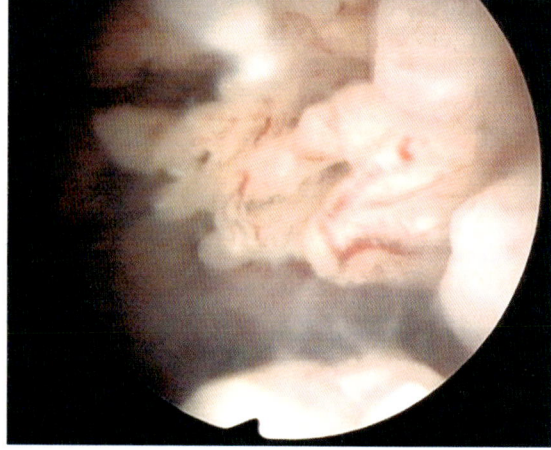

Fig. 24.1f: Friable, surface irregularities

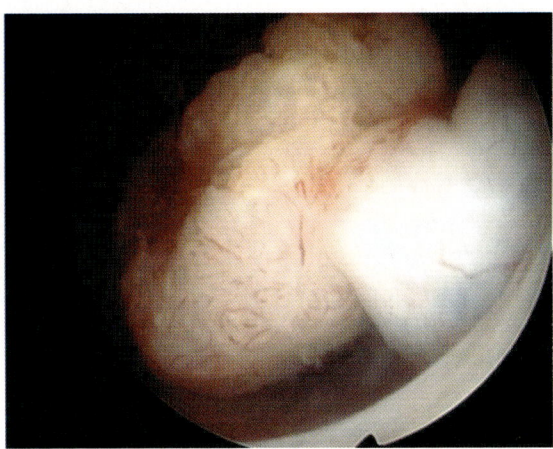

Fig. 24.1g: Gray lumps. Hysteroscopy in the treatment of endometrial cancer

directed biopsy is more advantageous compared to traditional uterine D&C.[2] Hysteroscopy is more accurate for the diagnosis of endometrial cancer and precancerous lesions.[3] Studies have shown that the accuracy and specificity of hysteroscopy in the diagnosis of endometrial cancer are higher than traditional D&C (endometrial cancer 99.5% *vs* 89.8% and endometrial dysplasia 89.1% *vs* 72.7%). Despite the fact that hysteroscopy is highly effective in the diagnosis of endometrial hyperplasia and cancer, histopathological examination is still irreplaceable.[4] In the modern cancer treatment, preoperative or peri-operative stage is crucial to ensure that the surgery matches the individual patient's disease stage. Therefore, the method must be highly accurate. Studies have demonstrated that hysteroscopy-directed biopsy could determine the grade of tumor with an accuracy of 97%.[5] In terms of accuracy, hysteroscopy-directed biopsy is more superior than traditional biopsy. It allows gynecologists to acquire the biopsy sample from the cancerous spot, which results in an accurate diagnosis of the stage classification. Besides, it is more accurate than MRI or TVS in assessing cervical involvement.[6] MRI combined with hysteroscopy-guided biopsies was found with significantly higher accuracy (81%) than all other combinations of examinations for the evaluation of risks and stage classification.

B. Controversy on Hysteroscopy in the Diagnosis of the Malignant Endometrial Cancer

It is worth mentioning that although hysteroscopy is widely used in the diagnosis of endometrial hyperplasia and cancer, histopathological study is irreplaceable. Hysteroscopy does not show a perfect correlation with histopathologic diagnosis. The improvement of hysteroscopy depends on two techniques, namely the quality of the viewing field and the method of biopsy. In addition, a great controversy exists in the dissemination of tumor cells to the abdominal cavity. Although hysteroscopy is widely used for the diagnosis of endometrial hyperplasia and carcinoma, a clear statement regarding tumor cell disseminating into the abdominal cavity is still needed. The distention of the uterus by the irrigation pump during the hysteroscopy may cause tumor cell dissemination into the abdominal cavity in patients with endometrial cancer. Some studies pointed out that the fluid hysteroscopy facilitates the spread of endometrial cancer cells into the abdominal cavity.[7–13] In 2009, The FIGO international staging committee changed the staging system so that positive peritoneal cytology test does not alter the tumor stage.[14] Undoubtedly, the diagnostic accuracy of hysteroscopy in premalignant (atypical hyperplasia) or malignant focal lesions of the endometrium is higher than the traditional D&C. Another research indicates that hysteroscopy does not increase tumor dissemination into the abdominal or affect the prognosis.[16] Therefore, it has been widely accepted that hysteroscopy is an accurate method for the diagnosis of endometrial precancerous lesions and endometrial cancer and it does not affect the prognosis of endometrial cancer.

2. HYSTEROSCOPY IN THE TREATMENT OF ENDOMETRIAL CANCER

A. Hysteroscopy in the Treatment of Early Stage Endometrial Cancer

It is controversial to use hysteroscopic treatment in early endometrial cancer. However, it is feasible as a conservative method for early stage endometrial cancer in young patients with the need of fertility. Selection criteria for conservative treatment of endometrial cancer are: No myometrial invasion, no extrauterine involvement (no ovarian tumors or metastases, no suspected retroperitoneal lymph node metastases), strong fertility needs, no drug therapy contraindications and patient's understanding about the fact that research on cancer-related pregnancy outcomes are limited.[1,17] Although several protocols are used for conservative management of endometrial cancer, no one has been proven to be superior. A combination of hysteroscopic resection and oral progestin therapy has recently been suggested as a novel management option.[20,21] The principle of hysteroscopic resection includes several key points: The lesion is focal, well demarcated, and distinguished from the surrounding normal endometrial tissue; resection of the lesion itself instead of total endometrial resection; remove additional strips of tissue from the periphery of the lesion to determine tumor margins; have follow-up hysteroscopy examination, followed by a biopsy to assess the endometrial status and rule out recurrence. Complete endometrial resection may result in total obliteration of the endometrial cavity. As a result, it will deprive patients' opportunities for hysteroscopic follow-ups.[22] Mazzon et al introduced the three-step method of hysteroscopic resection of the lesion: Resection of the tumor, resection of the endometrium adjacent to the tumor, and resection of the myometrium underlying the tumor.

Hysteroscopy in the Treatment of Endometrial Cancer

Our experience in the management of different cases is discussed in (Fig. 24.2a to g).

B. Advantages of Hysteroscopy Combined with Medications for Endometrial Carcinoma Treatment

At present, the literature reveals that only 50% endometrial cancer cases respond to progestin therapy, meaning that half of the young women treated conservatively will fail and require hysterectomy. The combination of hysteroscopy with progestin may have more advantages over progestin therapy alone.[20]

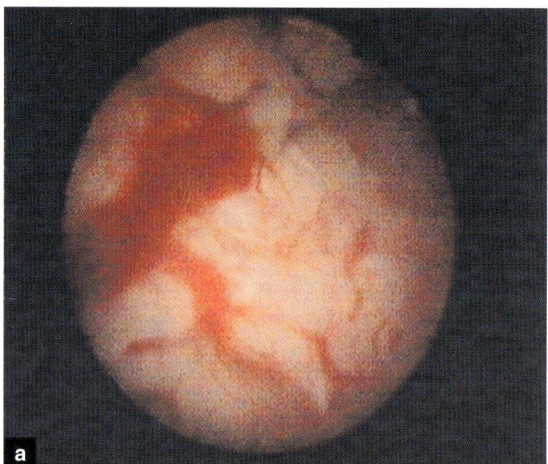

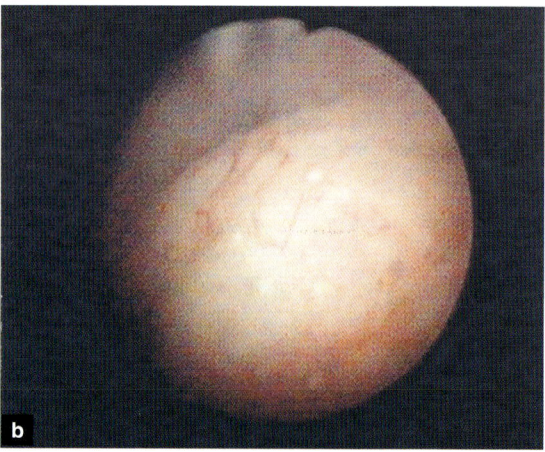

Fig. 24.2a and b: Low grade endometrium cancer before focal resection

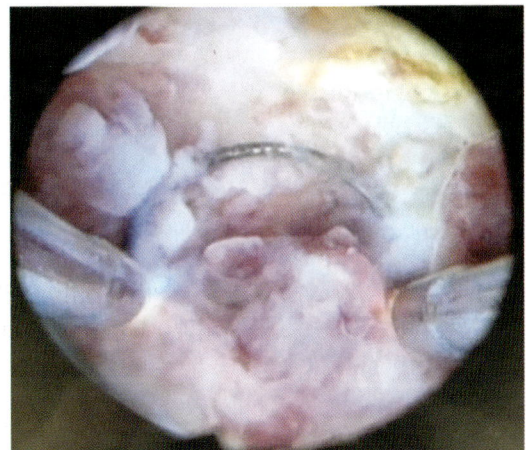

Fig. 24.2c: During focal resection with hysteroscopy

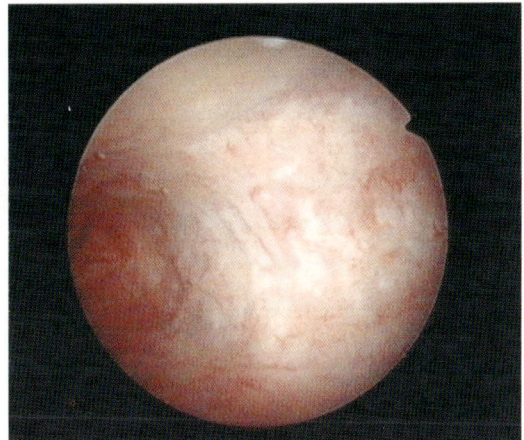

Fig. 24.2d: Medroxyprogesterone 160 mg/day treatment for 36 days after local focus resection

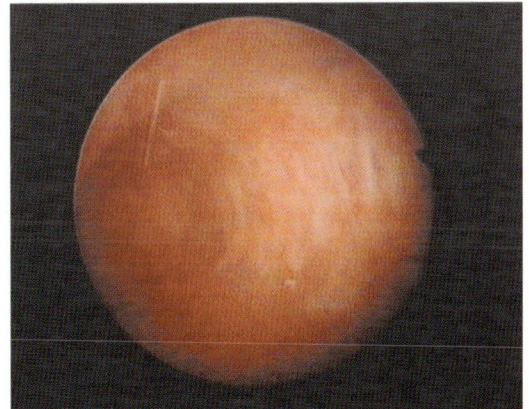

Fig. 24.2e: Medroxyprogesterone 160 mg/day treatment for 70 days after local focus resection

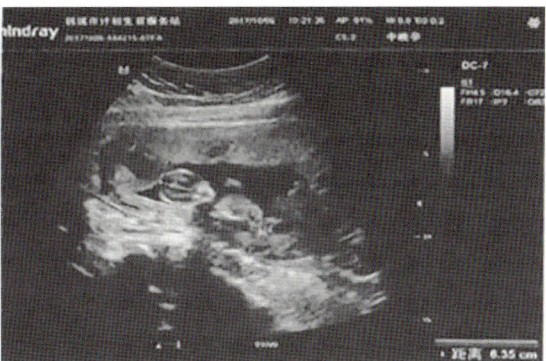

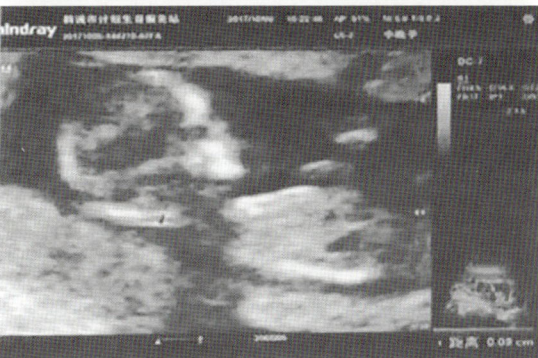

Fig. 24.2f: IVF pregnancy after resection for 7 months and was 13 weeks pregnant now

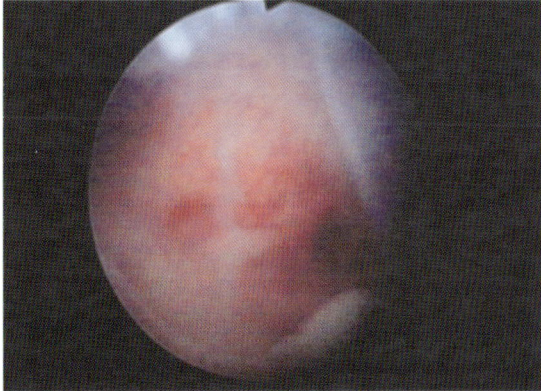

Fig. 24.2g: Postpartum 3 months

First, conservative management is usually reserved for early-stage endometrial adeno-carcinoma with no myometrial invasion. Hysteroscopic resection of the lesion and myometrium below allows for both a therapeutic effect of excising the tumor and an additional benefit of pathologic assessment of the depth of invasion. The accuracy of MRI for detecting myometrial invasion is uncertainty. In terms of therapeutic benefit, a complete excision of the tumor results in better outcomes. The response rate of the combination of hysteroscopic resection and progesterone can reach 100%. Secondly, hysteroscopic resection of tumor before treatment with high doses progestin therapy could shorten the course of treatment, as well as allow a quicker regaining of fertility. The latter benefit is an appealing feature of this method. Besides, a decreased interval between treatment and conception is beneficial for managing the risk of recurrence or progression. Last but not the least, a complete excision of the malignant tissue may decrease the possibility of recurrence. Further studies will be needed to verify this statement. Currently, there are evidences supporting the use of levonorgestrel intrauterine system (LNG-IUS) in treating the endometrial cancer. However, it is not conducive to follow-up and conceiving in a short time. The combination of hysteroscopy and medication in treating endometrial cancer requires a multidisciplinary collaboration to thoroughly assess patients, in which close follow-up is necessary. Although hysteroscopy may lead to an increasing risk of peritoneal dissemination of cancer cells, it does not necessarily correlate to poor prognosis, especially at early stages. Conservative management is a safer choice for young women with early-stage endometrial cancer with fertility needs. The conservative management with hysteroscopy will not only beneficial to decrease the recurrence rate in women with fertility needs, but will also lead to a faster remission and regaining of fertility. Gestation is a natural treatment method for endometrial complications. The key factors to success include an interdisciplinary approach to evaluate patients and a team with excellent expertise in hysteroscopic resection. It is surely needed to perform further studies with larger numbers of patients and longer follow-up to evaluate the role of hysteroscopy in the fertility-preserving management of endometrial cancer as well as to acquire consensus guidelines for the management of early-stage endometrial carcinoma in young women with fertility needs.

SUMMARY

The accuracy of the hysteroscopy-directed biopsy is high for endometrial cancer and premalignant lesion. However, hysteroscopy cannot replace the histopathological diagnosis of endometrial lesions. The accuracy of hysteroscopy-directed biopsies for determining tumor grade including atypical endometrial hyperplasia is superior to that of traditional endometrial biopsy. Compared with D&C, hysteroscopy will not lead to an increased intrabdominal tumor cell dissemination, alteration of tumor stage or worse prognoses. In recent years, a combination of hysteroscopic resection and oral progestin therapy has been recommended for early stage endometrial cancer and hyperplasia patients. However, further studies are required to enroll larger numbers of patients and longer follow-up to evaluate the role of hysteroscopy in the fertility-preserving management of endometrial cancer cases.

References

1. ACOG Practice Bulletin clinical management guidelines for obstetrician-gynecologists Endometrial Cancer[J]. Obstetrics & Gynecology, 2015, 125(4).
2. Garuti G, Cellani F, Garzia D, et al. Accuracy of hysteroscopic diagnosis of endometrial hyperplasia: a retrospective study of 323 patients[J]. J Minim Invasive Gynecol, 2005, 12(3):247–53.
3. Clark TJ, Voit D, Gupta JK, et al. Accuracy of hysteroscopy in the diagnosis of endometrial cancer and hyperplasia: a systematic quantitative review[J]. JAMA, 2002, 288(13):1610–21.
4. Lasmar RB, Barrozo PR, de Oliveira MA, et al. Validation of hysteroscopic view in cases of endometrial hyperplasia and cancer in patients with abnormal uterine bleeding[J]. J Minim Invasive Gynecol, 2006, 13(5):409–12.
5. Cutillo G, Cignini P, Visca P, et al. Endometrial biopsy by means of the hysteroscopic resectoscope

for the evaluation of tumor differentiation in endometrial cancer: a pilot study[J]. Eur J Surg Oncol, 2007, 33(7):907–10.

6. Ørtoft G, Dueholm M, Mathiesen O, et al. Preoperative staging of endometrial cancer using TVS, MRI, and hysteroscopy[J]. Acta Obstet Gynecol Scand, 2013, 92(5):536–45.

7. Obermair A, Geramou M, Gucer F, et al. Does hysteroscopy facilitate tumor cell dissemination? Incidence of peritoneal cytology from patients with early stage endometrial carcinoma following dilatation and curettage (D & C) versus hysteroscopy and D&C[J].Cancer 2000;88(1): 139–43.

8. Arikan G, Reich O, Weiss U, et al. Are endometrial carcinoma cells disseminated at hysteroscopy functionally viable?[J]. Gynecol Oncol, 2001, 83(2):221–6.

9. Plent HA, Friedman EA. Lymphatic System of the Female Genital Tract[M]. Philadelphia: Saunders, 1971:116–52..

10. Boronow RC,Morrow CP, Creasman WT, et al. Surgical staging in endometrial cancer: clinico-pathologic findings of a prospective study[J]. Obstet Gynecol,1984;63(6): 825–32.

11. Bettocchi S. Abdominal dissemination of malignant cells with hysteroscopy: Letter to the editor[J]. Gynecol Oncol, 1997,66:165.

12. Baker VL, Adamson GD. Threshold intrauterine perfusion pressures for intraperitoneal spill during hydrotubation and correlation with tubal adhesive disease[J]. Fertil Steril, 1995,64(6): 1066–9.

13. Cicinelli E, Tinelli R, Colafiglio G, et al. Risk of long-term pelvic recurrences after fluid mini hysteroscopy in women with endometrial carcinoma: a controlled randomized study[J]. Menopause, 2010, 17(3):511–5.

14. FIGO Committee on gynecologic oncology. Revised FIGO staging for carcinoma of the vulva, cervix, and endometrium[J]. Int J Gynaecol Obstet, 2009,105:103–4.

15. Loverro G, Bettocchi S, Cormio G et al. Diagnostic accuracy of hysteroscopy in endometrial hyperplasia[J]. Maturitas, 1996,25(3):187–91.

16. Selvaggi L, Cormio G, Ceci O, et al; Hysteroscopy does not increase the risk of microscopic extrauterine spread in endometrial carcinoma[J]. Int J Gynecol Cancer, 2003, 13(2):223–7.

17. Erkanli S, Ayhan A. Fertility-sparing therapy in young women with endometrial cancer: 2010 update[J]. Int J Gynecol Cancer, 2010, 20(7):1170–87.

18. Gunderson CC, Fader AN, Carson KA, et al. Oncologic and reproductive outcomes with progestin therapy in women with endometrial hyperplasia and grade 1 adenocarcinoma: a systematic review[J]. Gynecol Oncol, 2012, 125(2): 477–482.

19. Koskas M, Uzan J, Luton D, et al. Prognostic factors of oncologic and reproductive outcomes in fertility-sparing management of endometrial atypical hyperplasia and adenocarcinoma: systematic review and meta-analysis[J]. Fertil Steril, 2014, 101(3):785–94.

20. Mazzon I, Corrado G, Masciullo V, et al. Conservative surgical management of stage IA endometrial carcinoma for fertility preservation[J]. Fertil Steril, 2010;93(4): 1286–1289.

21. Laurelli G, Di Vagno G, Scaffa C, et al. Conservative treatment of early endometrial cancer: preliminary results of a pilot study[J]. Gynecol Oncol, 2011, 120(1): 43–46.

22. Vilos GA, Ettler HC, Edris F, et al. Endometrioid adenocarcinoma treated by hysteroscopic endomyometrial resection[J]. J Minim Invasive Gynecol, 2007, 14(1): 119–122.

23. Arendas K, Aldossary M, Cipolla A, et al. Hysteroscopic Resection in the Management of Early-stage Endometrial Cancer: Report of 2 Cases and Review of the Literature[J]. J Minim Invasive Gynecol, 2015, 22(1):34–9.

Safe and Patient-friendly Hysteroscopy

Pain Management in Hysteroscopy

Carugno Jose, Palin, Alonso Luis

INTRODUCTION

Hysteroscopy is an indispensable tool in modern gynecology.[1] Diagnostic hysteroscopy is considered the gold standard for the study of intrauterine pathologies. Operative hysteroscopy is becoming more proliferative with each passing year with procedures including: Endometrial polypectomy, endometrial ablation, removal of intrauterine devices, treatment of uterine morphological anomalies and leiomyomas among other pathologies. These advancements have also facilitated the growth of hysteroscopy in modern gynecology as a whole.[2] Traditionally women undergo hysteroscopy in the operating room; however, with recent advances in gynecologic instrumentation and improvements in operative techniques, women can now undergo hysteroscopy, diagnostic or operative, in the office setting.[3–5] Hysteroscopes, some as small as 3.5 mm, obviate the need for cervical dilation almost completely and operative techniques that decrease manipulation of pelvic organs increase patient tolerance to in-office hysteroscopy. Moreover, there is solid data showing that in-office hysteroscopy is just as efficacious as hysteroscopy performed in the operating room. In a systematic review of over 26,000 procedures a failure rate of 3.6 percent was reported with 4.2% in the outpatient setting and 3.4% in the inpatient modality.[6]

The goal of hysteroscopy is to perform a successful procedure as well as providing a positive patient experience. Success is closely related to having adequate visualization and effective instrumentation. If practitioners are able to accomplish both with in-office hysteroscopy, it is beneficial to both the doctor and the patient. A successful procedure in the office avoids the risks of anesthesia and the time spent recovering from a procedure performed under general anesthetic. One randomized control trial showed women recovering from in-office hysteroscopy to preoperative levels in just 2 days versus 3 days for traditional operating room hysteroscopy.[7] The patient also has the additional benefit to skip additional waiting times for scheduling with a hospital or surgery center. This extrapolates to great savings to the health care industry and society at large. Patients who choose to undergo in-office procedures cite privacy as another important factor for choosing a familiar, less-exposed office setting in lieu of an operating room.[8] Additionally, women avoid pre-operative medical optimization for comorbidities, which are becoming an ever-greater obstacle to routine surgery. In an effort to decrease cost and facilitate patient access, hysteroscopic procedures are increasingly migrating from the operating room to the office. The Centers for Medicare and medicaid services have endorsed a substantial increase in reimbursement for certain office-based hysteroscopic procedures.[9] Practitioners need to be able to effectively perform these procedures in the office to keep up with the newest standards for patient care as well as to help their practice flourish.

The keys to effective in-office hysteroscopy are threefold:

1. Good patient selection
2. Adequate pain management
3. Creating the correct environment for patient comfort.

Pain and inability to access the uterus are often cited as the main reasons to abort a hysteroscopic procedure.[10] However, with good pain control, there is no difference in outcomes between in office and operating room hysteroscopy. A randomized control trial of 400 women with abnormal uterine bleeding found that outpatient procedures including outpatient hysteroscopy were well tolerated, with good patient acceptability.[11]

There is no consensus in the literature as to the optimal method of pain relief. It is important to establish evidence-based pain management protocols to decrease pain associated with office hysteroscopy, which will reduce the rate of failed procedures. If practitioners can reliably perform procedures in the office, it will decrease the cost, time, and risk associated with performing the procedure in the operating room without decreasing patient satisfaction. The focus of this chapter is to address different available modalities for pain management for patients in the outpatient setting and to outline effective pain control regimens that could be used as a guide to manage pain when performing in-office diagnostic and operative hysteroscopy.

THE ANATOMY OF PAIN

The experience of pain associated with hysteroscopy, as any other pain eliciting procedure, is influenced by many factors related to the patient and the operative technique. Let us begin with a review of the anatomy of pain.

Pain most frequently occurs at five points throughout hysteroscopic procedures:

1. Insertion of the speculum
2. Placement of the tenaculum
3. Dilation of the cervix
4. Insertion of the hysteroscope into the cervix
5. Distension of the uterine cavity

A number of nerves and nerve plexuses are therefore, taken into consideration when contemplating pain management. The pudendal nerve innervates the bottom two-thirds of the vagina and vulva. This area is most significantly affected during placement of the speculum and manipulation of the speculum throughout the procedure. The lower uterine segment, the cervix and the upper third of the vagina are innervated by parasympathetic fibers from S2 to S4 that travel through the cardinal ligament. These fibers are responsible for sensation during tenaculum placement and dilation of the cervix. Lastly, sympathetic fibers from T10 to L2 innervate the fundus of the uterus. The inferior hypogastric plexus enters the uterus through the uterosacral ligaments and the other sympathetic fibers enter via the infundibulo pelvic ligament creating the ovarian plexuses at the bilateral cornua.[12] These are affected during distension of the uterine cavity and manipulation of the uterus itself. The basal third of the endometrium is also innervated (Fig. 25.1).

During operative procedures, pain is therefore experienced when the myometrial-endometrial interface is manipulated. This includes procedures such as polypectomy, endometrial biopsy, myomectomy, curettage, ablation or tubal sterilization.

Anatomy and innervation have been the focus of pain management and rightfully so. Increasingly, anxiety and environmental factors have begun to also be considered in patient perception of pain. We will consider

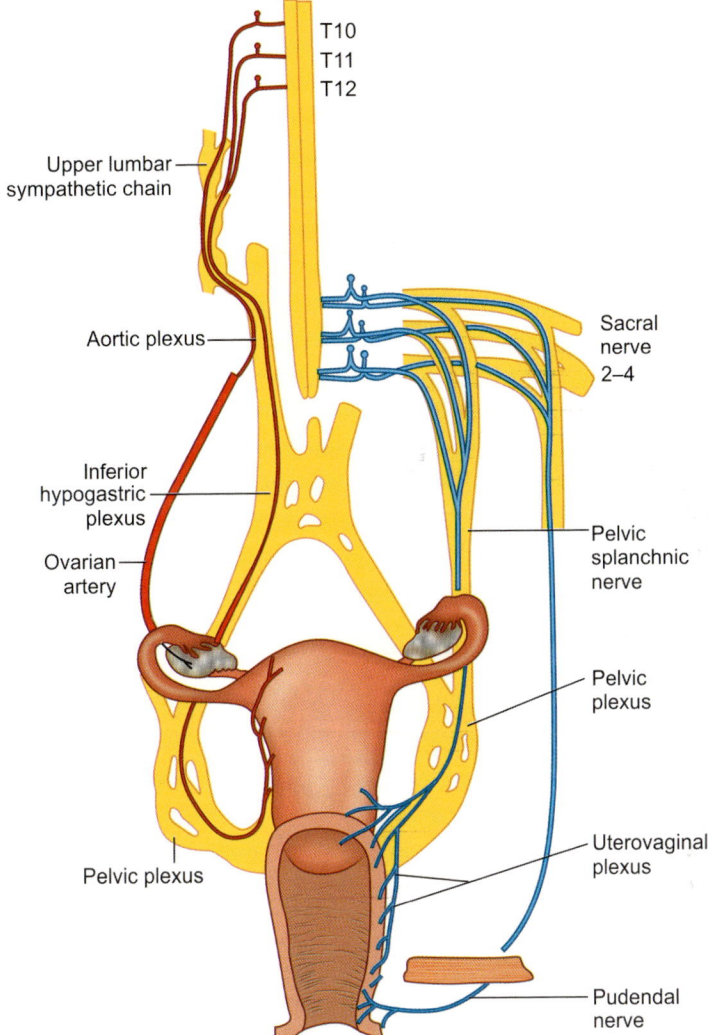

Fig. 25.1: Schematic view of the neuroanatomy of the uterus and vagina

both when determining patient eligibility for in-office versus operating room hysteroscopy.

PATIENT SELECTION FOR IN-OFFICE HYSTEROSCOPY

Adequate patient selection for in-office procedures is extremely important. Some patients will only tolerate the procedure if performed under general anesthesia. Providers should screen each patient to ensure that she is a good candidate for in-office performance of the needed procedure.

Patient related factors associated to pain perception during hysteroscopy

a. Parity: There is conflicting evidence regarding the influence of prior vaginal delivery and the pain reported during office procedures. Although some research shows that nulliparity does not increase reported pain during office hysteroscopy. Mazzon et al[13] published a prospective observational study revealing that the number of spontaneous vaginal deliveries is inversely correlated with pain intensity during hysteroscopy. This is concordant with findings published by Van Dongen et al[14] who reported that nulliparous women have a 27% higher risk of perceiving pain at visual analog scale (VAS) >5 during hysteroscopy when compared to women who have had vaginal deliveries. It is speculated that the more dilated multiparous cervix will require less force to introduce the hysteroscope as opposed to a nulliparous cervix that will pose more resistance.

b. **Menopausal status:** In an observational study of over 200 patients, Carta et al[15] described menopause status as a specific risk factor associated with pain >4 in VAS (OR, 2.81; 95% CI, 1.10–7.40). On the other hand, Török P et al[16] in a study evaluating pain level during office hysteroscopy according to menopausal status, parity, and size of the instrument, found no correlation between menopausal status and pain during office hysteroscopy.

c. **Cervical canal:** Mazzon et al[13] evaluated the correlation between pain perceived during hysteroscopy and the characteristics of the cervix, specifically the angle and morphology of the cervical canal. They concluded that the anatomy of the cervical canal does not seem to play an important role for pain. However, the presence of cervical adhesions and the resulting force needed to enter the uterine cavity is a major factor generating pain during hysteroscopy. In a recent video-article publication Bettocchi et al described different techniques to overcome the difficult cervix in over 30,000 in-office hysteroscopy procedures, demonstrating that the surgical technique and gynecologist experience is an important factor to reduce pain during in-office hysteroscopy.[17]

d. **History of chronic pelvic pain and/or dysmenorrhea:** There is solid, consistent evidence suggesting that a history of chronic pelvic pain or dysmenorrhea is associated with increased chance of unacceptable pain during hysteroscopy. Data from Tokushige et al revealed that women with a diagnosis of endometriosis were more likely to have small nerve fibers throughout the basal and functional layers of the endometrium leading to a greater perception of pain with endometrial manipulation.[18] A prospective case-control study of 198 women showed that those with a known history of endometriosis or adenomyosis had greater numbers of nerve fibers and that those women had higher reported pain levels.[19]

Table 25.1: Risk and protective factors associated with pain perception during in-office hysteroscopy

Increased pain	Decreased pain
Nulliparity	History of vaginal delivery
Postmenopausal status	High volume hysteroscopist
History of chronic pain/ dysmenorrhea	Short procedure
Anxiety	Low distension pressures
High level of anticipated pain	Small diameter hysteroscopes

APPROPRIATE PAIN MANAGEMENT

Pain is the most commonly cited reason for termination of hysteroscopic procedures. The options for anesthesia and pain management are ubiquitous; they will be divided into two larger categories: Procedural and medical options for pain management.

1. Procedural: Local Anesthesia

The use of local anesthesia is a common practice to decrease pain when performing in-office procedures. The administration of local anesthesia in gynecologic procedures can be performed using different modalities: Topical, intrauterine, intracervical, and paracervical. Safe use of anesthetic drugs requires a complete understanding of the potency, avoiding toxicity, and early recognition of potential complications.

a. Topical Agents

i. **Uterine cervix:** There is conflicting data to evaluate the use of topical anesthetics on the cervix to decrease pain during

Table 25.2: Clinical characteristics of local anesthetics

Agent	Onset	Duration	Maximum dose	Maximum dose with epinephrine
Bupivacaine	5–10 min	200 min	2.5 mg/kg	3 mg/kg
Lidocaine	2 min	30–60 min	3 mg/kg	5 mg/kg
Mepivacaine	3–5 min	45–90 min	6 mg/kg	5 mg/kg
Ropivacaine	5–15 min	200 min	3 mg/kg	3 mg/kg

hysteroscopy. Wong et al[20] found no benefit using lignocaine gel applied on the cervix before the procedure, whereas Soriano et al[21] demonstrated substantial reduction in pain associated with the use of lidocaine spray. Anesthetic agents delivered by sprays, gels and creams provide anesthesia to superficial pain receptors. A later published meta-analysis concluded that topical cervical anesthesia was not effective in decreasing pain during hysteroscopy when compared to placebo (20.32; 95% CI, 20.97 to 0.33).[22]

ii. **Uterine corpus:** Another commonly used modality is the administration of intrauterine local anesthesia. This technique has been investigated in several trials. A review published by Cooper et al[22] concluded that intracavitary anesthesia was not effective (20.11; 95% CI, 20.31 to 0.10). Moreover, a systematic review of the use of intrauterine anesthesia for different gynecologic procedures concluded that intrauterine anesthesia is an effective method of pain management for some gynecologic office procedures but not for all.[23]

b. Injectable Agents

The most common local anesthetics used in the office are lidocaine and bupivacaine. The maximum dose of lidocaine without epinephrine should not exceed 4.5 mg/kg. A dose of 200 mg of lidocaine (20 ml of 1% lidocaine) is often used for paracervical block and is well below the threshold of toxicity. At low serum levels of lidocaine, patients may experience

tinnitus and numbness of the mouth. This is not uncommon when using paracervical blocks. At higher levels of lidocaine, patients may experience visual disturbances, confusion, seizure, or cardio-respiratory arrest. Techniques to lower the risk of lidocaine toxicity include adding vasopressin or epinephrine to reduce systemic absorption and aspirating before injecting to reduce the risk of intravascular instillation.

i. **Paracervical block:** Although the paracervical block has been shown to be effective for many gynecologic procedures, performing the block itself causes considerable patient discomfort. There is no consensus on the proper technique to perform a paracervical block with great variability in the location and depth of injection as well as type and dose of anesthetic used. However, regardless of the technique, an extensive systematic review of local anesthesia during gynecologic in-office procedures concluded that there is significant reduction in pain associated with the use of paracervical anesthesia (21.28; 95% confidence interval [CI] 22.22 to 20.38).[24]

2. Systemic Medications

Office-based analgesia/anesthesia is typically limited to the provision of moderate sedation or less, but most providers restrict their practice to minimal sedation using a combination of oral anxiolytics and analgesics with local anesthesia. Minimal sedation is defined as a drug-induced state during which patients respond normally to verbal commands.

Although cognitive function and coordination may be somewhat compromised, ventilation and cardiovascular functions are not affected.

Moderate sedation, also known as conscious sedation, is defined as a drug-induced depression of consciousness during which patients are able to respond to verbal commands, either alone or accompanied by light tactile stimulation.

a. **NSAIDs:** Nonsteroidal anti-inflammatory drugs (NSAIDs), such as ibuprofen, are commonly used prior to and after gynecological procedures to reduce pain. Their mechanism of action involves the inhibition of cyclooxygenase, which results in a reduction of the amount of circulating prostaglandins. A recent study found that ibuprofen 600 mg, given 30 minutes preoperatively, improved pain control and decreased postoperative pain when compared to placebo in patients undergoing uterine aspiration for first trimester abortions.[25] NSAIDs have also been combined with misoprostol in an effort to decrease pain. Li et al[26] compared misoprostol alone versus misoprostol combined with diclofenac for women having abortions between 7 and 12 weeks of gestation. They found a small decrease in pain during the procedure among multiparous subjects only (mean 58 vs 63, P 5.06, median 51 vs 68). NSAIDs have not been shown to interfere with the action of exogenous prostaglandins such as misoprostol.

b. **Opioids:** The use of opioid drugs has been mainly studied during abortions and uterine aspiration procedures. In 2011, a systematic review and meta-analysis of pain management for office gynecologic procedures identified only 1 placebo-controlled RCT evaluating opioid drugs.[27] This study evaluated the use of sublingual buprenorphine for hysteroscopy and concluded that this medication did not decrease pain but substantially increased side effects including nausea, vomiting, and drowsiness.

c. **Benzodiazepines:** Benzodiazepines are anxiolytic medications that have been shown to be safe for use to decrease pain during first-trimester uterine aspiration. However, there is no data suggesting this type of oral medication decreases procedural pain for other gynecologic procedures.[28]

d. **Misoprostol:** Misoprostol has been studied for cervical ripening prior to hysteroscopy. One meta-analysis of 10 studies concluded that misoprostol leads to greater preoperative dilation, decreased need for additional dilation, and reduced rates of cervical laceration in premenopausal women.[29] The greatest benefits were seen in nulliparous women and with operative hysteroscopy. However, women treated with misoprostol had higher rates of side effects and minor complications such as transient vaginal bleeding, cramping, and preoperative fever. The optimal dosing regimen for cervical ripening before hysteroscopy is unclear. In premenopausal women, studies have found either 200, 400, or 1000 g of vaginal misoprostol or 400 g of oral misoprostol given at least 9 to 12 hours preoperatively to be superior to placebo.[30] Most of these studies focused on nulliparous women. There are a few trials comparing routes of administration, dosage, and interval to procedure. Batukan C et al[31] compared 400 mcg of oral vs vaginal misoprostol given 10 to 12 hours before operative hysteroscopy in a double-blinded, placebo-control trial. The authors found vaginal misoprostol to be superior in baseline cervical dilation and decreased time required for cervical dilation. Other trials evaluating vaginal misoprostol for shorter intervals, 4 to 6 hours preoperatively, have not shown evidence of any effect. With the current evidence we can conclude that misoprostol has greater effect

Table 25.3: Recommendations and suggested pain management protocols

Medication	Dosage	Time course
Regimen 1		
Preprocedure		
Misoprostol	400 mcg PO	Night before
Ibuprofen	800 mg PO	Night before
Procedure		
Paracervical block	20 ml Lidocaine 1%	
Postprocedure		
Ibuprofen	400 mg PO	PRN pain
Regimen 2		
Preprocedure		
Ketorolac	30 mg IM	1 hour before
Ibuprofen	800 mg PO	1 hour before
Procedure		
None		
Postprocedure		
Oxycodone	5 mg PO	PRN pain
Regimen 3		
Preprocedure		
Ketorolac	30 mg IM	1 hour before
Procedure		
Paracervical block		
Postprocedure		
Ibuprofen	400 mg PO	PRN pain

in pregnant and premenopausal patients. For postmenopausal women the data is conflicting, and most studies do not show a benefit from misoprostol. Misoprostol's actions on the cervix may require endogenous estrogen. It is not known if more intensive dosing regimens would affect the postmenopausal cervix.[29]

3. Environmental

A blossoming area of study is the environmental factors that play into pain perception and the pain response during in-office procedures. A number of specialties have begun to study the effect of environmental factors that increase anxiety and procedure length, many of which are found to decrease patient satisfaction.

a. Procedure/Technique Factors

i. **Experience of the operator:** Hysteroscopist experience has been shown to be associated with patient's perception of pain during hysteroscopy. Experts tend to perform the procedure more quickly and smoothly, thereby causing less discomfort to the patient.

ii. **Distension media:** Hysteroscopy requires distension of the uterine cavity to allow adequate visualization. It is well accepted that the use of normal saline is associated with less pain than carbon dioxide. An important, frequently neglected, factor that generates pain and discomfort is the filling pressure utilized during the procedure. Higher uterine filling pressures cause excessive pain, which can result in failed procedures. The optimal filling pressure to provide adequate visualization without causing excessive pain is around 50 mmHg.

iii. **Hysteroscope size:** In the last two decades, a new generation of "mini" hysteroscopes that are 1 to 3 mm smaller than the conventional 5 mm instruments have hit the market. These small scopes have made more feasible to perform in-office hysteroscopy as they require less dilation of the cervical canal, cause less trauma, and thereby decrease the pain experienced during the procedure. A systematic review of 8 studies including 2322 patients who underwent office hysteroscopy without anesthesia concluded that 3.5 mm rigid mini-hysteroscopes are associated with significantly less pain than conventional 5 mm hysteroscopes.[32–33]

iv. **Use of flexible hysteroscopes:** The incorporation of fiber optic technology has produced flexible hysteroscopes with the ability to accommodate the pathway of the cervical canal. One prospective, randomized clinical trial of 142 women showed that pain was lessened with the use of flexible hysteroscopes but visualization was superior and more rapid procedures were performed with rigid hysteroscopes. However, there is insufficient evidence at this time to encourage the use of flexible over rigid instruments.[34]

v. **Vaginoscopic approach:** In 1997 Bettocchi and Selvaggi[4] presented a revolutionary approach to hysteroscopy advocating the "vaginoscopic approach" for diagnostic hysteroscopy, which avoids the use of a speculum and tenaculum. They presented a series of 1200 hysteroscopy, of which 680 were performed using the vaginoscopic approach and were found to be associated with significantly decreased rates of patient's discomfort. This technique soon became widespread and is currently the preferred approach of most expert hysteroscopists. A RCT from Sagiv et al[35] compared the vaginoscopic approach without anesthesia to the traditional approach with intra-cervical anesthesia. Eighty-three women underwent hysteroscopy without use of a speculum, tenaculum, or anesthesia. Forty-seven women received intracervical anesthesia with 10 ml of 3% mepivacaine hydrochloride solution. Hysteroscopy was performed using 0.9% saline solution as distension media and a rigid 3.7 mm hysteroscope in both groups. Both mean pain scores during the examination and after completion of the procedure were significantly lower in the group without use of a speculum, tenaculum, or anesthesia (p = .008). We strongly encourage the use of vaginoscopy whenever possible.

b. *Anxiety*

It is reasonable to assume that reducing pre-procedure anxiety has a positive impact on the patient's experience of pain during the procedure. Unfortunately, a systematic review of anxiety and pain perception found that only 13% of studies (9 out of 70 studies performed) evaluated patient anxiety. In the studies that did evaluate for it, elevated levels of anxiety were reported in patients waiting for hystero-scopy. In a large study of over 500 patients interviewed by a physician before undergoing hysteroscopy, 65% reported anxiety.[36] Other evaluations of patient perception of pain reveal that pain perception both during and after hysteroscopy was affected by patient state anxiety levels at the time of procedure.[37] Ideas for how to combat this anxiety in an effort to improve patient pain levels, thereby improving outcomes of hysteroscopy, are important for success in office-based procedures.

i. **Procedure time/wait time:** A study that evaluated waiting time to procedure found that pain was "significantly associated with waiting time of 60 minutes or longer."[15] Duration of the procedure is considered a limitation when performing in office procedures. Longer procedures and more difficult to tolerate. There is conflicting evidence suggesting that severe or intoler-able pain is more frequently reported in procedures lasting longer than 2 minutes. A prospective study including 558 patients reported that the duration of the procedure was significantly longer in patients who reported having experienced severe pain during the procedure.[38] How-ever, based on our personal observation, shorter procedures tend to be better tolerated.

ii. **Improving patient coping skills:** Studies have been done evaluating language used during gynecologic procedures. The use of positive suggestion during procedures has been shown to decrease anxiety. Positive suggestion includes describing procedural steps in a positive light that help to boost patient coping skills.[39] Instead of stating, "this will cause pain and cramping" the practitioner would instead say, "this is distension material that allows for good visualization of the uterine cavity." There has been evidence that adequate consent and explanation of the procedure help the patient to cope with pain.[40] One study even went as far as to offer an emotional support person to help ease the stress of the procedure, though that was in reference to abortion procedures and not hysteroscopy.[41]

iii. **Music therapy:** Music is being studied as a method with which to decrease anxiety and reduce pain perception during many types of office-based procedures. There is no consensus as to whether or not music is efficacious in reduction of pain perception. A single blind prospective randomized controlled trial of 82 patients showed that there was no effect of music when utilized in a multi-modal approach.[42] However, many other studies disagree. A prospective study of 356 patients divided women into a music and non-music group and measured pain perception before, during and after surgery. The study found that there was a "significant decrease in both anxiety and pain scores" as well as decreased systolic blood pressure and heart rate measured during surgery in the music group.[43] It has been hypothesized that music is a distraction and decreases pain perception. In a study by Chan et al they segregated the data into that which affected pain and that which affected anxiety during colposcopy. They found that the women who had listened to music had significantly decreased anxiety scores and pain scores.[44] In a Cochrane review of music and pain relief, 51 studies were assessed and found patients who were exposed to music postoperatively had 0.5 units lower pain intensity than those not exposed to music and that this value was statistically significant.[45]

CONCLUSION

In-office hysteroscopy plays an important role in modern gynecology. The number of procedures that are being currently performed in an office setting is growing. Patient comfort directly affects the ability of the hysteroscope operator to safely complete a procedure. Adequate patient selection is a fundamental step to achieve a successful office-based practice.

References

1. Mazzon I, Favilli A, Grasso M, Horvath S, Bini V, Di Renzo GC, et al. Pain in diagnostic hysteroscopy: a multivariate analysis after a randomized, controlled trial. Fertil Steril. 2014;102(5):1398–403.
2. Cicinelli E. Hysteroscopy without anesthesia: review of recent literature. J Minim Invasive Gynecol. 2010;17(6):703–8.
3. Bettocchi S, Nappi L, Ceci O, Selvaggi L. Office hysteroscopy. Obstet Gynecol Clin North Am. 2004;31(3):641–54, xi.
4. Bettocchi S, Selvaggi L. A vaginoscopic approach to reduce the pain of office hysteroscopy. J Am Assoc Gynecol Laparosc. 1997;4(2):255–8.
5. Cicinelli E, Parisi C, Galantino P, Pinto V, Barba B, Schonauer S. Reliability, feasibility, and safety of minihysteroscopy with a vaginoscopic approach: experience with 6,000 cases. Fertil Steril. 2003;80(1):199–202.
6. Clark TJ, Voit D, Gupta JK, Hyde C, Song F, Khan KS. Accuracy of hysteroscopy in the diagnosis of endometrial cancer and hyperplasia: a systemic quantitative review. JAMA 2002; 288(13):1610.
7. Kremer C, Duffy S, Moroney M. Patient satisfaction with outpatient hysteroscopy versus day case hysteroscopy: randomized control trial. BMJ, 2000; 320(7230):279–282.
8. Dalton V, Harris L, Weisman C, Guire K, Castleman L, Lebovic D. Patient preferences, satisfaction and resource use in office evacuation of early pregnancy failure. Obstetrics and Gynecology. 2006; 108(1): 103–110.
9. Salazar C, Isaacson K. Office Operative Hysteroscopy: An Update. Journal of Minimally Invasive Gynecology 2018; 25(2): 199–208.
10. Ahmad G, Attarbashi S, O'Flynn H, Watson A. Pain relief in office gynaecology: a systematic review and meta-analysis. European Journal of Obstetrics and Gynecology and Reproductive Biology 2011; 155(1): 3–13.
11. Tahir M, Bigrigg MA, Browning JJ, Brookes ST, Smith PA. A randomized controlled trial comparing transvaginal ultrasound, outpatient hysteroscopy and endometrial biopsy with inpatient hysteroscopy and curettage. Br J Obstet Gynaecol. 1999; 106(12): 1259–1264.

12. Ireland L, Allen R. Pain Management for Gynecologic Procedures in the Office. CME Review Article 71(2).

13. Mazzon I, Favilli A, Horvath S, Grasso M, Di Renzo GC, Laurenti E, et al. Pain during diagnostic hysteroscopy: what is the role of the cervical canal? A pilot study. Eur J Obstet Gynecol Reprod Biol. 2014;183:169–73.

14. van Dongen H, de Kroon CD, van den Tillaart SA, Louwe LA, Trimbos-Kemper GC, Jansen FW. A randomised comparison of vaginoscopic office hysteroscopy and saline infusion sonography: a patient compliance study. BJOG : an international journal of obstetrics and gynaecology. 2008; 115(10):1232–7.

15. Carta G, Palermo P, Marinangeli F, Piroli A, Necozione S, De Lellis V, et al. Waiting time and pain during office hysteroscopy. J Minim Invasive Gynecol. 2012;19(3):360–4.

16. Török P, Major T. Evaluating the level of pain during office hysteroscopy according to menopausal status, parity, and size of instrument. Archives of Gynecology and Obstetrics. 2013; 287(5):985–8.

17. Bettocchi S, Bramante S, Bifulco G, Spinelli M, Ceci O, Fascilla FD, et al. Challenging the cervix: strategies to overcome the anatomic impediments to hysteroscopy: Analysis of 31,052 office hysteroscopies. Fertil Steril. 2016;105(5):e16–7.

18. Tokushige N, Markham R, Russell P, Fraser IS. High density of small nerve fibres in the functional layer of the endometrium in women with endometriosis. Hum Reprod. 2006: 21(3): 782–787.

19. Sardo A, Florio P, Fernandez L, Fuerra G, Spinelli M, di Carlo C, Filippeschi M, Nappi C. The Potential Role of Endometrial Nerve Fibers in the Pathogenesis of Pain During Endometrial Biopsy at Office Hysteroscopy. Repro Sciences, 2015; 22(1):124–131.

20. Wong AY, Wong K, Tang LC. Stepwise pain score analysis of the effect of local lignocaine on outpatient hysteroscopy: a randomized, double-blind, placebo-controlled trial. Fertil Steril. 2000;73(6):1234–7.

21. Soriano D, Ajaj S, Chuong T, Deval B, Fauconnier A, Darai E. Lidocaine spray and outpatient hysteroscopy: randomized placebo-controlled trial. Obstet Gynecol. 2000;96(5 Pt 1):661–4.

22. Cooper NA, Khan KS, Clark TJ. Local anaesthesia for pain control during outpatient hysteroscopy: systematic review and meta-analysis. Bmj. 2010;340:c1130.

23. Mercier RJ, Zerden ML. Intrauterine anesthesia for gynecologic procedures: a systematic review. Obstet Gynecol. 2012;120(3):669–77.

24. Lau WC, Lo WK, Tam WH, Yuen PM. Paracervical anaesthesia in outpatient hysteroscopy: a randomised double-blind placebo-controlled trial. Br J Obstet Gynaecol. 1999;106(4):356–9.

25. Wiebe ER, Rawling M. Pain control in abortion. Int J Gynaecol Obstet. 1995;50(1):41–6.

26. Li CF, Wong CY, Chan CP, Ho PC. A study of co-treatment of nonsteroidal anti-inflammatory drugs (NSAIDs) with misoprostol for cervical priming before suction termination of first trimester pregnancy. Contraception. 2003; 67(2):101–5.

27. Ahmad G, Attarbashi S, O'Flynn H, Watson AJ. Pain relief in office gynaecology: a systematic review and meta-analysis. Eur J Obstet Gynecol Reprod Biol. 2011;155(1):3–13.

28. Allen RH, Micks E, Edelman A. Pain relief for obstetric and gynecologic ambulatory procedures. Obstet Gynecol Clin North Am. 2013;40(4):625–45.

29. Crane JM, Healey S. Use of misoprostol before hysteroscopy: a systematic review. J Obstet Gynaecol Can. 2006;28(5):373–9.

30. Allen R, O'Brien BM. Uses of misoprostol in obstetrics and gynecology. Rev Obstet Gynecol. 2009;2(3):159–68.

31. Batukan C, Ozgun MT, Ozcelik B, Aygen E, Sahin Y, Turkyilmaz C. Cervical ripening before operative hysteroscopy in premenopausal women: a randomized, double-blind, placebo-controlled comparison of vaginal and oral misoprostol. Fertil Steril. 2008;89(4):966–73.

32. Paulo AA, Solheiro MH, Paulo CO. Is pain better tolerated with mini-hysteroscopy than with conventional device? A systematic review and meta-analysis: hysteroscopy scope size and pain. Arch Gynecol Obstet. 2015;292(5):987–94.

33. Cicinelli E, Rossi AC, Marinaccio M, Matteo M, Saliani N, Tinelli R. Predictive factors for pain experienced at office fluid minihysteroscopy. J Minim Invasive Gynecol. 2007;14(4):485–8.

34. Unfried G, Wieser F, Albrecht A, Kaider A, Nagele F. Flexible versus rigid endoscopes for outpatient hysteroscopy: a prospective randomized control trial. Human Reproduction, 2001; 16(1):168–171.

35. Sagiv R, Sadan O, Boaz M, Dishi M, Schechter E, Golan A. A new approach to office hysteroscopy compared with traditional hysteroscopy: a randomized controlled trial. Obstet Gynecol. 2006;108(2):387–92.

36. Tahir M, Bigrigg MA, Browning JJ, Brookes ST, Smith PA. A randomized controlled trial comparing transvaginal ultrasound, outpatient hysteroscopy and endometrial biopsy with inpatient hysteroscopy and curettage. Br J ObstetGynaecol. 1999; 106(12): 1259–1264.

37. Nichols, Halvorson-Boyd G, Goldstein R, et al. Pain management. In: Paul M, Lichtenberg ES, Borgatta L, et al. eds. Management of Unintended and Abnormal Pregnancy. Hoboken, NJ: Wiley-Blackwell: 2009.

38. de Freitas Fonseca M, Sessa FV, Resende JA, Jr., Guerra CG, Andrade CM, Jr., Crispi CP. Identifying predictors of unacceptable pain at office hysteroscopy. J Minim Invasive Gynecol. 2014;21(4):586–91.

39. Royal College of Obstetricians and Gynaecologists. Best Practice in Outpatient Hysteroscopy, 2011; 59.

40. Lau WC, Ho RYF, Tsang MK et al. Patient's acceptance of outpatient hysteroscopy. Gynecol Obstet Invest 1999; 47: 191–193

41. Chor J, Goyal V, Roston A, et al. Doulas as facilitators: the expanded role of doulas into abortion care. Journal of Family Planning and Reproductive Health Care, 2012; 38: 123–124.

42. Mak N, Reinders I, Slockers S, Westen E, Maas J, Bongers M. The effect of music in gynaecological office procedures on pain, anxiety and satisfaction: a randomized controlled trial. Gynecological Surgery, 2017; 14(14).

43. Angioli R, de Cicco Nardone C, Plotti F, Cafa EV, Dugo N, Damiani P, Ricciardi R, Linciano F, Terranova C. Use of music to reduce anxiety during office hysteroscopy: prospective randomized trial. Journal of Minimally Invasive Gynecology, 2014; 21(3):454–459.

44. Chan YM, Lee PW, Ng TY, Ngan HY, Wong LC. The use of music to reduce anxiety for patients undergoing colposcopy. Gynecologic Oncology, 2003; 91(1): 213–217.

45. Cepeda MS, Carr DB, Lau J, Alvarez H. Music for pain relief. The Cochrane Library 2006, Issue 2.

Complications of Hysteroscopy

Rahul Manchanda, Nidhi Chandil, Esha Sharma

Hysteroscopy enables visualization of the uterine cavity and allows the diagnosis and surgical treatment of intrauterine pathology. To achieve this, the uterine cavity needs to be distended by a medium which could either be fluid or carbon dioxide.[1] As bleeding during operative procedures obscures visibility, for this reason, CO_2 is no longer used for operative hysteroscopy. Fluid media are used for operative procedures, as they allow continuous irrigation giving a clear picture and enable use of both mechanical and electrosurgical instruments.

TYPES OF COMPLICATIONS

- Early complications
- Late complications

EARLY COMPLICATIONS

A. Complications Related to the Patient Positioning

- *Femoral neuropathy:* The necessary lithotomy position (Fig. 26.1) in itself can cause nerve

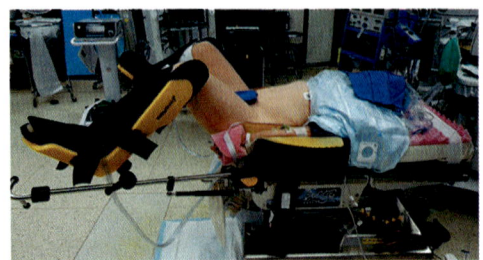

Fig. 26.1: Lithotomy position during hysteroscopy

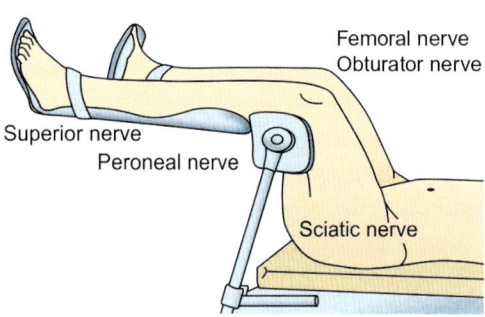

Femoral nerve
Obturator nerve
Superior nerve
Peroneal nerve
Sciatic nerve

Fig. 26.2: Nerve injury due to faulty position

trauma and direct injury to muscles.[2] Combination of excessive hip flexion, abduction and external hip rotation can cause extreme angulation of the femoral nerve result in femoral neuropathy as the nerve gets compressed and damaged. This injury resolves spontaneously in most cases over several months.

- *Sciatic and common peroneal nerve injury:* The sciatic nerve is located at the level of the neck of the fibula. Here sciatic nerve and peroneal nerves are fixed (Fig. 26.2). Excessive hip flexion with straight knees or too tightly fitted stirrup to the fibula results in nerve damage and foot drop or paresthesia over the lateral lower extremity.
- *Acute compartment syndrome:* Increased pressure in the muscle of an osteofascial compartment compromises local vascular

perfusion causing ischemia followed by reperfusion and capillary leakage within the ischemic tissue, and a further increase of edema leading to neuromuscular compromise. This causes rhabdomyolysis and possible serious sequellae including permanent disability.[3]

B. Anesthetic Complication

- Routine use of opiate analgesia before outpatient hysteroscopy should be avoided as it may cause adverse effects.
- Women without contraindications should be advised to take standard doses of non-steroidal anti-inflammatory agents (NSAIDs) such as 1000 mg paracetamol or 400 mg ibuprofen, around 1 hour before the scheduled outpatient hysteroscopy appointment with the aim of reducing pain in the immediate postoperative period.
- Operative hysteroscopy is usually performed under general anesthesia which is sometime related to certain complications are given below.

Allergic Complication

- Characterized by typical symptoms of agitations, palpitations, pruritis, cough, shortness of breath, urticaria, bronchospasm, shock and convulsion.
- *Treatment:* Administration of oxygen, isotonic intravenous fluid, intramuscular or subcutaneous adrenaline and intravenous prednisolone and aminophylline.

Cardiac Complication

- Impaired myocardial conduction includes bradycardia, cardiac arrest, shock and convulsion.
- *Treatment*—administration of oxygen, intravenous atropine (0.5 mg), intravenous adrenaline and the initiation of appropriate cardiac resuscitation.

Neurological Complication

- Paresthesia of the tongue, drowsiness, tremors and convulsions.

- Treatment-intravenous diazepam and respiratory support.

C. Complication Related to Instrumentation

   i. *Cervical laceration:* Routine cervical dilatation should not be done before office hysteroscopy.
- The cervix can be lacerated by the tenaculum used to stabilize it for the dilatation during operative hysteroscopy.

  ii. *Failed entry:* Causes are stenotic os, nulliparous cervix, menopausal flushed cervix, previous surgeries—cervical biopsy, cone biopsy, cryosurgeries, acute anteflexion or retroflexion, gonadotropin-releasing (GnRH) agonist use.

 iii. *False passage:* Occurs during dilatation of cervix without actually perforating the uterus (Fig. 26.3).

Measures to Reduce Cervical Injury

- The recommendation is always to use two tenacula; one at three and one at nine o' clock.
- The cervical canal has to be dilated with Hegar's progressively starting at four up to ten and a half. A certain amount of patience is necessary.

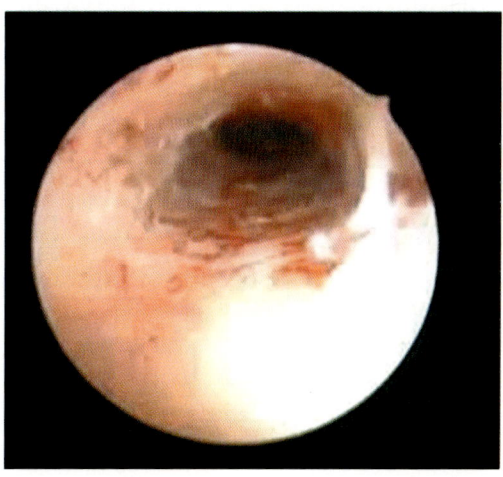

Fig. 26.3: False passage

- Misoprostol, a prostaglandin PGE_1 analogue is used as 400 µg vaginal suppositories 12 hours. before surgery associated with less intraoperative complications (cervical tears, creation of false passage, perforation, bleeding or simply difficulty in entering the internal os).[4]
- Adding vaginal 25 µg estradiol a day for 14 days even does reduce postoperative discomfort in postmenopausal women.[5]

D. Complications due to Distension Media

There are various types of distension media used in hysteroscopy (Flowchart 26.1).

Large volumes of distension solutions are being used during operative hysteroscopy for continuous irrigation, can lead to serious complications arising from significant fluid absorption through the opened blood vessels within the myometrium.

A fluid deficit of more than 1000 mL should be used as threshold to define fluid overload when using hypotonic solutions in healthy women of reproductive age.

A fluid deficit of 2500 mL should be used as threshold to define fluid overload when using isotonic solutions in healthy women of reproductive age (GPP).

- A decrease in serum sodium of 10 mmol/L corresponds to an absorbed volume of approximately 1000 mL when using 1.5% glycine.[6]
- However, in the elderly or those women with co-morbid conditions such as cardiovascular disease and renal impairment, lower thresholds should apply and it is suggested that upper fluid deficit levels of 750 mL for hypotonic solutions and 1500 mL for isotonic solutions.[7]
- Procedure should be abandoned once this threshold has achieved.

Factors Affecting Systemic Absorption

Absorption of distension media into the systemic circulation occurs by:
  i. Retrograde passage of the fluid through the fallopian tubes
  ii. Through the endometrium, and
  iii. via opened blood vessels and sinuses during resection of uterine tissue
- *Intrauterine pressure:* The higher the pressure, the greater the degree of absorption into the body; systemic absorption of fluid increases considerably when intrauterine pressure exceeds mean arterial pressure.[8] In addition, intrauterine pressures >75 mm Hg increases the volume of media passing back along the fallopian tubes and into the peritoneal cavity.[9]
- *Mean arterial pressure:* The lower the mean arterial pressure, the lower the intrauterine pressure required to cause passage of fluid into the systemic circulation. Caution is thus

Flowchart 26.1: Types of distension media

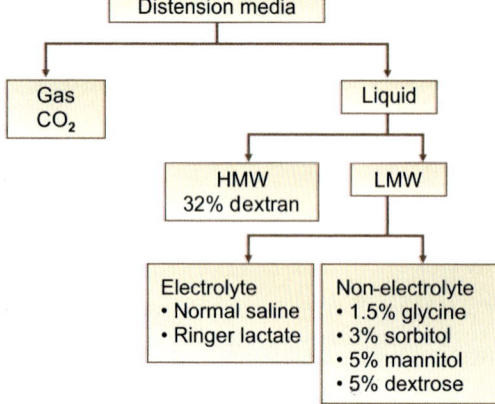

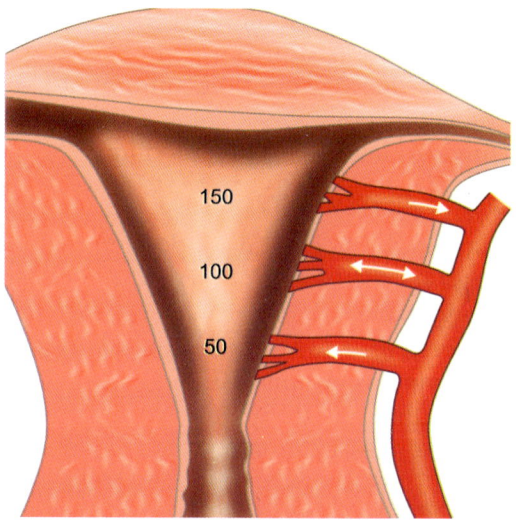

Fig. 26.4: Relation between intrauterine pressure and intra-arterial pressure

required in the elderly and those with cardiovascular co-morbidities.[10]

- *Depth of myometrial penetration:* When tissue damage extends into the deeper myometrium, instilled fluid can be rapidly absorbed through opened myometrial venous sinuses. The risk of fluid absorption is even greater during myomectomies where large blood vessels are breached facilitating the absorption of fluid under pressure.

- *Duration of surgery:* The longer the procedure the more time for fluid to accumulate within the body.[11]

- *Size of uterine cavity:* Larger cavities provide a greater endometrial surface area for fluid absorption and procedures will generally be longer. However, despite requiring more instilled fluid, high intrauterine pressures to allow adequate visualization are harder to achieve.[12]

- *Osmolality of distension fluid:* Hypotonic electrolyte-free solutions like glycine, mannitol and sorbitol can cause hyponatremic hypervolemia. If unrecognized and left untreated, bradycardia and hypertension can develop, rapidly followed by pulmonary edema, cardiovascular collapse and death.[13]

- *Menopausal status:* Premenopausal patients have a higher risk of developing neurological complications due to the suppressive effects of estrogen on the ATPase pump which regulates the flow of electrolytes through the blood–brain barrier.[14, 15]

- *Cardiovascular and renal disease:* Those women with known cardiovascular disease, renal impairment and the elderly are less likely to adapt to sudden significant increases in intravascular fluid such that complications from systemic fluid expansion and electrolyte imbalance are more likely at lower levels of fluid deficit.[16]

1. Electrolyte imbalance due to fluid overload with hypotonic fluid media

Glycine 1.5% (200 mOsm/L) and sorbitol 3% (165 mOsm/L) are the most common hypotonic electrolyte-free distending media used for operative hysteroscopy with monopolar electrosurgical energy. Moderate fluid overload causes hypervolemia and consequent dilutional hyponatremia. At this stage, despite the drop of sodium concentration, the osmolality of the blood is not greatly affected (normal osmolality, 280 mOsm/L). This asymptomatic hyponatraemia can be managed with fluid restriction and diuretics such as frusemide in the absence of a diuresis.

Symptoms usually develop when serum sodium concentration drops below 125 mmol/L. The most frequent symptoms are headache, nausea, vomiting and weakness. If further fluid intravasation occurs, reduction of the blood osmolality creates an osmotic gradient that moves water into the interstitial and intracellular space, leading to brain edema and increased intracranial pressure. The resultant cerebral edema may present with signs of cerebral irritation such as agitation, apprehension, confusion, weakness, nausea, vomiting, visual disturbances, blindness and headache. If significant, it can lead to brain stem herniation, coma and death.[17] A further fall of sodium below 120 mmol/L may lead to confusion, lethargy, seizures, coma, arrhythmias, bradycardia and respiratory arrest.

Management of fluid overload and electrolyte imbalance: Early recognition and treatment is essential to prevent cardiovascular complications and permanent neurological sequelae resulting from toxic hyponatremia.

- A strict fluid balance must be commenced in theatre and should extend into the postoperative period (Figs 26.5 and 26.6).

- An urinary catheter should be inserted and the electrolytes, urea and creatinine measured.

- A loop diuretic like frusemide should be given intravenously and the urine output measured.

Table 26.1: Management of suspected hypervolemic hyponatremia arising from fluid overload >1000 mL with hypotonic distension media

Acute hypervolemic hyponatremia[a]	Management
Asymptomatic hyponatremia and [Na⁺] ≥125 mmol/L	Fluid restriction (e.g. <1 L/day) and loop diuretics, e.g. 40 mg frusemide
Symptomatic hyponatremia and/or [Na⁺] <120 mmol/L	Hypertonic (3%,) saline (1 L = 513 mmol/L NaCl compared with normal saline where 1 L = 154 mmol/L), supplemental oxygen, indwelling urinary catheter, high dependency care and multi-disciplinary team involvement

[a]Normal serum sodium levels are approximately between 135 and 145 mmol/L

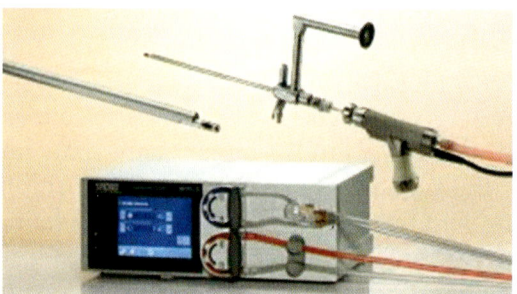

Fig. 26.5: Hysteromat with hysteroscope

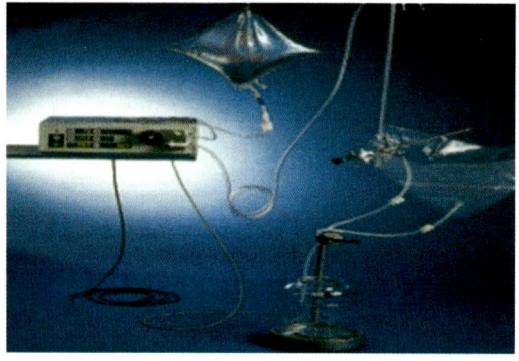

Fig. 26.6: Fluid delivery and collection system

- If the patient develops signs of cardiac failure or pulmonary edema a cardiac echocardiogram and chest X-ray should be undertaken with involvement of the physicians.

The management of symptomatic hyponatremia requires multidisciplinary involvement including anesthetists, physicians and intensivists in a high dependency or intensive care unit (Table 26.1).

- Hyponatremia below 120 mmol/L should be treated with a 100 mL bolus of 3% hypertonic saline over 10 min and this can be repeated up to three times, until serum sodium rises to 120 mmol/L, followed by an intravenous infusion of a slow 3% hypertonic sodium chloride infusion (typically 1–2 mmol/L/hr to prevent pontine myelinolysis) is indicated until serum sodium rises to 125 mmol/L.[12, 13, 17, 18]

- The recommended target increase of the serum sodium is 6 mmol/L over 24 h until 130 mmol/L is reached. Even a small increase in the sodium concentration can reduce the risk of cerebral edema and the risk of systemic complications.[19, 20]

- Oxygen saturations, urine output and serum electrolytes including potassium and calcium should be closely monitored.

- Sorbitol 3% is a hypotonic sugar solution and if excessive intravasation of sorbitol occurs, it can also lead to hyperglycemia and hypocalcemia. Consequent symptoms can develop quite rapidly, as myoclonus within an hour of the procedure has been described.[21, 22] In this situation, monitoring of the blood sugars is necessary and starting an insulin sliding scale if the blood sugar levels are high.

- Hypocalcemia should be corrected with 3 g of calcium gluconate over 10 min.[23] This should be given with advice from an intensivist.

2. Fluid overload with isotonic fluid media

Bipolar electrosurgery is conducted with electrolyte containing solutions such as isotonic saline. This medium reduces the risk of hypo-osmolarity and hyponatremia with excessive fluid absorption but does not eliminate the risk of congestive cardiac failure and pulmonary edema. Fluid restriction, diuretics and monitoring as described above is usually all that is required.

Estimation of Fluid Loss

- Closed systems should be used as they allow more accurate measurement of the fluid output.
- Drapes that contain a fluid reservoir should be used as they allow measurement of the fluid output.
- Urine output should be measured by catheterizing the bladder.
- Ultrasound is used to estimate the amount of fluid in the peritoneal cavity.
- Measurement of the fluid deficit should be done at a minimum of 10 min intervals during hysteroscopic surgery.
- Communication with the anesthetist is important to guide postoperative fluid management as they will also be aware of the amount of intravenous fluid given peri-operatively.

3. Air or gas embolism

- Although it is rare but can occur during a hysteroscopy with both gas (CO_2) or fluid distension media and in the outpatient as well as inpatient setting.[24, 25]
- Air can enter the uterine cavity during insertion of the hysteroscope if the inflow tubing is not primed with fluid or due to air bubbles within the distension medium potentially causing air embolism.[26]
- To minimise the risk of air embolism, the hysteroscope and inflow tubing should be primed with the fluid media to eliminate air bubbles before inserting the hystero-scope into the uterine cavity.[24]

- Gas embolism may arise from the combustion of gases produced during hystero-scopic electrosurgery.[27]
- The gases normally produced are primarily carbon dioxide (CO_2) as well as carbon monoxide and evaporative gases, the latter being easily soluble in blood and hence do not cause serious complications.[27]
- Isotonic electrolyte-containing distension media such as normal saline should be used with mechanical instrumentation and bipolar electrosurgery because they are less likely to cause hyponatremia if fluid overload occurs.
- Hypotonic, electrolyte-free distension media such as glycine and sorbitol should only be used with monopolar electro-surgical instruments.
- Carbon dioxide gaseous media should not be used for operative hysteroscopy.

Various Preoperative Measure to Reduce Fluid Absorption

- GnRH agonists can reduce electrolyte disturbance in premenopausal women by enhancing the action of the sodium-potassium ATP ase pump responsible for shunting sodium outside the cells. This pump is inhibited by female sex steroids making premenopausal women more susceptible to hyponatremic complications during hysteroscopic surgery.[2, 15]
- Studies have shown that giving pre-operative GnRH analogues when under-taking resection of the myoma or endo-metrium reduces the incidence of fluid overload.[28, 29]
- A distension medium is required to separate the uterine surfaces, for visualiza-tion of the uterine cavity needing an intrauterine pressure (IUP) between 70 and 100 mmHg. The pressure needed depends on the uterine size, muscle thickness and tone. The higher the IUP is, the higher the risk of excessive fluid absorption. The pressure within the venous

sinuses in the myometrium is thought to be around 10–15 mmHg.[30]

- Three studies have shown that intracervical injection of diluted vasopressin immediately before cervical dilatation is associated with reduced fluid absorption during operative hysteroscopy.[31–33]

E. Uterine Perforation

- Perforation may occur during dilation of the cervix, positioning of the hysteroscope, or as a consequence of the intrauterine procedure (Fig. 26.7).

- Incidence of perforation varies between 4% and 13% as reported in literature.[34]
- With complete perforation, the endometrial cavity typically does not distend and the visual field is generally lost.
- When perforation occurs during dilation of cervix, the procedure must be terminated but because of the blunt nature of the dilators, usually there are no other injury.
- If perforation occur by the activated tip of a laser, or electrode, there is a risk to injuries to the adjacent viscera. Therefore, operation

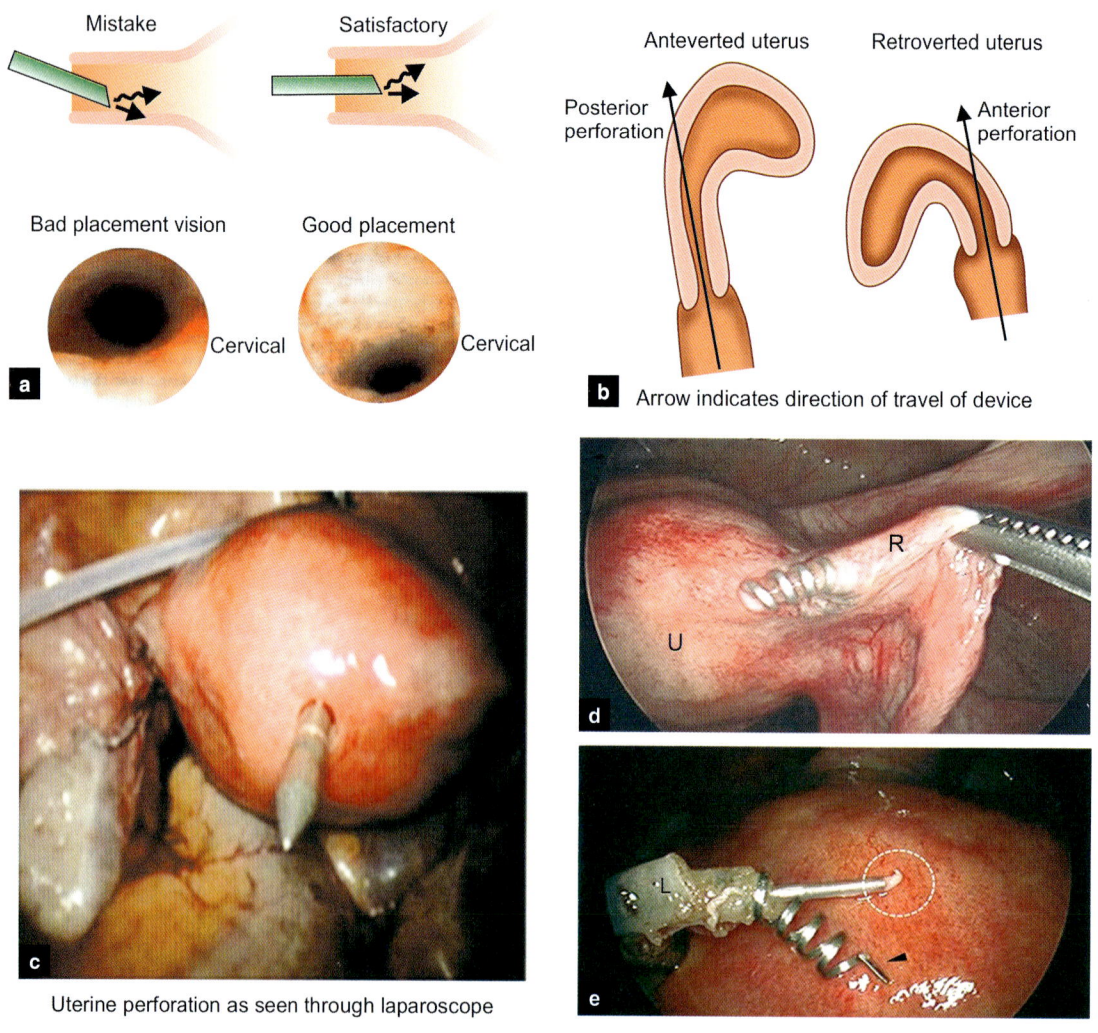

Fig. 26.7a to d: Perforation injury during hysteroscopy

must be stopped and laparoscopy or laparotomy should be performed.

- Perforation can occur with morcellators used in operative hysteroscopy. The device should never be activated outside the uterine cavity. A clear exposure by adequate expansion of the uterine cavity is mandatory when using the device.[35]

F. Bleeding

- Bleeding can occur during or after hysteroscopy generally result from trauma to the vessels in the myometrium or injury to the vessels in the pelvis.
- The risk for bleeding may be reduced by the preoperative injection of diluted vasopressin in the cervical stroma.[32]
- The risk of injury to branches of the uterine artery can be lowered by limiting the depth of resection in the lateral endometrial cavity near the uterine isthmus, where ablative technique should be considered.
- The ball electrode can be used to desiccate the vessel electrosurgically.
- Intractable bleeding may respond to the injection of diluted vasopressin (4 U or 0.2 mL in 60 mL normal saline) directly into the cervix 2 cm deep, at the 4 and 8 o'clock position or to the inflation of a 30 mL Foley catheter balloon or similar device in the endometrial cavity (Fig. 26.8).[36]

G. Infection

Endometritis following operative hysteroscopy is an extremely rare complication 0.01 to 1.42% except in the removal of IUCDs in postmenopausal patients except in the later routine antibiotic prophylaxis is not recommended for the general population.[37] Level B recommendation.

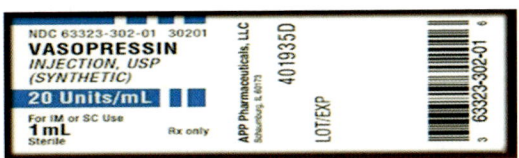

Fig. 26.8: inj. vasopressin

If patients present with a history of pelvic inflammatory disease (PID) the use of prophylactic antibiotics may be considered by ACOG and the Society of Obstetricians and Gynecologists of Canada. Level C recommendation.

H. Electrosurgical Complications

The important intraoperative or postoperative complications from electrosurgical devices are thermal injuries to viscera which can lead to peritonitis, sepsis and death. Thermal injuries usually follow perforation, however, thermal bowel injury in absence of uterine perforation has been reported.[38]

Electrosurgical thermal effects with monopolar current are complex and not fully understood. Undesired energy transfer from active electrode to viscera can occur due to faulty insulation, direct coupling and capacitive coupling.

Proper instrumentation and activation of electrode always under vision, will prevent this undesirable energy transfer but jumping of electrical energy due to capacitive coupling is beyond the control of surgeon. Fortunately, capacitive coupling is not reported with hysteroscopic surgery.

LATE COMPLICATIONS

I. Intrauterine Adhesions

- Postoperative adhesion formation is a problem in women of reproductive age seeking further pregnancies. One RCT on the effectiveness of preoperative treatment claims that the incidence of postoperative adhesions is of 3.6% after polyp removal, 6.7 % after resection of uterine septa, 31.3% after removal of a single fibroid and 45.5% after resection of multiple fibroids (Fig. 26.9).[39]

J. Hematometra

- Hematometra is a very unlikely complication and occurs only when the resection encloses the isthmus of the uterus causing occluding adhesions.

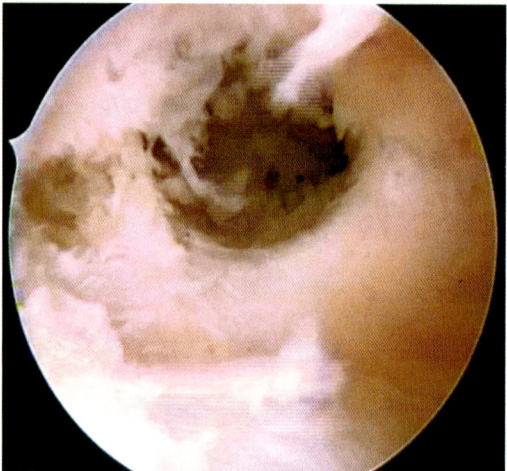

Fig. 26.9: Intrauterine adhesion following hysteroscopy

- Its incidence is 1–2%.[40]
- Most cases can be treated with dilatation of the cervical canal except for strong adhesions in the cornu. These need a repeat operative procedure.
- When endometrial patches remain in the cornu these can create a post-ablation tubal sterilization syndrome with symptoms of unilateral, bilateral cramping cyclic pelvic pains and vaginal spotting.

K. Unplanned Pregnancy

- An unplanned pregnancy may occur after hysteroscopic sterilization although it is very uncommon with the newer generation devices.
- Unplanned pregnancy may occur in post-endometrial ablation patients.

  In 2002, Cook et al reported 43 pregnancies and 17 over 20 weeks gestation.[41]

  In 2005, Hare et al reviewing the literature did find 70 reported pregnancies of which 31 viable with 12.9% perinatal mortality, a degree of 42% of prematurity, morbidly adherent placenta in 26% and a 17% of Cesarean sections for 31% of malpresentations.[42]

- The conclusion is that pregnancies after operative hysteroscopy have to be treated as high-risk pregnancies.

L. Dissemination of Cancer Cells

Recently a systematic review and meta-analysis did demonstrate a significant higher occurrence of malignant peritoneal cytology following hysteroscopy versus no hysteroscopy performed in women where the diagnosis of endometrial carcinoma had been made. (Odds ratio (OR) 1.8 at 95% confidence interval (CI) 1.1–2.8 P = 0.013 , 9 studies, 1015 women.) There was an higher rate of disease upstaging compared with no hysteroscopy (OR 2.6, 95% CI 1.5–4.6, P = 0.001, 9 studies, 1015 women). When normal saline is used there is an increase in the rate of malignant peritoneal cytology (OR 2.9, 95% 1.5–5.6, P = 0.002, 9 studies, 1015 women). The increase of the appearance of malignant cells in the peritoneal fluid does not seem to increase with increasing intrauterine pressure up to 100 mmHg (OR 3.2, 95% CI 0.94–11, P = 0.06).[43]

On the other hand from earlier studies it has been proven that there is not only the tubal passage but also other passageways for cancer cells as in some patients with previous blockage of the tubes cancer cells have been found in the peritoneal fluid and hence the intrauterine pressure to be aware off.[44]

References

1. Brusco GF, Arena S, Angelini A. Use of carbon dioxide versus normal saline for diagnostic hysteroscopy. Fertil Steril 2003;79:993.
2. Munro MG. 'Complications of hysteroscopic and uterine resectoscopic surgery'. Obstet Gynecol Clin North Am 2010; 37:399–425.
3. Dua RS, Bankes MJ, Dowd GS 'Compartment syndrome following pelvic surgery in the lithotomy position'. Ann R Coll Surg Engle 2002; 84:170–71.
4. Al-Fozan H, Firwana B, AlKadri H, Hassan S, Tulandi T. Cochrane Database Syst Rev 2015 Apr 23;(4):CD005998.
5. Casadei l, Piccolo E, Manicuti CL, Cardinale S, Collamarini M, Piccione E. Role of vaginal estradiol pre-treatment combined with vaginal misoprostol for cervical ripening before operative hysteroscopy in postmenopausal women. Obstet Gynecol Sci 2016;59(3):220–26.

6. Istre O, Bjoennes J, Naess R, Hornbaek K, Forman A. Postoperative cerebral oedema after transcervical endometrial resection and uterine irrigation with 1.5% glycine. Lancet 1994;344: 1187–89.

7. AAGL Practice Report: practical Guidelines for the Management of hysteroscopic distension media. J Minim Invasive Gynecol 2013;20:137–48.

8. Garry R, Hashamf, Kokrims, Mooney P. The effect of pressure on fluid absorption during endometrial ablation. J Gynecol Surg 1992;8(1):1–10.

9. Hasham F, Garry R, Kokri MS, Mooney P. Fluid Absorption during laser ablation of the endometrium in the treatment of menorrhagia. Br J Anaesth 1992;68:151–54.

10. Bennett K, Ohrmundt C, Maloni J. Preventing intravasation in women undergoing hysteroscopic procedures. AORN J 1996;64(5): 792–99.

11. Paschopoulos M, Polyzos NP, Lavasidis LG, Vrekoussis T, Dalkalitsis N, Paraskevaidis E. Safety issues of hysteroscopic surgery. Ann N Y Acad Sci 2006;1092:229–34.

12. Varol N, Maher P, Vancaillie T, Cooper M, Carter J, Kwok A, Reid G. A literature review and update on the prevention and management of fluid overload in endometrial resection and hysteroscopic surgery. Gynaecol Endosc 2002; 11(1):19–26.

13. Kaijser J, Roelofs HJM, Breimer LTM, Kooi SG. Excessive fluid overload with severe hypo-natremia, cardiac failure, and cerebral edema complicating hysteroscopic myomectomy. J Pelvic Med Surg 2007;13:367–73.

14. Taskin O, Yalcinoglu A, Kucuk S, Burak F, Ozekici U, Wheeler JM. The degree of fluid absorption during hysteroscopic surgery in patients pretreated with goserelin. J AmAssoc Gynecol Laparosc 1996;3(4):555–59.

15. Taskin O, Buhur A, Birincioglu M, Burak F, Atmaca R, Yilmaz I, Wheeler JM. Endometrial Na+, K+ ATPase pump function and vasopressin levels during hysteroscopic surgery in patients pretreated with GnRH agonist. J Am Assoc Gynecol Laparosc 1998;5(2):119–24.

16. Aydeniz B, Gruber IV, Schauf B, Kurek R, Meyer A, Wallwiener D. A multicenter survey of complications associated with 21676 operative hysteroscopies. Eur J Obstet Gynecol Reprod Biol 2002;104:160–64.

17. Baggish M, Brill A, Rosenweig B, Barbot J, Indman P. Fatal acute glycine and sorbitol toxicity during operative hysteroscopy. J Gynecol Surg 1993; 9(3):137–43.

18. Vachharajani TJ, Zaman F, Abreo KD. Hypo-natremia in critically ill patients. J Intensive Care Med 2003;18:3–8.

19. Verbalis JG, Goldsmith SR, Greenberg A, Schrier RW, Sterns RH. Hyponatremia treatment guidelines 2007: expert panel recommendations. Am J Med 2007;120(11):S1–21.

20. Verbalis JG, Goldsmith SR, Greenberg A, Korzelius C, Schrier RW, Sterns RH, Thompson CJ. Diagnosis, evaluation, and treatment of hyponatremia: expert panel recommendations. Am J Med 2013;126(10):S1-42.

21. Lee GY, Han JI, Heo HJ. Severe hypocalcemia caused by absorption of sorbitol-mannitol solution during hysteroscopy. J Korean Med Sci 2009; 24(3):532–34.

22. Almonti S, Cipriani M, Villani V, Rinalduzzi S. Reversible myoclonus in a patient undergoing transcervical hysteroscopic surgery. Neurol Sci 2013;34(10):1815–17.

23. Lee JW. Fluid and electrolyte disturbances in critically ill patients. Electrolyte Blood Press 2010;8(2):72–81.

24. Brandner P, Neis KJ, Ehmer C. The etiology, frequency, and prevention of gas embolism during CO_2 hysteroscopy. JAmAssoc Gynecol Laparosc 1999;6(4):421–28.

25. Brundin J, Thomasson K. Cardiac gas embolism during carbon dioxide hysteroscopy: risk and management. Eur J Obstet Gynecol Reprod Biol 1989;33(3):241–45.

26. Brooks P. Venous air embolism during operative hysteroscopy. J Am Assc of Gynecol Lap 1997; 4(3):399–402.

27. Imasogie N, Crago R, Leyland N, Chung F. Probable gas embolism during operative hystero-scopy caused by products of combustion. Can J Anaesth 2002;49:1044–47.

28. O'Connor H, Magos A. Endometrial resection for the treatment for menorrhagia. N Engl J Med 1996;335:151–56.

29. Muzii L, Boni T, Bellati F, Marana R, Ruggiero A, Zullo M, Angioli R, Panici PB. GnRH analogue treatment before hysteroscopic resection of submucous myomas: a prospective randomized, multicenter study. Fertil Steril 2010;94:1496–99.

30. Sethi N, Chaturvedi R, Kumar K. Operative hysteroscopy intravascular absorption syndrome: a bolt from the blue. Indian J Anaesth 2012; 556:179–82.

31. Corson SL, Brooks PG, Serden SP, Batzer FR, Gocial B. Effects of vasopressin administration during hysteroscopic surgery. J Reprod Med 1994;39(6):419–23.

32. Phillips DR, Nathanson HG, Milim SJ, Haselkorn JS, Khapra A, Ross PL. The effect of dilute vasopressin solution on blood loss during operative hysteroscopy: a randomised controlled trial. Obstet Gynecol 1996;88:761–66.

33. Goldenberg M, Zolti M, Bider D, Etchin A, Sela BA, Seidman DS. The effect of intracervical vasopressin on the systemic absorption of glycine during hysteroscopic endometrial ablation. Obstet Gynecol 1996;87(6):1025–29.

34. Grames DA. "Diagnostic dilatation and curettage a reappraisal". Am J Obstet Gynecol 1982;142:1–6.

35. Noventa M, Ancona E, Quaranta M, Vitagliano A, Cosmi E, D'Antona D, Gizzo S. "Intrauterine Morcellator Device: The Icon of Hysteroscopic Future or Merely a Marketing Image? A Systematic Review Regarding Safety, Efficacy, Advantages and Contraindications". Reprod Sci 2015 Oct; 22(10):1289–96.

36. Brill AI. What is the role of hysteroscopy in the management of abnormal uterine bleeding? Clin Obstet Gynecol 1995;38:319–45.

37. American College of Obstetricians and Gynecologists (ACOG). Antibiotic prophylaxis for gynecologic procedures. Washington (DC), 2009, ACOG Practice Bulletin no 14.

38. Kivnick S, Kante MK. Bowel injury from roller-ball ablation of endometrium. Obstel Gynecol 1992;79:833.

39. Taskin O, Sadi S, Onoglu A. "Role of endometrial suppression on the frequency of intrauterine adhesion after resectoscopic surgery". J Am Assoc Gynecol Laparosc 2000; 7:351–54.

40. Hill D, Maher P, Wood C. "Complications of operative hysteroscopy". Gynaecol Endosc 1992; 1:185–89.

41. Cook JR, Semal IE. "Pregnancy Following Endometrial Ablation: Case History and Literature Review" Obstetrical and Gynecological Survey 2003; 58–8:551–58.

42. Hare AA, Olah KS. Pregnancy following endometrial ablation: a review article. Journal Obstetrics and gynaecology 2009; 25:108–14.

43. Polyzos MP, Mauri D, Tsioras S. "Intraperitoneal dissemination of endoemtrial cancer cells after hysteroscopy. A systematic review and meta-analysis". Int J Gynecol Cancer 2010; 20:231–67.

44. Creasman WT, Lukerman J. "Role of the fallopian tube dissemination of malignant cells in corpus cancer". Cancer 1972; 29:456–57.

Hysteroscopy Redefined

Artificial Intelligence in Hysteroscopy

Péter Török

Thanks to Pantaleoni we have the opportunity to have been having an inner-view of the uterus for 150 years.[1] Using the continuously developed instruments and techniques better and better visualization of the intrauterine pathologies could be achieved. Beyond the improving diagnostic value, by more and more operative procedures these pathologies could be treated, as well.[2] Introducing video computer chip in 1986, projection of images onto television screens could be carried out, so more and more endoscopic operations were performed including hysteroscopies and laparoscopies instead of open surgery and laparotomy.[3] Advantages and disadvantages of the endoscopic method were described by several publication, leaving no doubt about the preferred minimally invasive procedures.[4] Besides its vast advantages, a serious drawback of endoscopy is lacking of most tactile information. Differentiating and identifying structures and tissues are very important step of the procedure to decrease complication rate, operative time and mortality, as well. It is also useful for avoiding or at least minimizing the rate of the complications. The position, color of the structures and their connections to other organs can lead us to identify structures. Frames, captured by high resolution endoscopic cameras letting us to examine the structures under magnification. Connecting these cameras

to a computer is giving us another huge opportunity. The capacity of a computer makes it possible to have it proceed millions of processing per seconds. With this property images of endoscopic surgeries could be analyzed very quickly, even during the procedure.

During hysteroscopy many types of intrauterine pathologies and various kinds of operative procedures could be observed. This new opportunity could help in many ways to the surgeon. By recognizing different types of tissue it can help in decision making in several aspects. As a proof of concept, first we tried two different image processing.

In first study, we used automatic segmentation of videos. On these images focal pathologies (polyps or fibroid-myometrial margin) were annotated manually. The pre-trained method was tested after on images, by the accuracy of recognition.

During second study endometrial pattern was analyzed by image classification algorithm. Endometrial receptivity has been researched for many years all over the word. Morphologic quality, histologic discrepancy, proteomic, lipidomic investigations have been running continuously. Trying to find and eliminate different obstructing factors (like chronic endometritis) success rate of *in vitro* fertilization could be improved. In this preliminary study, by having the endpoint if IVF treatment (intrauterine gravidity detected by sonography), due to the differences in endometrial features we tried to find some correlation.

In the past years, deep learning-based techniques became the primary tools to handle digital image processing problems. Among them, perhaps the most versatile methods consider convolutional neural networks (CNNs). Originally, CNN architectures were created to solve image classification tasks.[5–7] Later on, they have been modified to handle more complex tasks like part/keypoint detection,[8,9] or the localization of objects by bounding boxes.[10,11] In 2015, a new variant of CNN models, called fully convolutional neural network (FCNN), was released, which is able to make a pixel-wise prediction in order to solve semantic segmentation tasks.[12]

Gold standard method for treatment of submucous fibroids is hysteroscopic resection.[13] Independently the instrument (monopolar resectoscope, bipolar resectoscope, LASER, cold-loop technique), that is used for the main point is to respect the pseudocapsule. Following this principle damage of the healthy myometrium can be avoided. Resection of the myoma only decreases the rate of complications (uterine perforation, adhesion formation, fibroid regrowth).[14] Differentiating healthy myometrium and myoma is very important, but challenging problem. Computer analyzation of endoscopic images therefore could be a good assistance in this question.

Among intrauterine pathologies lying in the background of heavy menstrual bleeding or infertility, in most of the cases polypoid growth can be visualized by hysteroscopy.[15] Polypoid pathologies could be histologically proved to be endometrial polyp, endometrial cancer or hyperplastic endometrium, as well. Differentiating them by the visual information could help in choosing the proper therapeutic method.

1. Our approach for the extraction of the myomas or polyps from the background is

based on fully convolutional neural networks (FCCNs). As for methodology, FCNNs are used for the automatic segmentation of the video frames to determine the region of myomas or polyps. Using these types of architecture, we can create a pixel-level probability map for the input image regarding the question which pixels belong to myomas or polyps. Our main contribution in this field is that we raised segmentation accuracy using ensemble-based approaches in two stages. First, after splitting a video frame into sub-images, we aggregate the predictions of an individual FCNN for the overlapping regions. As the applied FCNN models require input image size of 500×500 pixels, we have partitioned our original full HD (1920×1080 pixels) resolution video frames to overlapping sub-images. We chose this option, because the resizing of the ROI of the pictures would smooth the small differences and decrease the segmentation accuracy. By combining these fragments, we can get the predictions for the whole input images. Then, the final segmentation result is composed as a weighted combination of the outputs of three FCNNs in both uses cases (myomas and polyps segmentation). For the visual explanation of how these three outputs are aggregated to gain a final segmentation with a weighted ensemble-based approach (Fig. 27.1).

For the training of the FCNNs, the gynecologist manually marked the region of interest (ROI) for recognition during the operation. Annotation happened by the same expert gynecologist with more than 1000 operative hysteroscopies, who performed the operation. These manually drawn binary images where white/black pixels belonged to the myoma or polyps/healthy parts of the image.

Considering the case of myoma segmentation problem we collected 6288 sub-images have been collected from hysteroscopic videos recorded during the same number

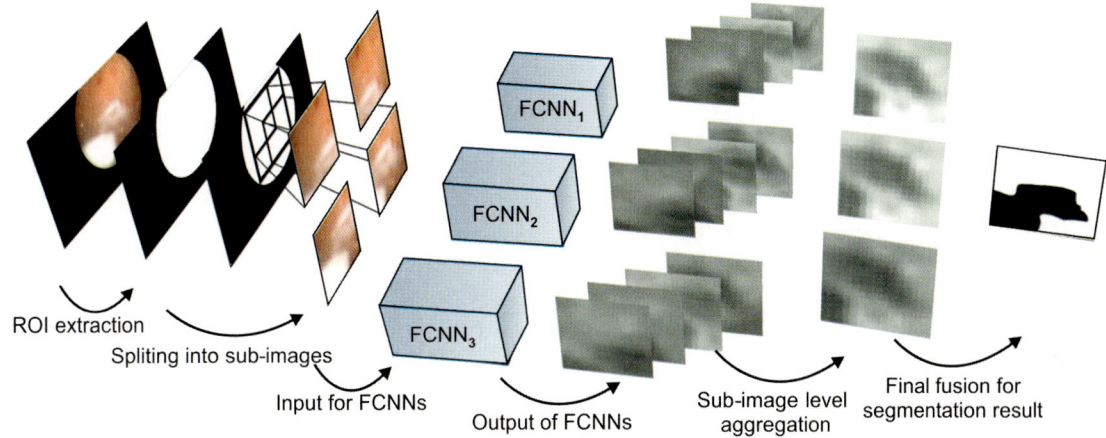

Fig. 27.1: Flowchart of the proposed ensemble-based system

of gynecologic surgeries. On the images myoma/myometrial margins were drawn and annotated manually. The image set is divided into two parts as training and test set which contain 4688 and 1600 images, respectively.

For the polyp segmentation task, to provide the ground-truth for training/testing, gynecologist revised the video frames (extracted from 12 videos) and collected those ones, where polyps were visible, in this way we extracted 4220 sub-images.

During the time-demanding training phase, the applied FCNN networks automatically extract the features of the different classes of the pixels and after that it can segments the region of myomas/polyps from the background as it can be seen in Fig. 27.2.

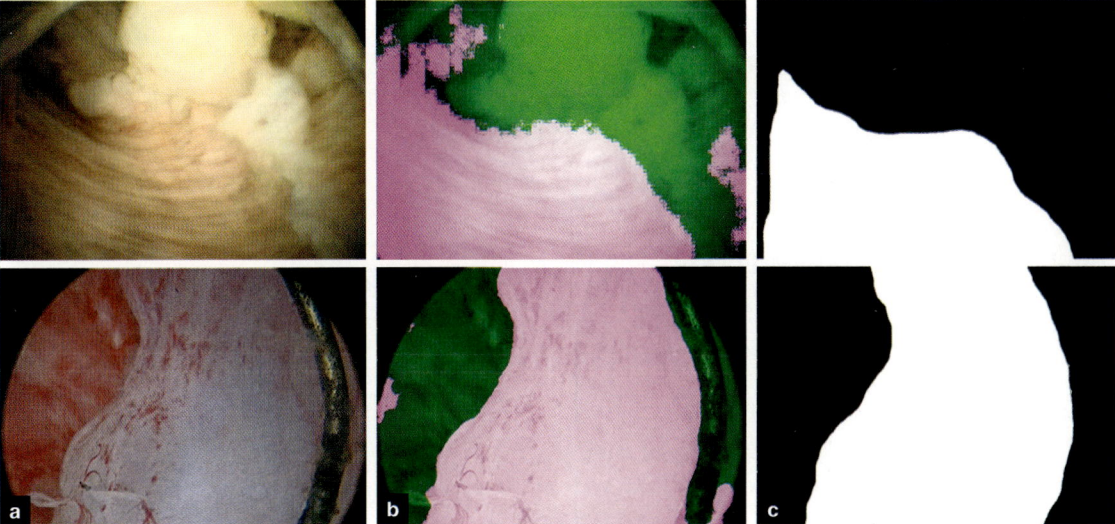

Fig. 27.2a to c: (a) Sample images for myoma/myometrium (1st row) and polyp (2nd row) segmentation; (b) Result of automatic segmentation where the green/pink color shows the healthy/unhealthy regions; (c) Manual drawn ground-truth

For measuring the performance of the segmentation accuracy, we considered the following notions, a true positive (TP) denotes such a pixel that is labeled as myoma/polyp both in the prediction and the ground-truth images, while a pixel is a true negative (TN), if it is part of healthy tissue and also labeled so by its prediction. False positive (FP) and false negative (FN) cases represent the incorrectly predicted pixels. In the case of myoma/polyp segmentation the achieved results which is determined as (TP + TN)/(TP + TN + FP + FN).

With the test set accuracy in myoma series was: 0.8619. Accuracy in cases with polyps was: 0.7925.

2. Our second aim is to create a decision support system in order to provide additional information in connection with the receptivity of endometrium based on image classification algorithm. For this purpose, the local gynecologist recorded several video streams about the uterine cavity and the fundus before the procedure of implantation. The annotations for these video were labels according to the performed *in vitro* fertilization was successful or not. Our framework evaluates these video frames using deep learning-based approaches and try to predict the receptivity of uterus. Recently, in the field of natural image classification, several CNN architectures have been published, like AlexNet,[5] GoogLeNet,[6] VGGNet,[7] beside others. Some of these architectures are available as pre-trained models initially trained on approximately 1.28 million natural images from the dataset ImageNet.[16] Thus, we can use the weights and biases from these pre-trained models and can connect them to be trained together to take advantage of their joint behavior. In this investigation, we would like to classify endoscopic images about uterine cavity as healthy with high receptivity or diseased with low one. For the evaluation of the classification performance of our method, we used our dataset has been collected during gynecology operations performed in the Department of Obstetrics and Gynecology of the University of Debrecen. The 24 videos were recorded by a full HD 1-MOS camera attached to an endoscope at resolution of 1920 × 1080 pixels and 30 frames/sec. We have extracted 6800 images for the training of CNNs and 600 images for the performance evaluation. Each involved individual CNN and their ensemble have been evaluated by measuring the accuracy, sensitivity, and specificity which have been calculated at the confidence threshold 0.5. In this way, our proposed approach has reached 64, 5% final accuracy beside 0.825 sensitivity and 0.285 specificity regarding this binary classification task.

CONCLUSION

Using the new development of the computer science in endoscopy could help the everyday work of the gynecologists. By applying deep learning methods complication rates could be decreased while success rates could be improved. Since all endoscopic tower involves computer as a part of the image transfer system, costly investments are not needed for benefiting from these techniques. In the future we plan to continue these studies on a bigger dataset.

References

1. Tarneja P, Duggal BS. Hysteroscopy: Past, Present and Future. Med J Armed Forces India. 2002; 58:293–4.
2. Sutton C. Hysteroscopic surgery. Best Pract Res Clin Obstet Gynaecol. 2006; 20: 105–37.
3. Stellato TA. History of laparoscopic surgery. Surg Clin North Am 1992; 72:997.
4. Kadar N. Surgical anatomy and dissection techniques for laparoscopic surgery. Curr Opin Obstet Gynecol 1996; 8:266–77.
5. A. Krizhevsky, I. Sutskever, and G.E. Hinton, "ImageNet classification with deep convolutional neural networks," in Proc. of the 25th International Conference on Neural Information

Processing Systems, Lake Tahoe, 2012;1:1097–1105.

6. C. Szegedy, W. Liu, Y. Jia, P. Sermanet, S. E. Reed, D. Anguelov, D. Erhan, V. Vanhoucke, and A. Rabinovich, "Going deeper with convolutions," arXiv, pp. 1409.4842, 2014.

7. K. Simonyan and A. Zisserman, "Very deep convolutional networks for large-scale image recognition," arXiv, pp. 1409.1556, 2014.

8. J. Long, N. Zhang, and T. Darrell, "Do convnets learn correspondence?," in Proc. of the 27th International Conference on Neural Information Processing Systems, Montreal, vol. 1, pp. 1601–1609, 2014.

9. N. Zhang, J. Donahue, R. Girshick, and T. Darrell, "Part-based r-CNNS for fine-grained category detection," in Proc. ECCV 2014, Part I, Lecture Notes in Compter Science, 2014;8689:834–49.

10. P. Sermanet, D. Eigen, X. Zhang, M. Mathieu, R. Fergus, and Y. LeCun, "Overfeat: Integrated recognition, localization and detection using convolutional networks," in Proc. International Conference on Learning Representations, CBLS, 2014.

11. R. Girshick, J. Donahue, T. Darrell, and J. Malik, "Rich feature hierarchies for accurate object detection and semantic segmentation," in Proc. IEEE Conference on Computer Vision and Pattern Recognition, Columbus, 2014; 580–87.

12. J. Long, E. Shelhamer, and T. Darrel, "Fully convolutional networks for semantic segmentation," arXiv, 2014;4038:1411.

13. Mazzon I, Bettocchi S, Fascilla F, DE Palma D, Palma F, Zizolfi B, DI Spiezio Sardo A. Resectoscopic myomectomy. Minerva Ginecol. 2016 Jun;68(3):334–44.

14. Tinelli A, Malvasi A, Hurst BS, Tsin DA, Davila F, Dominguez G, Dell'edera D, Cavallotti C, Negro R, Gustapane S, Teigland CM, Mettler L. Surgical management of neurovascular bundle in uterine fibroid pseudocapsule. JSLS. 2012 Jan-Mar;16(1):119–29.

15. Deutsch A, Sasaki KJ, Cholkeri-Singh A. Resectoscopic Surgery for Polyps and Myomas: A Review of the Literature. J Minim Invasive Gynecol. 2017 Nov–Dec;24(7):1104–10.

16. J. Deng, W. Dong, R. Socher, et al, "ImageNet: A Large-Scale Hierarchical Image Database", 2009 Conf Comput Vision and Pattern Recogn (CVPR), 2009;248–55.

Debunking Hysteroscopy: Facts and Fiction Regarding Intrauterine Surgery

Osama Shawki, Yehia Shawki

The development of hysteroscopy is rooted in the work of Pantaleoni, who first reported uterine endoscopy in 1869. And since the late 19th century progressing up to the present day, medicine has excelled at optimising the intracavitary view of body organs to allow for minimally invasive solutions for surgical diseases.

1. Pressure Conundrum

Without doubt, the most controversial talking point in hysteroscopy today is the fluid pressure dilemma. Ever since fluid media replaced CO_2 gas as a distension medium in the 1980s; faculties have argued over the adequate pressure to be used to expose the uterine cavity.

Initially fluid bags were merely hanged from a height with the column of fluid providing the only pressure, gradual progression to syringe injection, pressure cuff and eventually fluid pressure pumps were devised by leading endoscopy manufacturers.

The question remains, what pressure is optimal for viewing the cavity?

Authors have debated that the pressure should not increase above mean arterial blood pressure to minimise intravasation and avoid the most serious of hysterocopy complications, namely fluid overload.

This begs to question a key fundamental fact: How can the pressure inside the cavity according to the pressure pump be greater than the MAP and yet still not be enough to stop bleeding from minute capillaries in the endometrium and myometrium?

It is logical to assume that once the pressure provided is greater than MAP, that not a single drop of blood would be seen. The answer lies in the difference between actual intrauterine pressure and the pressure pump reading. The explanation lies in 2 parts:

A. The uterus is a vascular contractile organ which alternates pressure vastly from one patient to the other and from one instance to another. Compounded by the fact that each uterus will have 3 channels to release fluid (2 tubes and the cervix) which means that there is always a source of leakage and a constant alteration in the actual intrauterine pressure.

Compared to laparoscopic insufflation where there is no means of gas leakage and the pressure remains fairly constant and the difference is magnified.

B. The channel of the hysteroscope you are using limits the flow of fluid media based on the diameter of the sheath. For example, when utilising an office 3.4 mm sheath with pressure setting at 150 mm Hg, you will have a different intrauterine pressure than when using the 26 Fr resectoscope at 150 mm Hg. In the same way that flow rate through a veress needle cannot compare to that of the primary tracer in laparoscopy and thus insufflation with the needle takes a longer time. The problem with the uterine cavity is that due to constant leakage, you will always need high flow rate to maintain intrauterine pressure and thus the larger sheaths give a more accurate representation of pressure pump numbers.

Here begs the question: So how do we identify what pressure is needed to perform operative hysteroscopy?

The answer is simply that there is no fixed figure. Rather a "Proper Pressure" is required which entails expansion of the cavity and tamponading any small bleeding capillaries. A shift from fluid pressure to fluid deficit is what should be used to avoid fluid overload.

2. Hysteroscopy *vs* Intrauterine Surgery

There is no clear line of demarcation between the different surgical levels required for hysteroscopic surgery. In truth, certain procedures performed require a vastly different skill set, equipment and experience level.

Breakdown: "Hysteroscopy" by definition is the visualization of the uterine cavity. In order to perform spot diagnostic procedures, extract missed IUCD, cut minute filmy adhesions or grasp a small polyp; the surgeon needs only basic equipment.

Requirements here are:
- 30° 2.9 mm optic lens
- Office sheath
- Basic office instruments such as hysteroscopic scissors and grasper
- Basic camera, screen and light source
- Pressure cuff

This tool set is relatively economic and could realistically be owned by all gynaecologists wishing to provide office/outpatient hysteroscopy at their place of work (Fig. 28.1).

Experience level here is modest and the procedures will have close to no complications. In the 21st century, the value of "hysteroscopy" is endless for the modern day gynecologist as the main applications of diagnostic hysteroscopy focus on infertility and bleeding which constitute 80% of practice. Therefore, advocation of all gynecologists owning/ having access to a basic hysteroscopy set is crucial and training to perform these simple procedures does not require a long time.

Moving on to "intrauterine surgery" and the equipment + skill level here changes drastically.

Requirements here are:
- 30° 2.9 mm optic lens
- Office sheath
- 30° 4 mm optic lens

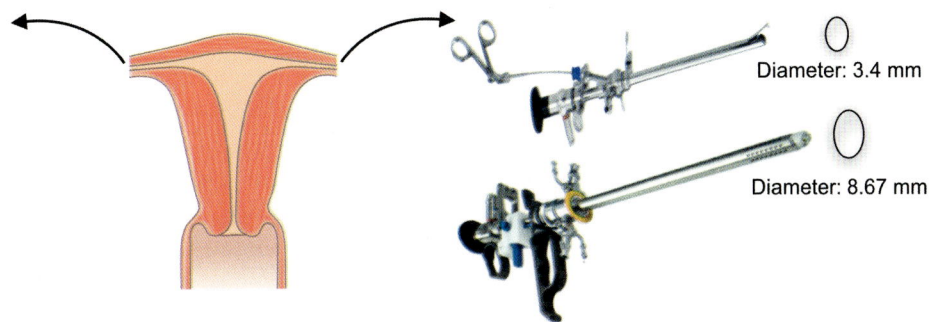

Diameter: 3.4 mm

Diameter: 8.67 mm

Fig. 28.1: Instruments of hysteroscopy

- Hysteroscopic scissors and grasper
- Operative resectoscope (inner sheath, outer sheath, working element)
- Inserts (loop, collin's knife, roller ball)
- Advanced camera system providing much higher quality images
- Advanced light source
- Endoscopy monitor
- Pressure pump

This equipment is far less economical and should not realistically be owned by individual gynecologists. Procedures to be performed here include:

- Congenital uterine anomalies metroplasty
- Intrauterine synechiae (asherman) adhesiolysis
- Organic causes of AUB management such as submucous fibroids, large polyps, transcervical
- Resection of endometrium
- Hysteroscopic tubal occlusion
- Amongst other miscellaneous uses.

Skill level here is far greater and experience enthrals a much longer learning curve and dedication to mastering the surgical technique.

Complications also arise in this category as fluid overload is more likely during these longer procedures and perforations by electrocautery are far more dangerous than those done by cold energy or the scope itself.

It is not required by all gynecologists to be intrauterine surgeons in the same way that all Ob/Gyns are expected to perform routine NVD and CS but not all are performing cesarian hysterectomy for placenta percreta.

All gynecologists should be performing hysterectomy but not all should handle grade IV. Endometriosis with extensive bowel involvement or oncology radical procedures.

CONCLUSION

Hysteroscopy is a wonderful surgery (one must start doing it to benefit all phases of women). One should be judicial and sceptical in applying it on various problems of females of all ages.

Index